PSYCHEDELIC INJUSTICE

Pitchstone Publishing
www.pitchstonebooks.com

Library of Congress Cataloging-in-Publication Data

Names: Hatsis, Thomas, 1980- author.
Title: Psychedelic injustice : how identity politics poisons the psychedelic renaissance / Thomas Hatsis.
Description: Durham, North Carolina : Pitchstone Publishing, [2025] | Includes bibliographical references. | Summary: "Psychedelic Injustice offers a history of psychedelic use, discusses the benefits of psychedelic medicines, and analyzes the ways in which critical social justice ideology is harming psychedelic culture"— Provided by publisher.
Identifiers: LCCN 2024062023 (print) | LCCN 2024062024 (ebook) | ISBN 9781634312783 (paperback) | ISBN 9781634312790 (ebook)
Subjects: LCSH: Hallucinogenic drugs—Social aspects. | Hallucinogenic drugs—History. | Social justice.
Classification: LCC HV5822.H25 H38 2025 (print) | LCC HV5822.H25 (ebook) | DDC 306/.1--dc23/eng/20250218
LC record available at https://lccn.loc.gov/2024062023
LC ebook record available at https://lccn.loc.gov/2024062024

PSYCHEDELIC INJUSTICE

How Identity Politics Poisons the Psychedelic Renaissance

Thomas Hatsis

Pitchstone Publishing
Durham, North Carolina

Contents

Preface: Everybody Needs a John

Friendship

While I typically eat a healthy diet, every few months I get a hankering for fried chicken (especially if I've been rewatching *Breaking Bad*).

The cure for my cravings comes in the form of dinner with one of my closest friends, John, who lives down the block from George's—a small dive bar that just so happens to have (in our mutual opinion) the best fried chicken in the city of Portland. John is a musician, an intellectual, and a pillar of the Portland visionary art community. He is even-keeled, considerate, kind, honest, and you'd be hard-pressed to find someone who doesn't like him. During the six-year tenure of our friendship, I have never once seen him put himself before someone else. I've never heard him talk down about anybody (even those who have wronged him). He loves people. He loves our city. He works hard to make it all happy and beautiful.

But John also satisfies another craving I have—one more necessary than the taste of George's delectable fried chicken. Despite our closeness, John and I don't agree on everything. Our fried chicken dates double as debate nights on social issues. We are both moderates who lean more left or right depending on the topic. John is one *very* persuasive son of a bitch. While I do not always see eye to eye with him, I always learn something from him during our friend chicken dates. He has told me the same.

I am very fortunate. The importance of having a close friend who can discuss complex issues without judgment seems to be missing for a lot of folks (so far as I can tell). Social media has locked us all in echo chambers, talking to "friends" we've never even met, and few rarely get away from their computers or phones these days.

For me, John is an oasis.

And then there is Chris.

Chris and I used to be very close. He, too, is a psychedelic historian—and a damn good one. We used to speak on the phone or message each other practically every day—sometimes for days on end (especially if we had books due to our respective publishers). His research abilities are dogged and difficult to match. While most of us are content with writing books a couple hundred pages in length, Chris produces 600-page mammoths. His keen eye at evaluating source material is commendable. While Chris does not have even an undergraduate degree, his research abilities far surpass many with PhDs.

I miss Chris every day. Unlike John, Chris is ideologically captured by extreme leftist politics. For all his insights and intelligence, Chris finds it *very* difficult to change his mind—perhaps a curse for those who are *usually* correct. That is to say, his remarkable intellectualism has also rendered him quite incapable of hearing when and if he is wrong about this or that topic. He's simply too used to being right.

And so it happened that he took the far-left narrative when it came to a shooting incident that occurred a few years ago. The specifics of the incident are irrelevant to our purposes here. What is relevant is that our legacy media rushed to paint the shooter as a "white supremacist." As more and more of the facts came out, it was revealed that said individual was not a white supremacist. When the shooter was exonerated, I (perhaps stupidly) took to Facebook and made a short post, which read, "Always remember: the media lies, forensic science does not."

Due to his politics, Chris had been very invested in a guilty verdict. Ignoring all the facts of the case, all the testimonies, and all the cell phone video evidence, Chris had decided since day one that the shooter was not only guilty, but also a member of some radical right-wing militia. The media told him so. And he believed it.

After calling me all the usual names one would expect in that kind of situation, he, naturally, blocked me on all social media platforms.

Since that day a few years ago I have reached out to Chris several times. He simply won't talk to me. For Chris, the shooter was a bigot, and I was defending his bigotry.

Thank Gaia, I have John. John can admit when he's wrong and will change his mind to conform to the evidence.

Everybody needs a John.

Part I

Narratives

I

Captured by Ideology: Two Culture Wars

I saw the best minds of my generation destroyed by madness.

—Allen Ginsburg, "Howl"

Wounds

We are all wounded somewhat. And those wounds sometimes make it difficult to hear ideas that we might not like. When we are wounded, we do not listen with our heart; instead, we filter messages, even those made with good intention, through our wounds. I am sensitive to this truth. And so I ask something mighty of both of us, dear appreciated reader. I ask that we both access our heart beyond our wounds.

In this book I am going to gently try to reach past your wounds. As you read, I ask that you do the same for me.

Critical Social Justice

The United States and larger Western Civilization are currently embroiled in two culture wars. On the first frontline we find critical social justice (or CSJ[1]), a perspective that sees racism and sexism as ever-preset and ordinary, carefully curated in Western society through governments, free markets, and the university and justice systems.[2] One need only fix a CSJ lens within the frames of her rose-colored glasses, and she would see the world for what it really is: a social binary separating the oppressors from the oppressed. Here, a person's intersectionality points (i.e., how many perceived social grievances she can stack in her favor) push her into either the oppressor or oppressed category. Social value depends upon acceptance of this ideology. Those who uphold the ideology are righteous. Those who question the ideology are bigots.

To be clear, my critique of critical social justice will not ignore the fact that racist and sexist people exist. When I use the term critical social justice throughout this book, I am not discounting the terrible ways minority populations have been treated historically. Rather, I am referring to a perspective that herds people into either the oppressor or oppressed group based not on the oceanic depths of individual behavior, but instead anchored in the shallows of identity politics.

Psychedelia

The second frontline, psychedelia (or what some insiders affectionately refer to as the "psychedelic Renaissance"), aims to address societal problems through the careful incorporation of plant and mushroom medicines used to heal the traumas that come with human existence. Since the 1950s, psychiatrists, psychologists, and a host of physicians holding different specialties have known that LSD, psilocybin (or "magic") mushrooms, mescaline, and other psychedelic medicines can alleviate depression, anxiety, and post-traumatic stress disorder (PTSD) in some people. And here it is conservative ideology, not critical social justice, that presents a sizeable stumbling block to reintroducing these extraordinary medicines to the masses. Conservative views of psychedelic medicines are roundly mistaken and profoundly outdated.

---

1. This term has been popularized by culture writer Helen Pluckrose. See, for example, her book *The Counterweight Handbook: Principled Strategies for Surviving and Defeating Critical Social Justice—at Work, in Schools, and Beyond* (NC: Pitchstone Publishing, 2024).
2. Richard Delgado and Jean Stefancic, *Critical Race Theory: An Introduction* (NY: New York University Press, 2017), pp. 3, 8.

These two seemingly separate culture wars have, in recent years, collided. Critical social justice enjoys much prestige within the ivy-strewn halls of the psychedelic Renaissance, as leaders of both brigades have cooked their arguments in the same university cauldron for the last few decades. Leaders of the psychedelic movement largely believe that university approval will axiomatically bestow the keys to the halls of mainstream acceptance. Only, the very ideology that has compromised our institutions of higher learning has filtered into the psychedelic Renaissance.

Brave New Woke

Broadly speaking, critical social justice ideology takes on three general forms. There is the violent kind of activist that dominated the news between 2017 and 2020. The popular name for this group of ideologues is "Antifa," which is short for "anti-fascist." Antifa is not an official organization, but rather an umbrella term for a variety of unaffiliated pseudo-revolutionary groups largely comprised of middle-class white Americans. Some of them call people "Nazis" while behaving like the actual Nazi Storm Division, Hitler's hit men who would disrupt speeches of opposing views, burn down buildings, and beat, rob, and maim those who did not follow in goosestep with their perspectives—just like Antifa does. They are far more *Pro*fa than *Anti*fa and will be referred to as such for the remainder of this work.

In this book we will meet Psymposia, a nonprofit leftist psychedelic media outlet. Some of the organization's members align with the views of Profa.[3] Fans of so-called cancel culture, Psymposia's writers engage in unethical journalistic practices, slandering anyone ever so slightly right of Chairman Mao. Their activities have been noticed by others in the field, resulting in Psymposia's staff getting banned from the Wonderland conference in Miami, Florida, in 2022.[4] Psymposia promotes a culture of

3. See David Nickels, "We Need to Talk about MAPS Supporting the Police, the Military, and Violent White Supremacism," *Psymposia* (July 17, 2020); Brian Pace, pers. comm.

4. James Kent, "Wonderland Miami Exposes Growing Rift in Psychedelic Community," *Psychedelic Spotlight*, November 8, 2022.

fear rather than one of compassion.[5]

There is also the intellectual kind of critical social justice ideologue, the Theorist. This class is largely made up of well-compensated therapists and humanities professors who believe they can detect a pervasive racism in everything said and done. Theorists favor an authoritarian form of indoctrination as a tactic, hoping that with their careful instruction a person can be reeducated to a higher version of race consciousness. It is a most sinister form of alchemy, one which renders gold into lead. Theorists seek real power, even as they denounce the very idea of hierarchy based on merit and the power structures that inevitably follow. They have no real wish to end racism holistically; they only concern themselves with eradicating certain kinds of racism.

For our purposes, we need look no further to find psychedelic Theorists of this kind than Chacruna Institute, another nonprofit psychedelic organization founded by anthropologist Dr. Beatriz "Bia" Labate and therapist Clancy Cavnar. Those affiliated with Chacruna Institute are active on social media, publish impressive amounts of articles, and speak at and host psychedelic conferences that focus on systemic oppression, decolonization, and gender issues. Chacruna Institute's Instagram and LinkedIn pages promise "high-quality research on plant medicines and psychedelics."

We shall put that claim to task.

Still, there is a third kind of critical social justice ideologue, who is less radical and thankfully seems to make up the majority, which I call the psychedelic social justice warrior (or psychedelic SJW).[6] This individual truly believes she is doing good work and seeks to correct what she believes are real injustices. She is honest, kind, smart, and reliable. But she is also wholly misguided and ignorant. She doesn't even know where the ideas she believes come from. She has never questioned them. I have a specific friend of mine in mind as I write these words who is fairly representative of this group.

5. ". . . I admit, too, that it was also fear, knowing that any critical take on psymposia's conduct was being met with immature, reactionary, and even violent recourse from them. And that I just didn't have the capacity to get in the pen with rabid (watch)dogs and keep myself afloat in the rest of my life." James W. Jesso, Facebook post, April 6, 2021.

6. While I know the term "SJW" is ever more passé these days, I am at a loss to come up with a better term. As such, it seems we are stuck with it for the while.

I wrote this book for her and the many like her in the psychedelic Renaissance. It is my belief that once all the facts have been laid bare, anyone with an open mind will be able to see critical social justice for what is: a collection of shallow and divisive ideas. I will be careful to note, however, where I find agreement with Team CSJ.

Chacruna Institute, Psymposia, and other independent psychedelic SJWs push what we shall call in this book "The Narrative." The Narrative comes in many forms, but all versions boil down to the same point; namely: all Europeans and their white American descendants are evil, racist, misogynist colonizers (especially heterosexual men); and all non-European peoples and their descendants are righteous and innocent victims.[7] How a person actually *behaves* is not relevant through the critical social justice narrative; perceived levels of grievance (real or imagined) are all that matter. Admittedly, this jousting with narratives puts me in quite an awkward position—as I'm going to narrate these narratives with my own narrative! So let me be clear from the outset. The narrative I will tell in this book is not meant to be complete. Rather, it is to show the incompleteness of the other narratives, despite the fact that there are some truths to them. It's the divisive exaggerations of these narratives, and their seemingly carved-in-stone nature (which psychedelic SJWs hold as above reproach) that I feel needs addressing. While I do not pretend to have all the answers (I mean, who does?), I do hope to open a civil, fried chicken-like dialogue about how these societal fractures influence (and ultimately corrupt) the psychedelic Renaissance.

While cooler heads recognize a broad agreement among CSJ activists, liberals, and conservatives (and any perspective among or between them), which professes that no person should be held back, discriminated against, or otherwise disadvantaged in life due to her immutable characteristics, critical social justice narratives can, at times, take that moral decency too far.

And in the process, the narratives become indecent.

---

7. I should note that this latter group also includes transgender white Americans.

While I believe that critical social justice ideologies are ignorant, I don't believe psychedelic SJWs are disingenuous (for the most part). As such, I do not intend to reduce those who align with critical social justice into a simple abstraction. At times this will be difficult to manage because the ideology demands a total acceptance of all its precepts (recall my former friend Chris mentioned earlier). Even evolutionary biologist Richard Dawkins, once a darling among the critical social justice crowd for his contributions to atheism, has felt the brunt of the ideology because he recognizes biological sex as a natural fact.[8] Critical social justice necessitates a person suspend all nuanced thinking and toe the line without asking any questions, giving a religious aspect to the narratives.[9] And so I find myself in a conundrum. While I (and I imagine most people) can accurately predict what a CSJ activists will say in most any given situation—indeed, they all seem to be reading from the same script—I also recognize that people are far deeper and more complex than any ascribed labels. I will do my best to moderate those polarities as we move forward.

This book will focus on the ways critical social justice narratives manifest in the psychedelic Renaissance and outline why it is crucial to uproot them before they corrode the reentry of psychedelia into mainstream culture. I focus on critical social justice because at the moment radical right-wingers, who are no doubt just as susceptible to identity politics, aren't much involved in psychedelia. That is not to say that some radical right-wingers don't enjoy LSD or mushrooms from time to time. Maybe some do. I wouldn't know—not my crowd. It is to say that these people have no major platforms or influence in the psychedelic Renaissance of which to speak. They do not present at public psychedelic forums, they do not write books on psychedelia, and I am unaware of any truly influential radical right-wing psychedelic media outlets. In fact, I've never even heard of a radical right-wing psychedelic media outlet. Like those who adopt CSJ ideology, those who adopt radical right-wing identity politics are not a simple, singular abstraction. While I abstain from iden-

8. Alison Flood, "Richard Dawkins Loses 'Humanist of the Year' Title over Trans Comments," *The Guardian* (April 20, 2021).
9. See John McWhorter, *Woke Racism: How a New Religion has Betrayed Black America* (NY: Portfolio/Penguin, 2021).

tity politics of all kinds, I find that people on both sides of these extremes are trying to fill a void. I reckon they are seeking purpose and connection. And that warrants more compassion than it does judgment. Rest assured, if the radical right was to one day appear in the psychedelic Renaissance in a noticeable way and undermine its core values—i.e., mental health, cognitive liberty, and spiritual autonomy—as critical social justice has, I'll be writing a book about that too. For now, within psychedelic culture, critical social justice provides one of the biggest stumbling blocks for a unified movement.

Radical right-wingers aside, mainstream conservatives typically shun both—critical social justice and psychedelia—seeing the former as the tantrums of wealthy students at elite colleges and the latter as a fool's escape from reality. While I find agreement with mainstream conservatism's regard to critical social justice (though, I'm not much interested in "owning the libs"), I find that the right has unfairly rejected the benefits of psychedelic medicines, which, coupled with other positive reinforcing behaviors,[10] can have remarkable, lifechanging effects on a person. Psychedelics are less an escape from reality than they are a confrontation with ultimate reality. An ultimate reality where the very God to whom many conservatives pray may appear before their bemushroomed eyes.

Conservatives also overlook that there was a time in America's history when psychedelia was, well, *conservative*—the 1950s, for example. Throughout that decade, conservative public figures, Hollywood elites, and academics in the highest institutions of learning, Church, and State endorsed psychedelics. We will explore the history of psychedelic conservatism more fully later. For now, we might consider a list of social values that many mainstream Americans embrace: seeing wisdom in tradition, being goal-oriented, seeking self-improvement and spiritual fulfillment, building strong families and communities, maintaining clean and orderly cities and neighborhoods, and pursuing happiness. Mainstream American values those are indeed, but they are also the values of the psychedelic Renaissance. Psychedelic medicines have been used for myriad reasons in a variety of places all over the world and throughout history. Western Civilization is no exception. Along the centuries that

10. That is, meditation, martial arts, painting, music, gardening, foraging mushrooms, learning a new language or craft, etc.

merged the foundational roads of Athens and Jerusalem, psychedelics have appeared scattered throughout the cobblestones. At different points in history, Greeks, Romans, Hebrews, and Christians all incorporated mind-altering plants into their understanding of religious mythopoetics. We will explore that history in chapter 4.

I live in Portland, Oregon, a bastion of both critical social justice activism and psychedelic culture. It is my dedication to the latter that allows me to endure the former. But there are other things to love about Portland besides its liberal stance on psychedelia. The people are generally sweet, the food is excellent, summers are gorgeous, bike-riding is abundant, dogs are seemingly everywhere, and the urban mushroom foraging is more fruitful than in any other city in which I've lived. I've got great friends and a great community and enjoy a very active social life in a city with a vibrant artistic pulse.

Outside Portland, I am surrounded by other cities whose residents have a large interest in psychedelia, down the coast to Los Angeles and up the beautiful Cascades to Vancouver, British Columbia. Some of those cities are also quite absorbed in critical social justice politics (San Franscisco to the south; Seattle to the north).

For the last twenty-odd years, I have been on the liberal side of psychedelic research. I still am today. I will be tomorrow. I know the healing qualities of psychedelic medicines. I have seen them firsthand in myself and in others and there is a growing body of literature that supports such assertions (which we will meet later). But I wonder how much it's all worth when some stewards of the movement have edited a message of hope with a militant quill.

Historically, psychedelic experiences have given people healing, spiritual exaltation, and a sense of stability in an uncertain world. They also have been used towards truly dreadful ends like torture and human sacrifice. Psychedelics are what LSD researcher Stanislav Grof called "non-specific amplifiers"—whether horrific or pleasurable.[11] A person may "fathom hell or soar angelic" as one psychedelic psychiatrist re-

11. See Stanislav Grof, *LSD Psychotherapy: The Healing Potential of Psychedelic Medicine* (CA: Multidisciplinary Association for Psychedelic Studies, 2008).

marked in 1957.[12] Psychedelics are not magic bullets. They will reveal all the hidden aspects of a person's character—the good, the bad, and the ugly. Extreme care and caution must be taken when working with psychedelics, otherwise a person can do more harm than good. So I'm not here to tell you that psychedelics are all love and light. I am here to tell you the truth about these extraordinary medicines, their history, and what we stand to lose or gain from their use. Of first importance, we will explore whether or not critical social justice is aligned with the core values of the psychedelic Renaissance: mental health, cognitive liberty, and spiritual autonomy.

A Note on Terminology

As I will later argue that "race" is a myth, I purposefully misuse the word "ethnicity" when referring to immutable regional traits in various peoples. However, when speaking of "race" as a myth, I retain the term. I also debated whether to use descriptors like "black" and "white" when discussing people, both individually and in groups. I'm not much of a fan of either term, and I cringe when writers capitalize the "B" in "black" and "W" in "white." But I also recognize that referring to a person as either black or white remains common parlance. I therefore settled on "black American" and "white American" for this book. If I was going to use black and white as descriptive terms to satisfy contemporary national colloquialisms, I wanted something that reminded readers that there is far more that binds us than separates us. I retain this phraseology for other ethnicities as well (e.g., Chinese American, indigenous American, Latin American, etc.). Further, "American" isn't an ethnicity; it's a philosophy that anyone can adopt. In this book, "American" simply refers to a person who believes in the common values of life, liberty, and the pursuit of happiness, no matter their ancestry.

I also use the terms "substantia" (coined by Phonomantic magician Sean Manseau) and "plant medicine" to encompass a variety of psychedelics. For example, while cannabis and ayahuasca are certainly plant-based, peyote is a cactus and *Amanita muscaria* is a mushroom; however,

12. Quoted in Michael Horowitz and Cynthia Palmer, *Moksha: Aldous Huxley's Classic Writings on Psychedelics and the Visionary Experience* (VT: Park Street Press, 1999), p. 107.

when I use the term "plant medicine" throughout this book, consider it a shorthand term that includes peyote and mushrooms every bit as much as it does cannabis and ayahuasca. I also employ the word "entheogen" from time to time. Entheogen was coined by Boston University classics professor Carl Ruck in 1979 and means to "generate divinity from within."[13] The idea behind "entheogen" is that these plant medicines have a divine nature to them that can awaken the sacred in a person. Entheogenic refers, more or less, to having a specifically *spiritual* or *religious* experience with psychedelics. Those having an entheogenic experience will claim to have talked to God, danced with angels, or embodied some kind of religious revelry and awe through substantia. They might feel like they saw—even for a brief moment—what Heaven must be like. These experiences can be very deep and powerful and can sometimes turn even the staunchest of atheists into an even stauncher theist.

The following chapters will deal with delicate subjects about decolonization, racism, and gender ideology—both how they affect the culture at large and how they present themselves in and influence the psychedelic Renaissance more specifically.

Please read carefully.

---

13. Robert G. Wasson et al., *Persephone's Quest: Entheogens and the Origins of Religion* (CT: New Haven, 1986), p. 30.

2

The Racist Library Near My House: Foundations of CSJ Psychedelia

This used to be a very civil town.[1]

—Portland resident

Unrest

Following the death of George Floyd (1973–2020) in May 2020, the cities of America erupted in protest. My home city of Portland, Oregon, was no different, even earning a reputation for responding to the tragedy in a particularly radical style. I attended several of the mostly peaceful riots that occurred in Rose City simply to observe. During one march through my neighborhood, Woodstock, on 5 June 2020, a young woman yelled that we needed to burn the library around the corner from my house to the ground. The library, she informed the crowd, was "a symbol of white supremacy."

A library? I thought. Curious, I spoke up: "How would we make books accessible to those who can't afford them?" I asked.

Her answer: we would burn down the library and rebuild a new antiracist one in its place. City planners had built the library back in

1. Quoted in Douglas Murray, *The War on the West* (NY: Broadside Books, 2022), p. 45.

the 1950s, during the age of Jim Crow, and so it served as an emblem of systemic oppression. Burning down the library would cleanse the building of its racist bricks and mortar. Library visitors, specifically black Americans, would *now* feel comfortable studying, reading, and borrowing books without feeling racially traumatized.

"And how will the book exchange work in the new antiracist library?" I asked.

She looked at me incredulously—like I was an idiot.

"Same way it does now! Library cards!" she shrieked in my face.

"So we should burn down the library, rebuild it, restack the shelves with books, and use library cards to borrow them for a defined period of time? Isn't that exactly how that library operates right now?" I asked.

"Yes," she replied.

"Then why should we burn it down?" I followed up.

"Because it's racist."

When I first moved to Portland at the end of 2014, I had no idea that the city planners had built a racist library near my house. While there certainly was a time in this country's history when all buildings in the United States were racist in a very ugly systemic way, I had never heard of a racist building—library or otherwise—existing in my lifetime. I'd lived in New York most of my life and had never heard of a racist library; neither had I heard of one when I lived in St. Louis throughout most of 2014. Finding myself calling the West "home" for the first time, however, I decided to keep an open mind. I visited the library near my house often and never once heard someone call it racist. There are no signs reminiscent of a deplorable past instructing certain visitors to use the back doors or not enter the library at all. No signs over water fountains indicating who was and who was not allowed to quench their thirst. I've seen mothers, fathers, grandparents, guardians, and children of many ethnicities in the library who all seemed to be enjoying themselves (notwithstanding the students wrapped up in busy work). In some way that had not yet been made clear to me, the library nonetheless represents only a small part of a broader scheme of white supremacy.

The Woodstock Boulevard protest was not the only march and rally I attended that year. Earlier that spring, I had joined protestors at (the appropriately titled) Revolution Hall down on SE Stark Street.

We arrived at Revolution Hall in the early evening, where a large crowd had gathered to listen to speakers list a battery of grievances coated in buzzwords like "power structures," "systemic oppression," and "white supremacy" that we were all obligated to applaud. Qualifications to speak before the crowd were not based on any kind of expertise in any given area. A young woman stood on stage and informed us that the African continent was a veritable utopia before Europeans ever stepped one buckled boot on its soil. Institutions like slavery, governmental oppression, and more individual atrocities like rape and murder did not exist in Africa . . . not until the Europeans imported them with sword and Bible, she proclaimed. She then informed all the white Americans in the crowd that we were no longer allowed to smoke cannabis, as that plant was "stolen" from Africa. (As we will see in later chapters, cannabis not only has a long history of use in Europe but was also introduced to the Americas via Spanish trading companies bringing the plant to Mexico.)

Historical truth mattered not. The crowd cheered in a somewhat nervous chorus of ignorance and fear.

We then marched west on SE Stark Street towards the Burnside Bridge, which would take us downtown to Pioneer Square. We were led by a truck that had amplifiers and a few people in the bed; a young lady sitting in the bed spoke into a microphone, informing us that when (not *if*) the police started firing their guns, we (the mostly white American crowd) needed to form a perimeter around the protest organizers. Her *ad hoc* theory held that since police don't shoot white Americans, our "white privilege" would protect us. There was a certain irony to her theory. The police had already been ordered to back off from the protest marchers (which struck me as odd in a supposedly white supremacist country). Further, as we will see later, plenty of white Americans are shot by the fuzz.

When we arrived at Pioneer Square we listened to more speakers—this time professors, writers, and professional activists—offer creative interpretations of history, statistics, and sociology much the same way the unprofessional ones had done at Revolution Hall. We then marched back to Revolution Hall. Once arrived, the amplifiers that had earlier projected factually untenable remarks about insurrection and systemic oppression now pumped dance music. Cases of beer were brought in and opened, and people got high on one thing or another. The protest turned into a party. Everyone forgot about George Floyd as they threw an illegal soirée that I would have imagined a white supremacist country would have stopped immediately. But the protestors knew they weren't really in any danger.

This was political LARPing with a keg party finale.

BLM's position, which holds that black Americans (specifically men) are the target of racist police officers, occupies one aspect of the larger critical social justice perspective that sees the world as a binary, an insidious chasm between the oppressors and the oppressed. Because George Floyd was a black American he was "oppressed." Because Derek Chauvin is a white American (and a police officer) he is an "oppressor." Through the critical social justice perspective, Chauvin the individual represents a larger, ever-present systemic racist oppression in the United States, to which every white American allegedly contributes. He is, in fact, a stand-in for all white Americans—every bit as much as Floyd is a stand-in for all black Americans. The lens by which CSJ ideologues view this binary is called critical race theory (CRT), a legal philosophy which is very important to the story of psychedelic injustice.

Let's briefly explore its origins.

Marxism

Karl Marx (1818–1883) was a political and economic theorist who believed he could ignite a proletarian revolution against the shackles of capitalism. With the rise of the Industrial Revolution, a major financial gap continued to widen between the haves and the have-nots. Marx hoped his revolution would level the paying-field[2]—laborers would overthrow the bourgeoisie. This revolution would not be localized to Western Europe but would eventually spill across borders, forming a new global paradigm. Along with his writing partner Friedrich Engels (1820–1895),

2. Pun intended.

Marx composed *The Communist Manifesto* (1848), which declared that all of human history represented a succession of class struggle. Their present struggle—that of Marx's and Engel's—would be the final showdown, the fiscal battle of Megiddo, where capitalism would fall for evermore in the West, followed by every other corner of the earth, making way for a kind of planetary utopian communism.

Whether one agrees with Marx's original vision or not is beside the point—it's simply an outdated model that could not work in a modern society. In Marx's day, class was very much dependent upon occupation. And while that is still true today it isn't *as true*. For example, in the mid-19th century when Marx lived, carpenters—across the board—were poor. No one had any difficulty deciding whether one carpenter was proletariat and another one was bourgeoisie—they were all proletariat. Today, that is no longer the case. There are low-income (i.e., "proletariat") carpenters and high-income (i.e., "bourgeoise") carpenters. The same rule applies to a host of other occupations (mechanic, plumber, teacher, and contractor, among others). Status in the United States is no longer contingent on being born into a specific class; it is about occupation.[3] A rich kid who squanders the family fortune is, at least culturally, seen as below the status of the kid born into humble beginnings who rises to the top of her field. Additionally, people marry across classes more often these days.[4] A low-income laborer might wed a high-income executive. Are the laborers supposed to overthrow their spouses?

This is not to suggest that I believe Marx and Engels were wrong about everything. To think so would simply mean that I deferred to an abstraction. There is, in fact, an area of their philosophy of which I find much agreement. We will further explore that space in a later chapter.

Neo-Marxism

Vulgar Marxism (i.e., the Marxism of Karl Marx based in economics) morphed into so-called Neo-Marxism in Germany after World War I. Marx's proletariat revolution had failed spectacularly, and his follow-

3. Alexander B. Dolitsky, "Opinion: Neo-Marxism Is a Threat to the Country," *Juneau Empire* (January 25, 2023).
4. Pavithra Mohan, "What It's Like to Date and Marry out of Your Social Class," *Fast Company* (October 22, 2018).

ers were left wondering why. In response to this cognitive dissonance, Marxist Carl Grünberg (1861–1940) founded the Institute for Social Research in 1923, later redubbed the Frankfurt School.

With the rise of Hitler's Reich, those German Marxists (who were almost all Jewish) fled to the United States, setting up camp at Columbia University in the early 1930s. It was in such lofty ivory towers that Max Horkheimer (1895–1973) developed the idea of Critical Theory, a philosophy that sought to forge society into a new Marxist vision. Critical Theory rested in three parts: affirming an "idealized vision of society"; theorizing why the idealized vision of society had not flowered; and promoting cultural upheaval to achieve the idealized vision of society.[5]

But there was a problem. The free market had not only brought prosperity to the United States but would also eventually spread to the rest of the West and would go on to raise the developing world out of poverty as well. Frankfurt School affiliate Herbert Marcuse (1898–1979), for example, noted how America had become "a well-functioning, prosperous society" that left the working class "[w]ell integrated and well rewarded."[6] The Marxists quickly learned that it is quite difficult to inspire someone to overthrow big business if said person can earn the requisite capital to buy shares in the company. It proved equally difficult to inspire someone to attack the bourgeoisie when so many of the financially destitute aimed at attaining just such a lifestyle.

Critical Theory

Instead of admitting defeat of the Marxian worldview, the Neo-Marxists sought a new proletariat to shape into social radicals. As it was no longer feasible to start a class war based in economics, they sought a social revolution based in identity politics.[7] Such moves saw the growth of what one writer calls "Identity-Marxism" (i.e., identity politics mixed with Marxism).[8] While our trusted friends at Wikipedia list Identi-

5. James Lindsay, *Race Marxism: The Truth about Critical Race Theory and Praxis* (FL: New Discourses, 2022), p. 94.
6. Herbert Marcuse, *An Essay on Liberation* (1969), pp. 39, 41.
7. Though the term "identity politics" did not exist yet, it is clear from the writings of Critical Theorists that this is what they had in mind.
8. Lindsay (2022), p. 9.

ty-Marxism as a "right wing conspiracy theory," there exists evidence to indicate otherwise. For example, Marcuse eschewed the proletariat and settled on a "new working class"[9]—two broad groups for the revamped revolutionary contingent: the leftist intelligentsia and black Americans, the latter he referred to as the "ghetto population."[10] To be fair to Marcuse, black Americans existed in a state of systemic oppression at the time. Their desire for social change was fully justifiable and necessary. However, such identity politics, while in the past were useful in some circumstances, are too divisive and lacking in nuance to serve as a preferable solution to our current societal fractures.

Critical Theory further evolved in the 1990s when critical legal scholars[11] wedged the word "race" between *critical* and *theory*—a strategy Marx, an unabashed racist himself, would have deplored.[12] The term critical race theory first appears in legal scholar Kimberlé Crenshaw's 1991 essay "Mapping the Margins." Crenshaw herself recognizes the Marxist roots of CRT even if Wikipedia does not.[13] While certainly having value in the 20th century and before, when black Americans experienced systemic marginalization, CRT seems vestigial today. As racism became less of a problem in America, Theorists started to court difficulty trying to find systemic oppression, which, by speaking against it, ultimately provides their bread and butter. With nowhere to turn, they decided that racism was now both *ever-present* and *invisible*, keeping residency only in the subconscious thoughts of white Americans.[14]

Questionable as this idea is, in recent years it has received support from a most surprising player—corporate America. This unholy alliance of business elites and Neo-Marxist CRT philosophy has drilled critical social justice deeper into the body politic.

---

9. Marcuse (1969), p. 41.
10. Marcuse (1969), p. 17.
11. Those who believe that laws are created and implemented to oppress marginalized peoples.
12. See Murray (2022), p. 177.
13. Kimberlé Crenshaw et al. (eds.), *Critical Race Theory: The Key Writings that Formed the Movement* (NY: The New Press, 1995), pp. xvii, xxiv.
14. Add intersectional feminism, indigenous activism, and gender studies to this perspective, and Critical Theory morphs into critical social justice.

The Most Pernicious Heist

In trying to make sense of corporate America's increasing promotion of Neo-Marxist ideas, I was scared that I was becoming a conspiracy theorist; but no explanation for what I was seeing and experiencing made sense to me other than the obvious one: old-fashioned greed.

Before we get there, let's travel back to September 2011. I still lived in New York, and a rumbling was in the air at my favorite open mic about some big protest that was erupting in the Financial District. Many of us from the mic community couldn't contain our interest and made our way downtown to Zuccotti Park to investigate the hubbub. We didn't realize it at the time, but we had just become a handful of the first one hundred or so people assembled to participate in what would come to be called the Occupy Wall Street movement. While the movement eventually decayed into shouting matches, gibberish, and ridiculous demands (e.g., abolishing student loan debt for obtaining useless degrees), the original message, articulated by local comedian Jon Savoy, bound as all in unity for a short while: "we are protesting corporations that hold more allegiance to foreign powers than they do to the American people."

That succinct explanation connected all of us—black, white, Asian, indigenous, Southeast Asian, Latin, and Middle Eastern Americans—into a common bond. We stood shoulder to shoulder; a beautiful medley of ethnicities, blue- and white-collar workers, and sexual orientations united by a mutual understanding of the way both corporate America and our government had betrayed our country. Through subprime mortgages, the suits in corporate banking boardrooms had tanked the American economy. Insulting as that was, the injury came when the US government bailed out the CEOs of those banks. The wealthy received bonuses, while those of us at the bottom struggled to keep our heads above water. It was a slap in the face to every mother working three jobs just to put food on the table. It was a kick to the balls of every father struggling in a soul-crushing job just to give his children a better life.

We were *pissed.*

And then, just a few years later, something happened that I couldn't quite understand. Our black American sisters started fighting with our Asian American brothers; our white American brothers quickly went for the figurative jugular of our Latin American sisters. We went from shoulder to shoulder to fist to face in only a few years. Something had poisoned us. And all those businessmen and bankers did was continue to count their profits as they watched us squabble in the streets from the safe vantage of their penthouses. We became the puppets of soulless corporations aimed at keeping us divided, lest they feel the brunt of our unity with another Occupy movement.

I have spent my career as a psychedelic historian debunking wild and baseless ideas. I detested conspiracy theorists as enemies of truth, and there I was forming my own little conspiracy about the Occupy movement and its downfall. The death of unity and the rise of critical race theory from an obscure legal theory to a widespread cultural paradigm seemed too odd a coincidence to me. But I didn't know enough about business culture to go any further than conspiratorially correlating causations. Turned out, my intuition was correct. *Woke Inc.* (2021) by Vivek Ramaswamy outlines the story with tremendous depth and personal knowledge into the inner workings of how corporate America bamboozled us all.

The cliff notes of "the most pernicious heist"[15] are easy enough to understand, and revolve around a single question: *how would these corporations make sure that another Occupy uprising would never seed and blossom*? The answer: *turn friends and allies into enemies.* Distracted and incensed with each other, we wouldn't notice our puppeteers who busily closed shady and exploitive business deals around the world. Jon Savoy's words proved fatidic. In recent years corporations have been opening new markets in the growing Chinese economy. Their allegiance is to the Chinese Communist Party (CCP) *not* the American people. In this way, Savoy anticipated the sentiments of AirBnB cofounder Nathan Blecharczyk, who, in response to concerns that too much personal user data was being shared with the CCP, reportedly stated quite bluntly to the company's "chief trust officer," Sean Joyce, "We're not here to promote American values."[16]

---

15. Vivek Ramaswamy, *Woke Inc.: Inside Corporate America's Social Justice Scam* (NY: Center Street, 2021), p. 7.
16. Quoted in Ramaswamy (2021), p. 162.

No longer would cultural uprisings pit the haves against the have-nots (which is bad for business). Instead, we would be divided based on race, gender, and sexual orientation—so-called Neo-Marxism—(which is good for business). Ramaswamy offers an eye-opening breakdown of this most pernicious heist:

> First, Black Lives Matter activists—or environmentalists or feminists or whoever—become the front for American technology companies to win consumer trust. Second, those companies monetize the trust by generating clicks, selling ads and charging fees—generating a treasure trove of sensitive personalized data about each of their customers. Third, the CCP demands access to that data as a condition of entry for companies to do business in China. Fourth, these companies supplicate to the CCP and make a killing while continuing to issue woke proclamations through their corporate megaphones. BLM wins. Silicon Valley wins. The CCP wins. The real losers of this game are the American people. . . . The deeper problem arises when the CCP flexes its muscle as a gatekeeper to the Chinese market to then convince corporations to *spread the CCP's own values abroad.*[17]

Major US corporations would ignore the blatant human rights violations perpetrated by the CCP (including concentration camps and genocide of the Uyghurs) while scolding Americans who refuse to comply with using the latest pronouns.

One example (among many) would point to toy manufacturer Mattel, whose executives decided to create a "Transgender Barbie" doll modeled after transactivist and actor Laverne Cox. Mattel hoped the doll would shine a light on "its commitment to continue to increase diversity and celebrates the impact [Cox] has had as an advocate for LGBTQ rights."[18] The executive vice president of the company, Lisa McKnight, boasted, "We are proud to highlight the importance of inclusion and acceptance."[19] The critical social justice ideologue celebrated this win for

17. Ramaswamy (2021), 163–64; *italics* in original.
18. Caitlin O'Kane, "Mattel's First Transgender Barbie Designed after Laverne Cox," *CBS New* (May 27, 2022).
19. Quoted in Monica Cole, "Mattel Pushes Transgender Barbie," *American Family Association* (June 24, 2022).

LGBT visibility.[20] But one need look no further than the bottom of the box that Cox (as Barbie) comes in, which reads, "Made in Indonesia," a country that passed a new criminal code in 2022 that outlawed same-sex marriage. The code also includes "curfews for females, [approval of] female genital mutilation, and mandatory hijab dress codes. Many of these regulations also discriminate against LGBT people."[21] Laverne Cox doesn't seem to mind, but it's also highly probable she isn't aware of any of it. Enamored with seeing herself in the form of a Barbie doll, she proclaimed, "I hope that people can look at this Barbie and dream big like I have in my career."[22] She also hoped the "doll will be a beacon of hope and possibility."[23] Indonesian people, apparently, do not count in Cox's big dreams of hope and possibility. But she need not worry. To avoid scandal, Mattel cleverly donated some funds in Cox's name to TransfamilySOS, a nonprofit transactivism organization. They can now feel good about themselves while the Indonesian LGBT community wallows in real systemic oppression.

The cosmic irony is not worth the terrestrial tragedy.

Serious issues aside, these virtue-signals can also lead to amusing contradictions. Take former San Francisco 49ers quarterback Colin Kaepernick, who in 2016 decided to take a knee during the National Anthem played before football games. Nike had planned to roll out a new sneaker in 2019 that featured the American flag coupled with a picture of flag-designer Betsy Ross. The idea was to promote and commemorate the many contributions women have made to the American experiment. So far, so good. But Kaepernick, who had earlier signed a deal with Nike, reportedly took issue with the sneaker. Using similar logic as the young lady who wanted to burn down the racist library near my house, Kaepernick apparently felt that since the flag had been designed while America was still truly a racist country, the stars and stripes could only serve as a

20. O'Kane, "Mattel's First . . ." (2022).
21. Human Rights Watch, "Indonesia: New Criminal Code Disastrous for Rights: Provisions Harmful to Women, Minorities, Free Speech" (December 8, 2022).
22. Quoted in O'Kane, "Mattel's First . . ." (2022).
23. Quoted in Cole, "Mattel Pushes . . ." (2022).

reminder that slavery used to exist in the United States.[24] White American women were never enslaved in the United States, so feminism would have to wait its turn.

Fair enough. Although it seems Kaepernick overlooked a few details in his lettered exposé of American history: the cameras that he loves to smile before were also invented when America was a racist country. The sports cars he enjoys driving and the airplanes in which he travels were invented during the age of Jim Crow. And where did his millions come from? Playing a sport whose modern incarnation formed over a decade before slavery ended in the United States. Will Kaepernick give up photo-ops, fancy cars, private jets, and all his wealth because they have roots in pre–Civil Rights America?

Of course not.

Colin Kaepernick presumably likes cameras, sports cars, and private jets. *Ipso facto*, those aspects of the racist American past can stay; they bring him comfort and status. Whereas flags, while they might make nice decorations for July 4th barbeques, do not provide him with any sense of status the way driving one of his several cars does. So the flag can go; but all his excessive creature comforts, also created at a time when America was a racist country, can stay.

Authoritarianism and Indoctrination

In line with the new critical social justice politic, one business after the next started to rivet DEI (Diversity, Equity, Inclusion) training sessions onto their employees. DEI has many overlaps with CRT, notably seeing the world as divided between oppressor and oppressed based on race and other immutable characteristics. CRT is mostly found in university settings, while DEI appears in corporate boardrooms, preschools, high schools, and churches. If CRT is the legal contingent of this indoctrination, then DEI is the social wing[25]—a form of office-space racism, instructing white American employees to disinter prejudices that they likely do not possess. One DEI training session organized by Coca-Cola reportedly had the white American men writing apology letters to imag-

24. Ramaswamy (2021), p. 220–21.
25. SpectraDIVERSITY, "CRT and DEI" (February 6, 2023).

inary black American women.[26] Theorist Dante King proclaims that "Whites are psychopaths, and their behavior represents an underlying biologically transmitted proclivity with roots deep in their evolutionary history."[27]

Black Americans take their hits from the other end of the DEI stick. They are told that this natural inhumanity of white Americans will cause them to perpetually discriminate against anyone with higher melanin levels. How can such brainwashing result in anything other than diminished ambition and resentment towards their white American peers? If black Americans believe the whole country—laws, culture, media, etc.—is stacked against them in a systematically racist way, why set goals? Why get an education? Why work for a better life? Such resentment quickly becomes a two-way street as non-racist white Americans will only look with disdain at people who hate them for no real reason. If one's goal was to slowly tear away the very fabric of common human decency, DEI seems an awfully good start.

Local governments started implementing DEI into public schools. Soon, even private schools fell in line, as happened at New York's Grace Church School. During one DEI struggle session, the facilitator showed a slide that listed "characteristics of white supremacy"—among them, *objectivity*. One math teacher in attendance, Paul Rossi, was confused by the slide. "Objectivity?" he questioned, "[h]uman attributes are being reduced to racial traits." The facilitator asked Rossi if he was experiencing "white feelings" over the slide. Rossi grew even more confused. "What makes a feeling white?" he asked. Two young women also spoke up, "The first step of antiracism is to racialize every single dimension of my identity," said one. "Fighting indoctrination with indoctrination can be dangerous," said the other.[28]

Despite the meeting operating under a confidentiality agreement,

---

26. Murray (2022) p. 56.
27. Dante King, "Diagnosing Whiteness and Anti-Blackness: White Psychopathology, Collective Psychosis and Trauma in America," lecture presented at UC San Francisco (February 8, 2024).
28. Quoted in Michael Powell, "New York's Private Schools Tackle White Privilege. It has not Been Easy," *The New York Times* (August 27, 2021).

someone reported Rossi's comments to school officials. Instead of considering his discerning objections, a Grace Church School spokesperson chastised Rossi for "creating a neurological imbalance" in the students.[29] One school official even claimed that Rossi's words might amount to "harassment."[30]

However, behind closed doors, the higher-ups at Grace Church, like Principal George Davison, agreed with Rossi. During a Zoom meeting with Rossi over his comments, Davison conceded that those brainwashing sessions were "demonizing white people" who hadn't done anything wrong.[31] The students' crime—the reason for their demonization? "Being born," Davison admitted. He also told Rossi that he had "grave doubts about some of the doctrinaire stuff that gets spouted at us in the name of antiracism. And so I don't disagree entirely with some of your points of view. . . . I think that one of the things that's going on a little too much . . . is . . . the attempt to link anybody who's white to the perpetuation of white supremacy." He also conceded that he was aware of other institutions that had already been "hollowed out" by antiracism.[32]

Davison presumably understood full well the kind of actual harm he was causing by having "a teacher, an authority figure, talk . . . endlessly, year after year . . . that because you [are white American] you are associated with . . . all these different evils."[33] Unfortunately, Davison took the coward's way out, opting to fire Rossi and deny any consensus with him. Thankfully, Rossi was a step ahead of Davison and recorded the conversation, which you can listen to at dailymail.uk.com. Davison, of course, laments that his words were taken out of context. Simply listen to the audio recording and decide for yourself. Grace Church School's Director of Communication, Topher Nichols, also took the coward's way out when confronted with the audio evidence: "At this point, we don't have a comment" is all we got from him.[34]

One could argue that Rossi got off easy. In Toronto, Principal Rich-

---

29. Quoted in Powell, "New York's Private Schools . . ." (2021).
30. Quoted in Murray (2022), p. 53.
31. Quoted in Shawn Cohen, "Headmaster of Elite NYC School Tells Colleagues he was 'Trapped by a Disgruntled Teacher . . .,'" *Dailymail* (April 23, 2021).
32. Quoted in Cohen, "Headmaster of Elite NYC School . . ." (2021).
33. Quoted in Cohen, "Headmaster of Elite NYC School . . ." (2021).
34. Quoted in Cohen, "Headmaster of Elite NYC School . . ." (2021).

ard Bilkszto also endured DEI indoctrination. When he questioned the instructor, he was belittled for having opened his mouth. The subsequent "workplace harassment and bullying" got too much for him, and Bilkszto killed himself.[35]

Social Justice

While social justice joins two words that sound nice individually, when put together they create a series of problems for both society and justice. Social justice works around group identity, not individual behavior. An extreme example of how wrong social justice can go can be found in Adolf Hitler's *Mein Kampf*, which targeted German Jews, who *die führer* blamed for social problems in Deutschland. The math is simple: one group (blonde-haired, blue-eyed, tall, attractive Germans—which ironically excluded Hitler himself) decided that another group (German Jews) was irredeemably guilty of societal subterfuge. Reading Hitler's disgraceful book, one instantly realizes that we need only replace the word "Jew" with the term "white people," and the chorus of contemporary critical social justice rhetoric embers from the ashes of the Third Reich. The math hasn't changed much today: one group (Team CSJ) has decided that another group (white Americans) is responsible for all the problems of society. Fanciful as this comparison might sound, a team of three scholars put this theory to the test with truly disturbing, albeit sometimes amusing, results.

Between 2017 and 2018, Helen Pluckrose, James Lindsay, and Peter Boghossian penned their infamous and eye-opening "Hoax Papers," a series of twenty academic articles filled with ludicrous ideas, including the possibility that penises contribute to climate change and how morbid obesity can be a form of body building. The papers were all written in a way that no rational, thoughtful person could ever take seriously. And yet, the critical social justice academics who oversaw the journals to which the hoaxers submitted these papers took them *very* seriously—one of which, submitted to the journal *Sociology of Race and Ethnicity*, saw the authors selecting passages from *Mein Kampf* and replacing the

35. Lee Harding, "Diversity Training Increases Prejudice an[d] 'Activates Bigotry' Among Participants, New Study Says," *ZeroHedge* (February 13, 2024).

word "Jew" with the term "white people." Not a single critical social justice scholar reviewing the paper noticed. In fact, they agreed with the premise. One reviewer said the paper was "refreshing"; another found "the article has potential to be a powerful and particular contribution to literature related to the *mechanisms that reinforce* . . . white supremacist perspectives."[36] The total lack of self-awareness is as astounding as it is disconcerting.

Backing up even further in history when the early modern period was feeding into the Renaissance (roughly 1450–1700 CE), we find another correlation between modern critical social justice and truly alarming authoritarianism. In those days, to be accused of witchcraft usually resulted in a death sentence. "Witch" wasn't just an accusation. It was a *label.* And one that proved quite inescapable once bestowed. In fact, the more a person denied any witchy inclinations, the more it demonstrated that she was certainly a witch. There simply had to be witches somewhere—how else to explain those mysterious epidemics, the famines, the child mortality? Conditions for common people were such that calamity and tragedy were part of everyday life. Cattle got sick, farm equipment broke, and children died quite often. A loving God would not allow such calamity, so the cleverest theologians reasoned, therefore witches were to blame. And these witches seemed to be everywhere. Therefore, the question for zealous theologians was not *did witchcraft take place*, but instead, *how did witchcraft manifest in that situation*? Inquisitors Heinrich Kramer (c. 1430–1505) and James Spranger (c. 1437–1495), authors of the *Malleus Maleficarum* (1486), open their infamous tome asking, "Whether the belief that there are such beings as witches is so essential a part of the Catholic faith that obstinately to maintain the opposite opinion manifestly savours of heresy[?]"[37] Roughly forty thousand people—mostly women—burned at the stake for imaginary crimes in the name of social justice.

We find similar authoritarian mind games, also phrased in question form, echoed by Robin DiAngelo, author of her own bestselling *kampf*, *White Fragility* (2018). At the 2014 Race and Pedagogy National Con-

36. Quoted in James A. Lindsay et al., "Academic Grievance Studies and the Corruption of Scholarship," *Areo Magazine* (February 10, 2018); *italics* mine.
37. Rev. Montague Summers (trans.), Heinrich Kramer and James Sprenger, *The Malleus Maleficarum* (NY: Dover Publications, Inc., 1971), p. 1.

ference, DiAngelo confirmed the CRT perspective that racism is present in every interaction. "The question is not 'did racism take place' but rather 'how did racism manifest in that situation?'" she instructed the audience.[38] Reading *White Fragility* really only demonstrates that DiAngelo is, herself, quite racist. This, of course, is not her fault. For in DiAngelo's bitter world, to be a white American (as she is) means "anti-blackness is foundational to our very identities as white people."[39] Her philosophy is similar to the playground taunt, "I know you are but what am I?" which she has modified to an even more childish verse, "I know I am, so you must be too."

DiAngelo is the kind of "thinker" shaping the critical social justice perspective today.

POSTMODERNISM

While the 1960s produced excellent strides in liberal culture (e.g., antiwar activism, the Civil Rights Movement, women's rights, and flower power), that decade also saw the birth of one of the greatest philosophical blunders in Western history: postmodernism.[40] The core and history of postmodern ideas are somewhat loopy, purposely dense, and reek of an intellectual pretense that goes far beyond the scope of this book. For our purposes, we need only understand the fundamentals: according to the postmodernist perspective, *truth* doesn't really exist (which is itself a truth claim, thereby crippling the entire philosophy right out the gate).

To their credit, the postmodernists were right to be skeptical of the kinds of scientific authoritarianism that launched the Holocaust. Similar—albeit less harsh—forms of bigotry existed in the United States in the manner of Jim Crow laws, to say nothing of Japanese Internment

38. Heather Bruce et al., "Between Principles and Practice: Tensions in Anti-Racist Education—2014 Race & Pedagogy National Conference," Race and Pedagogy Conference.

39. Robin DiAngelo, *White Fragility: Why It's So Hard for White People to Talk about Racism* (MA: Beacon Press, 2018), p. 91.

40. While postmodern art predates the philosophy by about twenty years, its assault on the humanities began in earnest in the 1960s. See Helen Pluckrose and James Lindsay, *Social Injustice: Why Many Popular Answers to Important Questions of Race, Gender, and Identity are Wrong—and How to Know What's Right* (NC: Pitchstone Publishing, 2022), p. 18.

Camps, and the abuse of First Nations peoples. So yes, the postmodernists were on to something when they spoke of unfettered oppressive power structures. We can agree there. But the postmodernists took these ideas into rather absurd places that are difficult to take seriously. Above all, the postmodernists were cynical, nihilistic, and skeptical of everything. And so, it was a short step from *scientific advancement can lead to oppressive authoritarianism* to declaring *science isn't real.* A heavy promoter of this idea was Michel Foucault (1926–1984), who conceived the idea of "power/knowledge," the belief that "truth isn't outside power. . . . Each society has its regime of truth . . . that is, the types of discourse which it accepts and makes function as true; the mechanisms and instances which enable one to distinguish true and false statements . . . the status of those charged with saying what counts as true."[41] For the pessimistic postmodernist, science is awash with notions of racism and sexism, and therefore not a legitimate method of finding objective truth, which they do not believe even exists.

In recent years, this curious mixture of Neo-Marxism, DEI, social justice, and postmodernism have seeded the psychedelic Renaissance.

41. Michel Foucault, *Power/Knowledge: Selected Interviews and Other Writings, 1972–1977* (Brighton, Sussex: Harvester Press), p. 131; see also, Lindsay (2022), pp. 25–6.

3

Hip Indoctrination: Praxis in Psychedelic Spaces

What would it mean if as a community we took these sacred medicines to break the system?

Dr. NiCole Buchanan, "Psychedelic Justice"

JEDI Mind Tricks

Psychedelic nonprofit Chacruna Institute has adopted DEI indoctrination (recently rebranded as JEDI by Stanford medical students in 2020), into its values.[1] Like DEI, the EDI in JEDI stands for "equity, diversity, and inclusion," with an additional J for "justice." Only we cannot take these words at face value. Here, "justice" should be read as "social justice," or, more correctly, Critical Social Justice, the political philosophy that translates to "guilt by association." "Diversity" should be interpreted as stacking as many people as possible with similar views on stage at public forums to agree with each other that they are oppressed (in some unspecified way); because diversity of *thought* is difficult to find at Chacruna Institute. Chacruna affiliates' use of "inclusion" can be read roughly

1. From the Community, "Opinion: Letter to the President and Provost: Action Items for Achieving Racial Equity," *The Stanford Daily* (June 19, 2020).

the same as "diversity." Speakers who promote approved rhetoric will be included. Any good-faith, dissenting voice will be excluded.

Let's now turn to the *E* in JEDI—equity.

Equity sounds similar to equality, but I find that most psychedelic thought-leaders do not consider the stark difference between the two. Equality, in this context, means "equal opportunity," a philosophy I hope we can all get behind. Thousands of kids living in depressed areas deserve the same chance to succeed in life as kids living in middle-class neighborhoods. They deserve good schools, stable homes, safe neighborhoods, and learning and career opportunities. However, when and if those things are not available (which has certainly been the case historically), some demand equity as a correction. Equity seeks to fix past systemic racism, not through "equal opportunity," but instead by trying to ensure "equal outcomes." A noble goal, perhaps, only it doesn't work.

In the early 2020s, some schools in California, Oregon, and Washington instituted "equity math" into their curricula.[2] They hoped such efforts would "dismantl[e] racism in mathematics." Because nothing screams "white supremacy" quite like times tables. "The concept of mathematics being purely objective is unequivocally false," say some of the drafters of Oregon's "Equitable Math" guidebook.[3] And whoever penned Seattle Public Schools K–12 "Math Ethnic Studies Framework" labels "Western mathematics" as uniquely "oppressive."[4] Supporters of equity math follow the postmodern line of Michel Foucault in their belief that mathematics represents a mere social construct used by oppressors to hold power over the oppressed. Equity math attacks reality at its most fundamental core. Only, mathematical reality is not born of "white supremacy," nor is it even Western; it is found throughout every human civilization in history (except the most prosperous, modern one, apparently).

Today, in the name of equity, too many American grade-schoolers are learning that 2+2 can equal, well . . . it depends on what kind of

2. "California Adopts New Mathematics Framework Focused on Equity and Social Justice," *Observer Newsroom* (July 14, 2023).
3. Sam Dorman, "Adding Wokeness: Oregon Promotes Teacher Program to Subtract 'Racism in Mathematics,'" *The New York Post* (February 12, 2021).
4. "Seattle Public Schools K–12 Math Ethnic Studies Framework" (August 20, 2019), p. 1.

"mathematical identity" the student adopts.[5] Equity math affirms what has been termed the "soft bigotry of low expectations." Although I find that there is nothing soft about hindering an entire generation of underserved kids through intellectual deterioration like equity math.

Additionally, some school districts have dropped honors classes "to increase equity."[6] Lowering standards in a highly competitive world will certainly not result in equal outcomes. But perhaps equal outcome is not the real goal here. If CSJ activists can convince someone that 2+2 equals anything but 4, said activists can convince that person of anything. And if said CSJ activists can convince a person of anything then they own her mind. All of the LSD in the world might not help her then. Equity math is a most sinister form of cognitive subjugation that is antithetical to the values of the psychedelic Renaissance. It, and the larger move towards equity education, will also do the job of which real white American racists have only dreamed. These kids will be intellectually crippled from the inside out.

It gets more troubling when we apply equity to the law.

OUT BY SUNDAY

Equitable policing, in theory, holds that toning down policing in favor of community solutions results in an overall better quality of life. I don't necessarily think that's a bad idea. However, there are two shortcomings with that remedy worth considering: first, for many people living in high crime neighborhoods, the solution to a better quality of life is more quality police officers who have good relationships with the communities they serve. This assures safer neighborhoods, and safer neighborhoods mean businesses invest in the areas and offer opportunities that begin the journey towards equal outcomes. Obviously, there is more that goes into each of our individual stories, but safe neighborhoods are a foundational starting point. And second, equitable policing in practice means considering ethnicity and historical discrimination while investigating a crime and granting leniency based on it—no matter how horrific the offense(s).

---

5. "Seattle Public Schools . . ." (2019), p. 3.
6. Sara Randazzo, "To Increase Equity, School Districts Eliminate Honors Classes," *Wall Street Journal* (Feb 17, 2023).

Jordan Henry basked in equitable policing. His rap sheet includes several felonies: carjacking, criminal robbery with a firearm, retail theft, a medley of traffic infractions, aggravated kidnapping with intent to inflict harm, aggravated battery, and violent aggravated criminal sexual assault.[7] For those unfamiliar with that last charge, it means not only that Henry raped a woman but also that he beat the shit out of her in the process. He also had a warrant in Indiana for theft. And yet, there he was, strolling through the Lincoln Park neighborhood in Chicago on a cold Midwestern day.

Approaching a 7-Eleven on 23 February 2022, Henry pulled an unregistered gun to a man's face hoping to carjack him. Thankfully, the victim was able to flee with both his life and car intact. Not so easily outdone, Henry then pulled his gun on a sixty-nine-year-old man who used his Volkswagen Jetta to drive for Uber. The man complied; Henry sped down the highway. The end result saw the car totaled after a police chase worthy of the Blues Brothers. Henry ran from the wreckage, even punching Hades, a police K-9, while trying to escape. As you can imagine, punching a pooch only intensified the officers' determination to catch Henry and take him down.

Eventually handcuffed and carted away in a police ambulance, Henry smiled at the officers and remarked, "I'll be out by Sunday."[8] And why wouldn't he be so cocky? Kimberly Foxx, District Attorney of Cook County, Chicago—where Henry mostly prowled—practiced equitable policing. Henry never faced proportional penalties for his violent crimes due to his ethnicity. DA Foxx had earlier tried to cut a deal with Jussie Smollett, the former *Empire* actor who disgraced his name by trying to reopen and capitalize on America's deepest wound.[9] Foxx presumably

7. James W. Glasgow, Will County Attorney, "Glasgow Announces Jordan Henry Sentenced to 22 Years in Aggravated Vehicular Hijacking on Diversey Parkway in Chicago" (March 2023).

8. Quoted in Glasgow, "Glasgow Announces . . ." (2023).

9. Smollett's poorly thought out plan also raises another issue. He tried to use his fabricated "attack" against his sexual orientation and skin color to gain prestige in Hollywood. But there is a major, telling flaw to his entire premise: wouldn't a white supremacist country simply shrug it off; perhaps even delight in the battery? What was the US population's overall reaction? A total outpouring of love and support. It isn't every day that A-list actors, the legacy media, a district attorney, and even the First Lady come to your defense—that's quite a privilege! Smollett's deception proved the opposite of what he

doesn't live in the kinds of neighborhoods that predators like Henry stalk and so practiced a contortionist-like leniency towards criminality—the kind of clemency that can only result in producing violent criminals like Jordan Henry.

But Henry messed up this time. The car chase took him into Will County, just outside the Windy City, where DA Foxx had no jurisdiction. Had he surrendered to the police in Cook County, where the carjacking took place, he might be on the streets today. Because police arrested him in Will County, Henry would face prosecutor James Glasgow, who was not going to further these egregious miscarriages of justice that DA Foxx had perpetrated on her own constituents by keeping Henry on the streets.

Glasgow secured a twenty-two-year stretch for Henry.

Chacruna Institute affiliates like therapists Monnica Williams, Sara Reed, and Jamilah R. George boldly claim: "At every level, the criminal justice system is heavily biased against Black people compared to White people."[10] While they are clearly wrong in Henry's case (and countless others excluded from this chapter so as not to belabor the point), they can at least rest easy knowing that Jordan Henry checked off every box for JEDI! *Justice* was finally served, after *equitable* policing had failed, resulting in Henry's arrest by a *diverse* force of police officers, so he can now be *included* in the prison population. Still, the question remains: how are we to ensure an equal outcome for someone like Jordan Henry?

Consummately, Chacruna Institute's JEDI initiative focuses on "the ways in which psychedelics influence and are influenced by factors such as social justice, privilege, and diversity and to better understand their reciprocal influences on psychedelic science, therapies, and praxis."[11] For

---

was trying to demonstrate—especially if he'd gotten away with it. His plan could not have possibly worked from the outset if the US was truly a racist country. What white supremacist nation cares about a gay black American man getting beaten up in the Chicago streets? It really doesn't make any sense if you think about it for two whole seconds.

10. Monnica T. Williams, Sara Reed, Jamilah George, "Culture and Psychedelic Psychotherapy: Ethnic and Racial Themes from Three Black Women Therapists," *Journal of Psychedelic Studies*, 4, 3 (2020), p. 128.

11. Chacruna Institute, "Diversity, Culture, and Social Justice in Psychedelics Course" (February 16, 2022).

those unfamiliar with that last term, "praxis" is a Marxist word that couples Theory with activism.[12] And in the true spirit of anticapitalism, Chacruna Institute charges $650 dollars a pop for such classes.[13]

Despite these Chacruna affiliates' insistence that we racialize every issue through JEDI training, they also recognize that "current research indicates that the experience of ongoing racism can indeed result in stress, traumatization, and even a formal diagnosis of PTSD."[14] Political scientist Wilfred Reilly, who has looked closely into this issue, feels differently. Says he, "the primary thing holding Black students back is not racism but rather the heartfelt belief that the 'white' world . . . is a pervasively racist place."[15] And Reilly is not a lone voice. Canadian professor David Haskell prepared a study for the Aristotle Foundation for Public Policy on the effectiveness of DEI and found such indoctrination "has been shown to increase prejudice and activate bigotry among participants by bringing existing stereotypes to the top of their minds or by implanting new biases they had not previously held."[16] Reilly and Haskell are supported by a battery of research papers that demonstrate how DEI is counterproductive to its stated goal of alleviating racism.[17] Perhaps it is no coincidence that one of the studies to expose DEI also found that such indoctrination "reduces sympathy, increases blame, and decreases external attributions for White people struggling with poverty." For Haskell, the reason was obvious: "[the indoctrinated were] even more hostile toward poor whites, because those people must be categorically lazy . . . [or] dysfunctional because they have privilege. Why are they not successful? . . . . White privilege completely ignores the thousands of other variables that go into every person, white or black or indigenous. There are so many things that can cause social and economic distress."[18]

We are left to conclude that Chacruna's affiliates exacerbate the

12. Pluckrose and Lindsay (2022), p. 233.
13. Chacruna Institute, "Diversity, Culture, and Social Justice . . ." (2022).
14. Williams et al., "Culture and Psychedelic Psychotherapy . . ." (2020), p. 128.
15. Reilly (2019), p. xix.
16. David Millard Haskell, "What DEI Research Concludes about Diversity Training: It is Divisive, Counter-Productive, and Unnecessary," *Aristotle Foundation for Public Policy* (February 12, 2024).
17. Lee Harding, "Diversity Training Increases Prejudice an[d] 'Activates Bigotry' among Participants, New Study Says," *ZeroHedge* (February 13, 2024).
18. Quoted in Harding, "Diversity Training Increases Prejudice . . ." (2024).

problem with JEDI mind tricks by creating, promoting, and recycling the very "ongoing racism" that leads to stress and PTSD—even if they don't intend to. Chacruna affiliates live in a world where "ongoing oppression"—an oppression that no one in their ranks can articulate[19]—must be tackled "as psychedelics go mainstream." To this end, Chacruna board members Dr. NiCole Buchanan and Jamilah R. George insist that black Americans face unique disadvantages in psychedelic spaces such as "barriers to access, criminalization of psychedelic use, and police surveillance,"[20] as if *all* inner-explorers do not face those challenges. At present, psychedelic medicines are still federally illegal for *everyone*, regardless of skin tone. And while it might be easy to assume that legal status doesn't matter if the police are all racist (meaning they leave white American substantia users alone), we will see in a later chapter that the narrative of an all-pervasive, all-powerful, racist police force doesn't stack up to the weight of the evidence. For now, take it in good faith that impoverished Americans from a wide variety of backgrounds have difficulty accessing these medicines. Perhaps we psychedelic researchers should work together to ensure that anyone who can benefit from these medicines has access to them, regardless of skin color.

Unconscious Bias

Chacruna Institute also pushes unconscious—or implicit—bias into psychedelic spaces. First developed by Anthony Greenwald and Mahzarin Banaji in 1998, unconscious bias is based in a hypothesis which holds that, despite a person having no racist thoughts in her daily life, there still exists a secret, malignant form of racism lurking in her unconscious mind. Obviously, we all have our biases. But as we will see in a moment, our biases are very much conscious and based on observational and environmental factors.

Greenwald and Banaji called the program they developed to mea-

19. I am not the first person to notice that this "oppression" is never defined. See Reilly (2019), p. 3.

20. Jamilah R. George and NiCole Buchanan, "Black Lives Matter and Psychedelic Integration: Pathways to Radical Healing Amidst Ongoing Oppression" (November 4, 2022).

sure such unconscious bias the Implicit Association Test (or IAT).[21] The IAT shows the test-taker a series of names that can broadly fit into certain ethnic stereotypes (e.g., Tyron and Latisha, or Brittany and Carson), alongside pleasant words (like love or friendship) and negative words (like hate or war). Test-takers are timed so as to gauge how quickly they associate certain words with ethnically white American names and other words with ethnically black American names. The longer it takes the test-taker to associate a black American ethnic-sounding name with a positive word is all the proof Greenwald and Banaji needed to cry racism. When the IAT was first launched in 1998, a press release from the University of Washington (of which Greenwald is affiliated) stated that the test uncovered implicit bias in "90 to 95 percent of people," including Greenwald and Banaji![22]

With results this eye-opening, the IAT has joined DEI training initiatives, which could be found in major universities like Harvard and Yale, private schools like Harvard-Westlake School (in Los Angeles) and the Brentwood School District (in Missouri), big tech companies like Google and Facebook, and various other institutions like the Department of Homeland Security, Cigna, and soda companies like Coca-Cola.

But there's a major problem with the whole concept of implicit bias. Anthony Greenwald later acknowledged that the link between implicit bias and discriminatory behavior is weak. Despite writing in his and Banajis' book, *Blindspot* (2013), that the IAT "predicts discriminatory behavior even among research participants who earnestly (and, we believe, honestly) espouse egalitarian beliefs," he later amended that claim to the peer-review board at the *Journal of Personality and Social Psychology*.[23] Therein, Greenwald affirms that the IAT is "problematic to use ... to classify persons as likely to engage in discrimination." He continues, "attempts to diagnostically use such measures for individuals risk un-

---

21. IATs are not limited to race, but have been developed for other unconscious prejudices too, like age or sexual orientation discrimination.

22. Joel Schwartz, "Roots of Unconscious Prejudice Affect 90 to 95 Percent of People, Psychologists Demonstrate at Press Conference," *University of Washington News* (September 29, 1998).

23. Quoted in Jesse Singal, "The Creators of the Implicit Bias Association Test Should Get Their Story Straight," *Intelligencer* (December 5, 2017).

desirably high rates of erroneous classifications."[24] In short, the IAT is bunk. Greenwald deserves credit for having the courage to admit he was wrong. We could all stand to be so genuinely humble.

Major corporations that had implemented the IAT soon dropped it. Facebook's diversity initiative barely made a noticeable impact on its day-to-day operations. Google admits that, despite its best efforts, it could not "show real results" with the IAT. Pinterest lost interest after the IAT training "didn't make a difference."[25] Maybe that is why Tiffany L. Green, professor of Health Sciences at the University of Wisconsin-Madison, remarked that use of the IAT "could cause more damage and exacerbate the very issues it is trying to solve."[26]

Perhaps Chacruna Institute ought to reconsider its strategy. If the very creators of the IAT (and subsequent major corporations that employed it) have realized the test's shortcomings, we mind-expanders shouldn't have much difficulty doing the same. Causing more damage and exacerbating rifts in society are antithetical to the values of the psychedelic Renaissance. The IAT (and larger unconscious bias movement) has proven to do both.

This does not mean that we don't have our biases. We all have basic survival equipment built into us through the noble sacrifices of thousands of our ancestors who miscalculated this or that situation and paid the ultimate price for their efforts. Though I'm still curious what DEI supporters think of the following hypothetical: suppose I am strolling down the sidewalk and see up ahead two groups of men on each side of the street. On my side of the street, a group of white Americans stands around the corner of the building, careful not to let the streetlights illuminate them too much. They sport shaved heads and have large swastika patches on their bomber jackets; leaning against the building is a placard that insists "God Hates Fags." I see the other group across the street is comprised of black Americans wearing ordinary clothing. I can hear them joshing each other, laughing, and making jokes.

You bet your sweet ass I'm crossing that street!

---

24. Quoted in Singal "The Creators . . ." (2017).
25. Olivia Goldhill, "The World is Relying on a Flawed Psychological Test to Fight Racism," *Quartz* (December 3, 2017).
26. Tiffany L. Green, "The Problem with Implicit Bias Training," *Scientific American* (August 28, 2020).

You'll have immediately noticed that the ethnicity of each group didn't factor into my decision. How they present themselves is all that matters to me. Being black American doesn't come with any intrinsic sinister implications.

Being a neo-Nazi does.

Still, the IAT has entered the psychedelic Renaissance through those like Dr. NiCole Buchanan, who offers implicit bias training through Chacruna Institute. She has even delivered TEDx talks on the topic at the university of her employment, Michigan State; on stage, Dr. Buchanan found herself in quite a unique position. She had to admit that, "Thankfully, we know that explicit bias—that old fashioned racism and sexism—that's been steadily decreasing over the past fifty years." But this presents a problem. Dr. Buchanan believes that racism is ever-present, despite her refreshingly honest acknowledgment to the contrary. Therefore, she promotes the idea of implicit bias, which, according to her, is "far more dangerous and insidious," and claims that it has grown over those same fifty-years.[27] Dr. Buchanan would like us to believe that the less racist people have become over time, the more racist they are today. Only she bases her conclusions on a test that has been discredited by its own creators. She is, in effect, making a faith-based appeal.

In the late 20-teens, I came face to face with implicit bias training in the psychedelic Renaissance. The Portland Psychedelic Society (PPS), which at the time had an uber-psychedelic SJW for the organization's president,[28] decided that anyone who hadn't participated in implicit bias training was barred from working with PPS. Since my business partner Eden and I hold no racist inclinations, we politely declined. We're workaholics who don't have time to waste signaling our purity to the larger Portland psychedelic community by taking a test that detects racism as

27. Buchanan, N. T., "Excising a Virus of the Mind: Individual and Institutional Responsibility for Reducing Implicit Bias," for TEDxMSU at Michigan State University, East Lansing, MI (January 20, 2017). See also, Buchanan N.T., "Bias and Its Role in Social Iniquity." Invited presentation for the forum, Sharper Focus, Wider Lens Symposium on "The Nature of Inequality," Michigan State University Honor's College (January 25, 2016).

28. In the spirit of fraternity, I withhold his name.

accurately as it measures the height of the Easter Bunny. We were immediately barred from working at any PPS events. We weren't even allowed to pay a vendor fee and set up a table to pass out harm reduction and educational literature. The former PPS president holds firm to the fantasy of implicit bias, allowing him to believe he has the moral high ground by "acknowledging" his own racism. Fair enough.

But then he demanded we admit guilt for a moral crime he committed.

Psychedelic Social Justice

Psychedelic social justice narratives are equally lacking in thoughtful discernment. Consider Chacruna Institute's Theorists' idea that black and indigenous Americans be paid for speaking engagements to the exclusion of others. At this point in the movement, few people get paid anything substantial to speak. If one is lucky, she might leave a conference with a $100 honorarium—most leave with nothing. Psychedelic "social justice" demands that *some* people get paid while others do not—and, of course, it is all based on melanin levels and outdated narratives.[29] Dr. Buchanan picks up this mantle. She, a well-compensated psychology professor at Michigan State University (who has received hundreds of thousands of dollars in research grants[30]), is to be paid for speaking engagements, even if everyone else must foot travel costs out-of-pocket, no matter their income.

Diné[31] speaker and author Belinda Eriacho has a short list of suggestions for any event organizer that hosts a First Nations speaker at a conference. Some of her suggestions, like having dinner with the speaker before the event to get to know each other, are certainly welcome! But others reek of preferential treatment in the name of psychedelic social justice. For example, an indigenous speaker should be given gifts and a welcome note upon arrival. All their expenses should be covered. They are to receive "the same offering or better" as non–First Nations peo-

29. See NiCole T. Buchanan, "Why Psychedelic Science Should Pay Speakers and Trainers of Color," in Labate and Cavnar (2021).
30. NiCole T. Buchanan, "Curriculum Vitae," p. 3–5.
31. Traditional name for "Navajo."

ples receive with regards to lodging (regardless of noteriety).[32] Eriacho also wants us to keep in mind that while an "academic or scientific psychedelic conference may not be the most ideal event for an Indigenous person to be a part of," organizers should make sure they are "included in the 'scientific' discussions." They are also to receive their own private rooms for "collective internal dialogue among themselves." First Nations speakers should also get the best speaking slots and car service to and from the venue. If they sit on a panel, they are to speak first. And never mind all the myriad activities that go into planning a conference, the organizers must put aside some time to learn all they can about the indigenous speaker's cultural history. However, the organizers must also be careful not to ask the speaker any questions about her culture. Instead, the organizers should hire a separate indigenous person to "support . . . in doing . . . research."

And always remember—"tokenization must be avoided"[!][33]

Let's admit right here that the US government has screwed over First Nations peoples. Reservations are littered with substance abuse, trauma, and a host of other social maladies that the government has mostly ignored. I suppose my point here is that we should give *those* people—the marginalized, the forgotten—preferential treatment; not the well-compensated speakers who advocate on their behalf. I don't want part of the price I pay for my ticket to an event to line Dr. Buchanan's pockets solely because she is an ethnic minority. She's doing just fine financially. I want my portion of the sale to go to those people who actually need it.

MICROAGGRESSIONS

Affiliates at Chacruna Institute also place their faith in the questionable social affront known as a "microaggression." Microaggressions, as defined by Kevin Nadal, psychology professor at John Jay College of Crim-

32. To clarify, there are many First Nations speakers who deliver eloquent—dare I say breathtaking—speeches. Unfortunately, that consideration comes secondary to identity politics.

33. Belinda Eriacho, "Considerations for Working with Indigenous People in Psychedelic Spaces and Guidelines for Inclusion of Indigenous People in Psychedelic Science Conferences," in Labate and Cavnar (2021), pp. 51–4.

inal Justice, are "everyday, subtle, intentional—and oftentimes unintentional—interactions or behaviors that communicate some sort of bias toward historically marginalized groups."[34] These are generally harmless questions like "where are you from?" that you might ask a new coworker or compliments like, "you speak [insert language] very well" to a foreign speaker. To interpret either as some semi-restrained aggression strikes me as odd. When I lived in Italy, it was obvious to everyone I met that I was not a native speaker. When asked countless times in myriad situations, *di dove?* ("where are you from?"), I felt no hostility emitting from the person to whom I was speaking. Turns out, I was wrong. The praxis of important microaggression work is to inspect everything a person says or does and *try to find* something with which to take offense. Robin DiAngelo phrases this idea in the form of a question: "Am I actively seeking to interpret racism in this context?"[35]

Chacruna board member Dr. Monnica Williams is a true-believer in microaggressions, bravely leading the charge against this windmill by producing almost 100 papers, presentations, and workshops on the topic.[36] Dr. Williams's apparent obsession with the inspired world of microaggressions might help explain why, as she laments, none of her white Canadian and American peers wish to collaborate with her.[37] Whilst Williams wonders why, sociologist Musa al-Gharbi of Stony Brook University knows the answer: "[JEDI and DEI] training also leads many to believe that they have to 'walk on eggshells' when engaging with members of minority populations. . . . As a result, members of the dominant group become less likely to try to build relationships or collaborate with people from minority populations."[38] Why would anyone put themselves in a situation where a person with whom they are in conversation is constantly scanning innocent words and phrases trying to parse out some fabricated example of "racism?" I certainly wouldn't. And I doubt any self-respecting person would. Microaggressions serve as the perfect way

34. Quoted in Andrew Limbong, "Microaggressions Are a Big Deal: How to Talk Them Out and When to Walk Away" (June 9, 2020).
35. DiAngelo (2018), p. 87.
36. Monnica T. Williams, "Curriculum Vitae."
37. Monnica T. Williams, "When Feminism Functions as White Supremacy: How White Feminists Oppress Black Women," in Labate and Cavnar (2021), p. 22.
38. Quoted in Harding, "Diversity Training Increases Prejudice . . ." (2024).

to keep peoples of various ethnicities looking askance at each other. They only further divide us.

Microaggressions aside, one of Dr. Williams's articles in Chacruna Institute's anthology of critical social justice essays, *Psychedelic Justice* (2021), is filled with bold claims about the world that rely more on abstractions and historical narratives than contemporary realities. Highlights include, "White feminists don't worry about going to jail, as they can afford good legal representation" and "White women have historically and currently used their sexuality to oppress men of color."[39] Let's take these broad assertions one at a time. Does Dr. Williams really believe that *all* white American women are rich and can afford quality legal counsel? Such a statement runs counter to available evidence presented by the Center of Budget and Policy Priorities, which places white Americans at the top of the list of welfare recipients. Accordingly, "6.2 million working-age whites" received government-assistance in 2014.[40] It's difficult to square that fact with the idea that millions of welfare-receiving white American women are also throwing fat stacks at high-power lawyers.

As for Williams's claim that in the past and presently white American women have and continue to oppress black American men through sex: historically, yes, Dr. Williams is correct—white American women certainly used their social status to oppress not "men of color" (which totally obfuscates the issue) but *black American* men specifically. From the Tulsa Race Massacre of 1921 to Emmitt Till's execution in 1955 (the examples Williams cites in her article[41]), I agree with her that perhaps the contemporary phrase "believe all women" is just a little too simplistic and can lead to terrible miscarriages of justice.

But notice that Dr. Williams has to dig back to the Tulsa Race Massacre and the murder of Emmett Till (when America was truly a racist nation) to make her case. One imagines that, should Williams have any evidence of this sort of grotesque form of racism going on today, she would have included it in her article. This is a Chacruna Institute

---

39. Williams, "When Feminism . . .," in Labate and Cavnar (2021), pp. 25 and 23.
40. Ryan Sit, "Trump Thinks Only Black People Are on Welfare, But Really, White Americans Receive Most Benefits," *Newsweek* (January 12, 2018).
41. Williams, "When Feminism . . .," in Labate and Cavnar (2021), p. 23.

sleight-of-hand trick: we can all pick numerous historical examples of ugly systemic racism in the United States; the real exercise is finding the Emmett Tills of today. Turns out, there aren't any. And while we might want to celebrate that fact, those who do will be called racist for acknowledging that lynching is no longer a problem in the United States.

Racist Medicine

Dr. Williams also finds racism within the American medical establishment because "[m]aternal mortality for Black women is four times the rate of White women" regardless of tax bracket.[42] While that is true, it is also true that the full reasons for this phenomenon are still not completely understood; nonetheless, we are instructed to attribute the disparity in maternal mortality between black and white Americans to racism alone. However, Dr. Williams has ignored a variety of factors that have begun to shine a light on this disparity. The three main causes of maternal mortality are hemorrhage, pregnancy-induced hypertension, and embolism.

Hemorrhages are caused by several factors including long-term alcohol and nicotine use, blood clotting disorders, cancer, viruses, injury from physical violence (e.g., a punch to the head), and other factors that are hardly the fault of doctors.[43] Black American women are nearly three times more at risk than white American women of suffering a hemorrhage.[44] The causes of pregnancy-induced hypertension are not yet fully understood. It may very well be caused by racism. It might also be caused by preexisting high blood-pressure.[45] It remains a mystery. Embolisms are caused by deep vein blood clots. How any of these conditions are the fault of a racist medical system is yet to be addressed by Dr. Williams.

Furthermore, 50% of all pregnancies across ethnicities in the United States are unplanned. Such pregnancies can be correlated with a higher possibility of either mother and/or infant dying. As the Centers for Disease Control (CDC) reports, "Lifestyle factors (e.g., smoking, drinking

42. Williams, "When Feminism . . .," in Labate and Cavnar (2021), p. 22.
43. Cleveland Clinic, "Hemorrhage" (2024).
44. See Mary Beth Flanders-Stepans, "Alarming Racial Differences in Maternal Mortality," *Journal of Perinatal Education*, 9, 2 (Spring, 2000).
45. "Causes of Gestational Hypertension," *Stanford Medicine* (2024).

alcohol, unsafe sex practices, and poor nutrition) and inadequate intake of foods containing folic acid pose serious health hazards to the mother and fetus and are more common among women with unintended pregnancies." Additionally, prenatal care is not pursued by 25% of these women during the first trimester.[46]

Obesity also has a role to play in the disparity of mother mortality between black and white American women. A study conducted in Pennsylvania (which has the sixth-largest state population in the United States), found:

> There is strong evidence linking prepregnancy obesity to adverse infant outcomes including infant mortality and stillbirth. . . . Non-Hispanic Black women carry the burden of the obesity epidemic in the U.S. . . . Stillbirth and infant death occurred at a rate two to three times higher in [Non-Hispanic] Black women compared with [Non-Hispanic] White women. . . . Compared with women without obesity, women with obesity had a higher rate of stillbirth and infant death.[47]

One might find this interesting in light of a video promoted by the Los Angeles Unified School District released in 2022. The video focuses on so-called "food neutrality" (or "food equity") and features three women who, in their own way, convey the idea that choosing healthy food options constitutes another of a seemingly endless array of "systems of oppression." One of these women, YouTuber Blair Imani, speaks of a "false standard of 'health.'" Another, Dr. Kéra Nyemb-Diop, who bills herself as "The Black Nutritionist," tells us that "fat phobia and systems of oppression have created false hierarchies of food and it shows up everywhere." They are echoed by Savage Fatty, who claims, "The only foods that are bad for you are foods that contain allergens (intolerants), poisons, and contaminants, or food that is spoiled or otherwise inedible."[48]

---

46. Flanders-Stepans (2000).
47. Lara S. Lemon et al., "Prepregnancy Obesity and the Racial Disparity in Infant Mortality," *Obesity* (Sliver Spring), 24, 12 (December 1, 2016).
48. LA Parent Union, "Food Neutrality" (September, 2022). In fairness to Savage Fatty, I do agree with her when she says, "we are incorrectly taught from a young age that our size and therefore the foods that we eat are markers of our self-worth." For certain, no one should gauge anyone else's self-worth based on diet. But to claim that there is no actual difference between healthy and unhealthy foods strikes me as just more postmodern

According to Dr. Nyemb-Diop's LinkedIn profile, she was a "Senior Scientist" in "Nutrition and Ingredient Research" at Mondelez, "one of the world's largest snack companies," which manufactures cookies and candies like Oreos and Sour Patch Kids.[49] Likewise, Blair Imani made a deal with Skittles.[50]

A candy-coated layer to a most pernicious heist.

Such is the moral compass of our Black Nutritionist and Blair Imani, warning kids about the nonsensical category of food equity at the expense of their health, while collecting a paycheck from candy companies. Since their advice unequivocally leads to a rainbow of health problems like diabetes, heart disease, cancer, and . . . *motherhood mortality*, might we safely conclude that neither Dr. Nyemb-Diop nor Imani care much about the black American lives they are harming with their message? Sadly, it is either that, or we might need to question whether they understand realities as basic as the difference between a carrot and a candy bar.

The convergence of arguments from Drs. Williams and Nyemb-Diop is self-refuting and vacuous: eating healthy food is white supremacy and then dying post-partum from eating unhealthy food is *also* white supremacy? Is anything reliant on individual choice anymore?

On the matter of motherhood mortality, most mindboggling is Dr. Williams's claim that "it's safer for a Black woman to have a baby in sub-Saharan Africa than in a modern hospital in Arkansas."[51] While it is true that Arkansas has a higher rate of mother and infant mortality than other states in the United States (33 to every 100,000 births),[52] it is nowhere near the level of sub-Saharan Africa, which sees around or over 500 deaths to every 100,000 births.[53] In 2017 alone, 300,000 African

---

relativistic nonsense that critical social justice ideologues smuggle into otherwise serious conversations.

49. Nicole Dominique, "Video Shared By LA School District Features Nutritionist Teaching Kids To Be Unhealthy—Turns Out She Works for Mondelez, a Company That Makes Junk Food," *Evie*, September 15, 2022; Mondelez International, "The Fifth Annual State of Snacking: Global Consumer Trends Study" (2024).

50. Anthony Myers, "Skittles Devotes its Platforms to Provide Visibility for LGBTQ+ Artists, Influencers, and Creators," *Confectionary News* (June, 2021).

51. Williams, "When Feminism . . .," in Labate and Cavnar (2020), pp. 22–3.

52. Alex Angle, "The Maternal Mortality Crisis in Arkansas," *KNWA Fox 24* (July 10, 2022).

53. Leah Rodriguez, "Why Maternal Mortality is so High in Sub-Saharan Africa," *Global Citizen* (August 6, 2021).

women died in labor or shortly thereafter.[54] In Arkansas that year, the number tops out at 304.[55] Sub-Saharan Africa is quite literally the best place on Earth to watch not only mothers but also children five years old and younger die. And the rest of the continent is putting up only slightly better numbers, where roughly 1 in 37 mothers die either during or after childbirth.[56]

How will Dr. Williams explain that? Equity math?

Try as Dr. Williams might to make this problem a race issue, the World Health Organization (WHO) disagrees. A recently published report by WHO opines that the problem isn't about black or white African doctors—the problem is a *lack* of doctors. Over the last twenty years, the African population, despite high infant mortality rates, has seen a steady increase. Unfortunately, there are not enough doctors (supply) to meet the needs of a growing population (demand). Racism has little, perhaps nothing, to do with any of it. Still, more problems persist with Dr. Williams's assessment. When it comes to mother mortality rates in the United States, the groups with the lowest are the Latin and Asian American populations. Somehow our racist Western medical system kills more white American women than it does Latin and Asian American women.[57]

Thankfully, despite Dr. Williams' dismissive claim that "no one seems to care" about this catastrophe among sub-Saharan African mothers and children, organizations like Pathfinder International exist, which "gives women and girls access to empowerment programs and reproductive health care that saves lives."[58] Pathfinder International does the real, on-the-ground work that most of us, myself included—and certainly not those whose work is based on abstractions and bad science—do not do.

---

54. Lisa Schlein, "UN: Most Child, Maternal Deaths Occur in Sub-Saharan Africa," *VOA News* (September 19, 2019).
55. National Center for Health Statistics, "Infant Mortality Rates by State," *Centers for Disease Control and Prevention* (2017).
56. "The State of Maternal Mortality in Sub-Saharan Africa," *Giving Compass* (August 9, 2021).
57. Eugene Declercq and Laurie Zephyrin, "Maternal Mortality in the United States: A Primer," Commonwealth Fund (December 16, 2020).
58. See https://www.pathfinder.org/about-us/our-history/. While the organization certainly had a racist past, it seems those days are over.

Psychedelic Misogyny

Perhaps tired from the good work Dr. Williams does for sub-Saharan mothers and children through her microaggression workshops, she finds it difficult "to muster up the energy to fight issues like the infamous wage gap."[59] But the so-called wage gap—really an "earnings gap"—is as factual as implicit bias, microaggressions, and food equity. That is, it doesn't exist in reality—or at least not nearly to the extent commonly believed. For those of us who prefer a nuanced assessment, we can see that the wage gap figures are misleading because, as commonly calculated, they account only for the total amounts earned yearly between women and men. This calculation does not account for the fact that men typically work more hours per week, seek jobs in STEM fields or dangerous—though lucrative—work, are more willing to relocate for a better position than are women, etc. When these other variables are factored in, "the wage gap narrows to the point of vanishing."[60]

Georgetown University's Center on Education and the Workforce released a study in 2014 based on college majors between the sexes. For petroleum engineering majors, men occupied 87% of the student body; electrical engineering majors were 89% male; naval architecture and marine engineering showed 97% male; mechanical engineering topped out at 90% male. On the other paw, humanities-based majors were dominated by women: early childhood education (97% female); counseling psychology (74% female), and human services and community organization (81% female).[61] All of these students were free to pick any major they desired. And yet, women still gravitated more towards social careers, while men floated towards STEM fields. All of this is not to say that women and men must or even should stay in these respective lanes. There are brilliant female scientists and wonderful male childhood educators. It is to say that when given the choice, more women tend to choose careers in the humanities and more men tend to choose dangerous or scientific careers. These choices, *not patriarchy*, account for payment differentials.

59. Williams, "When Feminism . . .," in Labate and Cavnar (2020), p. 26.
60. Christina Hoff Sommers, "6 Feminist Myths that Will Not Die," *Time Magazine* (June 17, 2016).
61. Christina Hoff Sommers, "The Gender Wage Gap Myth," *American Enterprise Institute* (February 3, 2014).

And, of course, no one is complaining that trash collection and coal mining are more often performed by men.

Once the abovementioned controls are entered into the wage gap, the entire argument falls to pieces. Dr. Williams is also perhaps not aware that younger, childless women earn more than their male counterparts. According to a study published by Reach Advisors, using numbers coming from the Census Bureau's American Community Survey in 2010, "in 147 out of 150 of the biggest cities in the U.S., the median full-time salaries of young women are 8% higher than those of the guys in their peer group." Moreover, the Bureau of Labor Statistics found that women today make up the *majority* of "highly paid managerial positions."[62]

How did the patriarchy not put a stop to this?!

Dr. Williams is quite successful herself. Having taught at both the University of Pennsylvania and the University of Ottawa, she is well published in academic literature, well respected in both the medical and psychedelic fields, sits on boards, and makes a very comfortable living. She has more status and privilege than most anyone of any ethnicity.

And Dr. Williams is far from the only person pushing a narrative of misogyny in the psychedelic Renaissance. A common trope advances the claim that there exists some barrier between women and psychedelic spaces. Consider the words of psychedelic therapist Veronika Gold: "As a female, I have been particularly attuned to the social, cultural, and political factors that have deterred women and other marginalized groups from entering the field of psychedelic research."[63]

Are women today really deterred from entering psychedelic spaces?

Back in 2018, an event organizer made a post on Facebook addressing the lack of women who submitted proposals to speak at previous conferences he'd held. He had performed a rudimentary statistical analysis to gauge the demographics of those who submitted proposals to his prior conferences and noticed fewer female than male applicants. Mind you, *anyone* can submit a proposal to speak; whether one gets

62. Belinda Luscombe, "Workplace Salaries: At Last, Women on Top," *Time* (September 1, 2010).

63. Veronika Gold, "Reflections on Personal Experiences in Psychedelic Training and Research," *Maps Bulletin*, Vol 29, No 1 (Spring 2019).

accepted is another matter. To balance the scales, the organizer stated in his Facebook post that he would favor submissions from women over men that year.[64] This person isn't a critical social justice activist. He's liberal and wanted more female representation at his conference (no issue there).

I always had a good time at this particular gathering and eagerly wanted to know who I'd see there. I reached out to three female friends of mine and asked if they were applying to speak. One asked for my help writing her proposal. My "help" included coming up with a topic and writing the proposal for her. The second friend said she wasn't much interested in attending the conference; after a long phone conversation, I convinced her to apply anyway. The third, knowing that the organizer would give women preferential treatment that year, said something to the effect that she didn't need to give her proposal much thought because she "ha[s] a vagina."

It's enough to wonder if academic standards matter to the psychedelic Renaissance anymore.

All three ended up speaking that year (as did Veronika Gold). Incidentally, this all took place a year *before* Gold wrote her article mentioning the undefined barriers women face in psychedelic spaces. Gold might consider that all three secured speaking roles after one white American man announced that he was actively looking for greater female representation and another white American man encouraged them to participate (even "helping" with the proposal of one of them).

But that's not the annoying part. The annoying part is that two of those speakers—the two for whom I did not write proposals—have made both public and private stinks about the lack of representation in psychedelic spaces if the female-to-male ratio is off ever so slightly. And yet, there they were doing their due diligence to avoid tipping the scales towards egalitarianism by shrugging off the application process.

It's easy to dismiss this as simply an experience I had—an anecdote that does not represent the breadth of the issue. Fair enough. But then how do we explain the numerous psychedelic organizations run by and

---

64. Meaning that if two proposals (one from a female, one from a male) equally "wowed" him, he would default to the former. Although, it might also be stated that this does not fix the problem of women not submitting proposals.

stacked with women? They produce large events, publish books, articles, and peer-reviewed studies. They work and teach at major universities and have thriving therapy practices. They serve on nonprofit boards and organize community spaces and public forums. If men are deterring women from psychedelic research spaces, as Veronika Gold suggests, where exactly is this happening? We are never told. Instead, we are offered abstractions built on outdated narratives pertaining to women in the sciences. There are many ethnically diverse women currently involved in a variety of psychedelic research fields and not a hint of anyone trying to stop them.

The Mushroom Classroom

In Oregon, psilocybin-assisted therapy is legal for therapeutic purposes.[65] Psilocybin is the active compound found in psychedelic mushrooms. Countless studies and personal testimonies support psilocybin's ability to treat depression, anxiety, and a host of other maladies.[66] Various psilocybin facilitator training schools have opened in Oregon, as well as some psilocybin service centers.

A friend and colleague of mine enrolled in one of the local 22-hour training programs through the Changa Institute. The majority of those 22 hours were spent discussing colonization and racism; the remaining class time was spent discussing proper psilocybin facilitation and safety protocols. One of my friend's teachers at this training school sounds like a walking DEI stereotype; "all white people are racist," she told the class of mostly white Americans. She would "invite conversation and then get super mad at anyone who said something that was not in line with her [rhetoric]," my friend revealed. At one point she made the extraordinary claim that "there are only two races: black and white." When a student

65. Somewhat. The Feds can crack down on this revolutionary treatment any time.
66. See Alan K. Davis et al., "Effects of Psilocybin-Assisted Therapy on Major Depressive Disorder: A Randomized Clinical Trial," *JAMA Psychiatry*, 78, 5 (November 4, 2020); Natalie Gukasyan, et al., "Efficacy and Safety of Psilocybin-Assisted Treatment for Major Depressive Disorder: Prospective 12–Month Follow Up," *Journal of Psychopharmacology* (February 15, 2022); Marija Bogadi and Snježana Kaštelan, "A Potential Effect of Psilocybin on Anxiety in Neurotic Personality Structures in Adolescents," *Croatian Medical Journal*, 62, 5 (October 2021).

honestly asked her what she meant by that, the teacher "got mad and attacked the whiteness of the person who asked the question and then shut down the conversation and moved on." (Recall the abuse that Paul Rossi and Richard Bilkszto endured for questioning their DEI overlords.)

Part of the facilitator class included having the students take the IAT. The teacher was trying to prove "that [the students] were all racist." When an older white American woman asked in honest humility what was meant by such a remark, the teacher "didn't want to explain the concept. She just wanted to get mad that we didn't understand it." For this JEDI knight, "even a question was threatening," my friend told me. However, one white American woman took the IAT and came back with no biases at all. One would think that in a world where all white Americans are considered racist it would have been nothing short of a miracle to find one who wasn't. Instead, "the facilitator got super mad [that a white American woman showed no racial bias] . . . her point had been undermined and she did not know what to do about it."

My friend's final thoughts on Changa Institute deserve to be quoted in full:

> We graduated not knowing the [psychedelic] territory, we do not know all the different dimensions of the mushroom head space, we do not know what dimensions someone else can go into, we have not been facilitated ourselves, we have not seen someone else facilitate, but we do know about abstract social justice things! It really annoys me because there is a conversation to be had. I'm a white [American] facilitator and if I have a black [American] client, it is important to think 'that client is now on mushrooms and might have a whole bunch of associations with my white face because of their own history of living in this country and there might be negative associations,' and I can understand that and I want to understand that better. That's an important part of my work, but we didn't cover that topic. We didn't focus on trauma (!)—I'm a fucking therapist and we didn't focus on any therapeutic concepts that have an obvious place in psychedelic facilitation. And it's just kinda terrifying. We have all these facilitators who are trained now, and who have not covered all these valuable topics. That's what I'm upset about—we didn't cover all these important topics . . . we just feel a sense of white guilt now. How is white guilt the only

> thing a [psychedelic] facilitator needs—surely there are other things to this job![67]

These psilocybin-facilitator training schools charge upwards of $15,000[68] and are churning out less-qualified facilitators than underground practitioners and regular therapists who have been secretly administering the medicine safely and successfully for years without any need for critical social justice.

Another friend and colleague revealed to me that he had spoken with an event organizer to discuss the possibility of presenting at the latter's psychedelic conference. He met all the criteria—that is, he had recently published a book, he hadn't spoken at the conference in several years, and he had what he was told was a very interesting proposal. Wondering how it was that he could meet all the criteria to speak and still be rejected, he finally asked the organizer straight out what the bias was against him.

The organizer's answer to my friend, verbatim, was "oh, there's no bias against you, it's just . . .. you're a white guy."

These might seem like small issues, but they indicate a larger problem. Adopting this critical social justice perspective begins the slow suffocation of the psychedelic Renaissance by causing unnecessary division through echoing obsolete narratives. These narratives are widespread in psychedelia, but only because no one has offered an alternative perspective. Like the crowd gathered at Revolution Hall during the Floyd uprisings, we psychedelic researchers, therapists, chemists, and otherwise are supposed to cheer for any ignorance we encounter, lest we be called "racist" for not playing along.

But how long can that really last? The psychedelic Renaissance is wrapped up with notions of mental health, honesty, individual autonomy, and authenticity. Critical social justice provides the perfect antitheses of those values: silencing, stereotyping, and repressing in service of

67. Pers. comm; my friend wishes to remain anonymous.
68. My friend's course cost $8,000.

the narrative (recall my friend's experience at Changa Institute). Perhaps most importantly, through the critical social justice perspective, there is no redemption. Only redemption is big in our Renaissance, coming with the (perhaps romantic) hope that psychedelic medicines, in conjunction with other positive behavior reinforcement efforts, can rehabilitate the distressed. Hurt people *hurt people*, we tend to say. Aggression, violence, narcissism, and distrust derive from trauma; healing the trauma heals the hurter. To date, psychedelic medicines seem worthy candidates for this kind of desirable transformation.[69]

I used to believe that psychedelia was immune to identity politics. That a tab of LSD was enough to see past our surface differences; that an eighth of mushrooms showed us the timeless connection of our human family; that a cup of ayahuasca could generate a feeling the size of a southwest noonday sunshine bursting in the heart, a radiance accompanied by choirs of angels reminding us of our common bond. I thought that the symphony of visions offered by psychedelics would guard us, that the medicine would keep us safe.

I was wrong.

Ideology is a powerful force—an egregore[70] that can grow so strong that even the loving embrace of Pachamama[71] offers no protection. Such is to be captured by ideology, whether on the extreme right or the critical social justice left. Psychedelics can potentially change the entire trajectory of a person's thinking and living for good or ill; it all depends on the preparedness of the mind. The conscientious person will ride the bursts of sunshine found on most any tab of LSD. The unprepared mind, whether inclined towards critical social justice or otherwise, will be limited by false cultural constructs that promote a disturbing and narcissistic neuroticism.

69. Amanda J. Khan et al., "Psilocybin for Trauma-Related Disorders," *Current Topics in Behavioral Neurosciences*, 56 (2022).

70. In occult circles, an egregore is an immaterial entity that culminates from groupthink and grows stronger the more people believe it.

71. That is, ayahuasca.

Turn on, Tune in, Help out

To overcome the as-yet-undetectable crises of sexism and racism in the psychedelic Renaissance, we are told to "do the work." In JEDI terms, to "do the work" means to uncover unconscious bias in the self. Only we explorers of the interior realms already have a version of "doing the work." Our work involves digging through the complex byways of our personality, traumas (and soul, if you believe in such things) to understand why each of us ticks the way we do and working—the so-called work—towards bettering ourselves for the sake of a better society. Medicine space[72] is a place to heal and see where past assumptions you've made were wrong so you can correct yourself and grow. If overcoming racism is a part of that work, so be it—and good on the person who sees and corrects it. But to default to such ideas as inherent and go looking for something that isn't there seems quite the folly.

Timothy Leary's adage of "Turn on, Tune in, Drop out" is a relic that doesn't represent the thrust of the psychedelic Renaissance today. While psychedelics are certainly still used recreationally at festivals and private gatherings *à la* the late 1960s, the real push of the psychedelic Renaissance is in treating personal and societal wounds with these medicines. Implanting and/or reinforcing the divisive ideas of JEDI, in combination with psychedelic medicines, will only serve to fracture us more. Psychedelics are powerful nonspecific amplifiers that can traumatize as much as they can heal. To bolster an oppression narrative to people seeking mental health alternatives seems suspect at best. At worst, it seems like cognitive and emotional abuse. How will highlighting outdated narratives play out in the mind of a person under a high dose of LSD who believes she's oppressed? It is my contention that psychedelic SJWs, yearning for the Beatific vision, have been sold a false promise of enlightenment.

And now psychedelic medicines, the greatest tools humanity has ever known for probing the subconscious mind, healing the wounded heart, and discovering the unexplored soul are being used to introduce undefined grievance and division into the psychedelic Renaissance through three heretofore unquestionable narratives of decolonization, race, and gender.

---

72. Places where people gather to consume substantia.

Part II

The Decolonize Narrative

4

Worse Angels: A Brief History of Prejudice

The Slave Trade is the Ruling Principle of my people.
It is the source . . . of all their wealth. . . .[T]he mother lulls
child to sleep with notes of triumph over an enemy reduced to slavery.[1]

—Ghezo, King of Dahomey, West Africa

We caught all the people. Not one escaped.
. . . [T]hese we killed and others we killed—
but what of that? It was in accordance with our customs.[2]

—Maori conqueror

The Decolonize Narrative

During his inaugural address on 14 March 1861, President Abraham Lincoln (1809–1865) had few thoughts on his mind other than preserving the fractured Union. He didn't want war; but his opponents didn't

1. Quoted in Hugh Thomas, *The Slave Trade: The Story of the Atlantic Slave Trade: 1440 –1870* (NY: Simon and Schuster Paperbacks, 1997), p. 673.
2. Quoted in Jared Diamond, *Guns, Germs, and Steel: The Fates of Human Societies* (NY: W.W. Norton and Company, 1999), pp. 53–4.

want compromise. And so, Lincoln tried to appeal to the universal traits present in every human heart—those characteristics dubbed "the better angels of our nature." Here, he referred to our ability to choose either good or evil as we move through life. When we choose good, we defer to our better angels. These better angels represent common truths found throughout time and place: honesty, integrity, compassion, fairness, hope, and a sense of justice (among others). All those attributes that we can properly call *human*. Ask anyone you know, and she will likely tell you that she possesses all those virtues.

And that's probably true.

Equally true, however, is the uneasy fact that we humans also have a capacity for entertaining the worse angels of our nature: greed, bigotry, dishonesty, and arrogance (among others). All those attributes that we can properly call *human*. For Theorists (psychedelic and OG), those evils corrupt the soul of only one civilization, that of the West, which exists in diametrical opposition to, say, First Nations peoples, who are seen as wise, compassionate, holy, and peaceful peoples—above reproach—in tune with nature and the Great Spirit, and far too noble and morally righteous to have exercised the worse angels of human nature. The historically wary among us recognize this as the "noble savage" stereotype—a racist perspective that infantilizes First Nations peoples.

The antidote to this inherent evil corroding the Western soul is decolonization (otherwise known as postcolonialism). To decolonize something means to strip any evidence of Western influence from it. And these days, everything must be decolonized. Like all the narratives we shall explore in this book, the Decolonize Narrative isn't totally wrong, it's just too narrow. Especially for those interested in mind-expansion.

So let's broaden the discussion.

Among the most famous of early postcolonial works was Palestinian American author Edward Said's *Orientalism* (1978). Some of Said's critiques of Western scholarship were quite necessary. For too long, Western scholars saw their methods as standard, while those of the East took a backseat. Postcolonial studies provided a much-needed correction to the Eurocentric model. However, postcolonial theory also came awash in claims of cultural relativism, the belief that no culture is better or worse than any other; they are all just different. Therefore, a prelude question we should ask is whether or not postcolonialists are responsive to evidence. The forecast is not promising. Postcolonial professor Linda Tuhiwai Smith tells us, "[T]he term 'research' is inextricably linked to European imperialism and colonialism. The word itself, 'research,' is probably one of the dirtiest words in the indigenous world's vocabulary."[3] Unencouraging as Professor Smith's perspective is, there is another concern upon which I think we ought reflect: if we are truly going to help people overcome trauma and addiction through psychedelic therapy then sound research is quite necessary.

Psychedelic postcolonialists reject this premise coming from the larger decolonization scholarship but replace it with an idea equally impractical. Researcher Paloma David wants us to "give indigenous expertise the space it deserves in scientific research. . . . it will be critical to give regard to knowledge that comes from different cultural and ethnic sources, bestowing upon them equal validity in the discussion of the adequate use of these substances"—otherwise, we risk perpetrating "intellectual violence" on First Nations peoples.[4] Putting aside that Western ideas are rarely considered part of this psychedelic knowledge diversity from postcolonialists, there is another issue: I thought David was opting for a *scientific* approach. Scientific validity requires better evidence, *not* identity politics or questionable allegations of intellectual violence. Otherwise, we are not engaging with scientific method. An idea cannot be accepted with "equal validity" simply because it comes from a First Nations medicine-worker any more than it can be accepted merely because it comes from an ancient Grecian oracle. However, a First Nations medicine worker with a proven track record of healing people's maladies through techniques unacknowledged by current scientific method is another story altogether. More on that later.

In recent years, the broader Decolonization Narrative has taken hold of both popular culture and the psychedelic Renaissance specifically. The

3. Quoted in Pluckrose and Lindsay (2022), p. 65.
4. Aref Touleimat, "Ayahuasca: A Plea for the Decolonization of Psychedelic Studies," *Open Foundation* (June 27, 2022).

prevailing postcolonial wisdom holds that colonization, slavery, bigotry, misogyny, and all the other worse angels of human nature were alien concepts to the good people living outside Europe, and only entered global consciousness during Europe's Age of Exploration. Recall that speaker mentioned during the BLM gathering at Revolution Hall in the second chapter—the one who was convinced that Africa was some kind of utopia before Europeans intervened. She might have just been one oblivious person at a rally, but she is not alone. Her ignorance aligns with that of author Michael Bradley, who writes, "Nuclear war, environmental pollution, resource rape . . . all are primary threats to our survival and all are the results of peculiarly Caucasoid behavior, Caucasoid values, Caucasoid psychology. There is no way to avoid the truth. The problem with the world is white men."[5]

In fairness, postcolonial Theorists have a point when they address the malicious ways Europeans (and later, white Americans) terrorized various indigenous peoples in the Americas. One Spanish explorer from the 16th century, Álvar Núñez Cabeza de Vaca (c. 1490–c.1560), recounts how "Christians had raided [native] land and had destroyed and burned villages and carried off half the men and all the women and children." And while de Vaca had been looking for those Christians to "tell them not to kill [the locals] or take them as slaves or remove them from their lands or harm them in any other way," we can all pick countless examples of gratuitous brutalities of colonialism quite easily.[6] Mistreatment of the locals got so bad that by 1542 Spanish King Charles V issued his "New Laws of the Indies for the Good Treatment and Preservation of the Indians"—sadly, to not much positive effect. The removal of the Cherokee from their land by President Andrew Jackson (1767–1845) was so vicious that even seasoned soldiers who walked the Trail of Tears with their First Nations sisters and brothers felt their "blood chill" on account of the horrors they saw. One militiaman who forced the Cherokee off their land later remarked, "I fought through the Civil War and have seen men shot to pieces and slaughtered by thou-

5. Quoted in Dinesh D' Souza, *The End of Racism: Principles for a Multiracial Society* (NY: The Free Press, 1995), p. 39.
6. Martin A. Favata and José B. Fernández (trans.), *The Account: Álvar Núñez Cabeza de Vaca's Relatión* (TX: Arte Público Press, 1993), p. 106.

sands, but the Cherokee removal was the cruelest work I ever knew."[7]

Postcolonial Theorists often maintain that America's sordid history is somehow covered up; as if you and everyone you know didn't grow up learning all about the horrors of this country's past in high school. *Of course we did.* What we didn't learn about were the ancestral sins of those who currently occupy the protected classes in the United States. Slavery serves as a perfect example. Leaving high school, I was all too aware that Europeans and white Americans practiced slavery. However, I graduated not knowing that Africans,[8] black Americans,[9] Asians,[10] Middle Easterners,[11] and First Nations peoples[12] also practiced slavery. I was never taught that some of the first slaves to arrive in North America were not Africans—but rather English and Irish.[13] I was never taught that there are more slaves in the world today than ever existed in the United States by the tens of millions. I was never taught that in some Arab areas today, the term "African" and "slave" *(Abeed)* are interchangeable.[14]

A World Away

Following the Reconquista (or "the Reconquest"), a grueling near-800-year war that saw the final expulsion of Islamic colonizers from Christian Spain in 1492, the Age of Exploration began. The ending of the Reconquista enabled the Spanish to sail into that oft-spoken mystery called the East (by way of the west) with two goals: opening new trade with nations found over the horizon and spreading the word of Christ.

---

7. Quoted in Dee Brown, "The Trail of Tears," pp. 170–1.
8. See Simon Webb, *The Slave Trade in Africa: An Ongoing Holocaust* (Pen and Sword History, 2023).
9. See Larry Koger, *Black Slaveowners: Free Black Slave Masters in South Carolina, 1790–1860* (NC: McFarland & Company, 2012).
10. See Titas Chakraborty and Matthias van Rossum, "Slave Trade and Slavery in Asia: New Perspectives," *Journal of Social History*, Vol. 54, Is. 1 (Fall, 2020): 1–14.
11. See Simon Webb, *The Forgotten Slave Trade: White European Slaves of Islam* (Pen and Sword History, 2021).
12. See Barbara Krauthamer, *Black Slaves, Indian Masters: Slavery, Emancipation, and Citizenship in the Native American South* (NC: University of North Carolina Press, 2013).
13. See Don Jordan and Michael Walsh, *White Cargo: The Forgotten History of Britain's White Slaves in America* (NY: New York University Press, 2007).
14. Murray (2022), p. 118.

They were ambitious goals and often needed one to stimulate the other. Inarguably the most famous of this new breed of explorers was Christopher Columbus (1451–1506), who set sail for God, gold, and glory the same year that saw the termination of the Reconquista. The voyage was taxing, taking roughly six months and almost ending in mutiny had land not been sighted that autumn of 1492. Relieved to step on solid ground again, Columbus and his crew set about exploring the small tropical island, which they named "Hispaniola."[15] For the postcolonial Theorist, this marked the beginning of the end, as wave after wave of European explorers and settlers imported to the Americas all the worse angels of human nature.

The Age of Exploration was launched by people fantastically ignorant about the world. Many contemporary Europeans believed that women from India could be born with the head of a dog; their brothers might leave the womb with both their feet facing backwards.[16] They reckoned that Satan caused earthly calamity. Fairies still danced in meadows. The Age of Exploration came at an odd time in Western history when the brightest people of the day straddled both the ignorance of yesteryear and a new, burgeoning scientific enlightenment. The scientific method introduced the world's first self-correcting system. It was never intended to be perfect; it need only recognize its own imperfections, account for, and correct them. Before that, our ancestors across the globe made their best guesses based on this or that "traditional" misapprehension about the natural world.

And Europeans were not alone in this ignorance. The various peoples they encountered on foreign soil held equally untenable claims about the nature of reality, some of whom believed that women could give birth to animals.[17]

Europeans of the time knew nothing of evolution or anthropology. Due to an overwhelming Christian perspective, most Europeans believed that all humans were the offspring of Eve and Adam. As such,

15. What we know today as Haiti and the Dominican Republic.
16. Konrad von Megenberg, *Buch der Natur* (Augsburg, Germany: Johann Bämler, 20 Aug., Montag vor S. Bartholomaeus, 1481), p. 396.
17. D' Souza (1995), p. 52.

all peoples presumably started building civilizations across the globe at the same point in time (or so it was believed). Therefore, it struck Europeans as odd that many of the peoples they encountered hadn't developed modern (for the time) commerce, large sailing ships, advanced metallurgy, art, and literature. Even the impressive empires of the Aztec, Inca, and Maya lagged behind the great cities of China, North Africa, Europe, Persia, and Southeast Asia. As just one example, while those latter civilizations employed the wheel for everything from gardening to military campaigns, the Maya saw no use for the wheel beyond parts for children's toys.[18]

What those latter civilizations had in common was that they all interacted with each other over millennia. The peoples of the Americas were cut off from those centuries of development that the larger Eastern Hemisphere undertook through war, trade, pilgrimage, colonization, and travel. Civilizations of the Eastern Hemisphere learned and shared and imitated. They conquered and they copied. Europeans brought to the Americas thousands of years of technological advancement courtesy of China, Persia, Southeast Asia, and elsewhere. Over time, a feeling of cultural superiority developed within all of those civilizations, which was roundly exported to all new areas in which they landed.

The Other

Much as the postcolonial psychedelic Theorists hesitate to admit, colonization has existed among nearly every advanced (and not so advanced) civilization of which we are aware. And in some cases, the West actually *improved* the lives of those it colonized.[19] Even still, the only colonization ambitions that we are allowed to acknowledge are those stemming from Europe and white America. But such a notion both flies in the face of history and smacks it along the way. Different peoples from different places all over the world have demonized, and subsequently colonized, the "other." Africans and First Nations peoples were no exception.

Where the postcolonialists are correct, however, are those occasions

18. Thomas Sowell, *Conquests and Cultures: An International History* (Basic Books, 1999), p. 251.
19. See Bruce Gilley, "The Case for Colonialism," *Academic Questions*, 31 (2008):167–185.

when otherizing was based solely on a biological idea created by the West, called "race." Race did not exist in the premodern world because evolutionary biology did not exist in the premodern world. Westerners—like everyone else—of course, recognized that different peoples from different places had different regional physical features. But such variances never amounted to discrimination or ideas of superiority. Greek writers, in fact, often commented on the nobility, good graces, and beauty of Ethiopians.[20] Sextus Propertius (c. 50 BCE–c. 15 CE) remarked "a tender beauty, white or dark, attracts."[21] Strabo of Amasia (c. 64 BCE–24 CE) commented on the "wretched" lives led by Ethiopians (due to lack of food in the area and poor diet) but says nothing disparaging about them due to any intrinsic ethnic failing.[22] On the other paw, he finds the Celts to be "complete savages." The reason they were so animalistic was obvious for Strabo: "because of the cold [weather]," he reasoned.[23] More than anything else, *environment*—not ethnicity—so the best thinkers of the ancient world believed, herded peoples into either "civilized" or "uncivilized," "human" or "subhuman," categories.

Middle Easterners also drew a sharp line between cultured and barbaric peoples based on climate. According to one Persian author, Africans were "distant from the standards of humanity." The problem? Too much sunlight. Likewise, the Islamic historian al-Masudi (896–956 CE) found Europeans to be the "ultimate barbarians [who] became paler, grosser, and dumber the further north one went."[24] The problem? Not enough sunlight. Middle Easterners were superior, neither black nor white, because they got the perfect amount of sunlight. For one 10th century Islamic author, such sunlight might directly affect the cooking process (so to speak) of an infant in the womb:

> The people of Iraq have sound minds, commendable passions, balanced natures, and high proficiency in every art, together with well-proportioned limbs ... and a pale brown color, which is the most apt and

20. D'Souza, (1995), p. 40.
21. Quoted in Frank M. Snowden, Jr., *Before Color Prejudice: The Ancient View of Blacks* (MA: Harvard University Press, 1983), p. 79.
22. "Ancient Sources on Nubia and Ethiopia."
23. Strabo, *Geography of Strabo*, Book II, Chap. V, Vol. I.
24. Quoted in D'Souza (1995), p. 45.

> proper color. They are the ones who are done to a turn in the womb. They do not come out with something between blond, blanched, and leprous coloring, such as the infants dropped form the wombs of the women of . . . light complexion; nor are they overdone in the womb until they are burned, so that the child comes out black, murky, malodorous, stinking, and crinkly-haired, with uneven limbs, deficient minds, and depraved passions, such as the Ethiopians and other blacks who resemble them. The Iraqis are neither half-baked dough nor burned crust, but between the two.[25]

Africans held similar views about Europeans, regarding themselves as "perfectly cooked but the white man is underdone because of a defect in the creator's oven."[26] Some African tribes, like the Zulu, turned their discrimination not to Europeans, but to other Africans, specifically the Sothos, who they believed had the skin color of "a yellowish claypot."[27] Even the Pueblos[28] of the southwest United States had a myth of "the Well-Baked Man." In the story, Man Maker tries to create humans by placing clay figures in an oven, but Coyote keeps tricking him. First Coyote tells Man Maker to take the figures out of the oven too soon. Man Maker removes them and is saddened to see that the figures are too pale, like Europeans. Man Maker again tries to bake two humans from clay. As he is about to remove them from the oven, Coyote tells him that they need to stay in longer—lest they come out undercooked again. When Man Maker finally pulls the figures from the oven, he is saddened to see that they are too dark, like Africans. Resolute, Man Maker fashioned two more clay figures, placed them in the oven, and admonished Coyote not to interfere. Man Maker waited for the proper time to cook the figures, eventually pulling them out of the oven. The figures "walked around, talked, laughed, and behaved in a seemly fashion. They were neither underdone nor overdone."

"These are exactly right," said Man Maker. "These really belong here; these I will use. They are beautiful."[29]

---

25. Quoted in D'Souza (1995), p. 33.
26. Quoted in Snowden (1983), p. 76.
27. D' Souza (1995), p, 30.
28. "Pueblo" does not refer to a single tribe, but several which, while different, share similar languages and customs.
29. "The Well-Baked Man."

The unspoken truth of postcolonialism is that all peoples in all places in all times have held shallow prejudices that they used to justify discrimination and abuse against the other. Such prejudices also provided a fitting excuse for why the other's land should be occupied. Discrimination, color-based or otherwise, is not the exclusive domain of Europeans. Like the better angels of our nature, the worse angels also have a place in every human heart.

The Noble Savage

Correct as the postcolonial Theorists may be to acknowledge the abuses that came with the colonization of the Americas, they never address what life was like *before* the European arrival or how those areas would have evolved had the Spanish stayed home. Accounts from early explorers and *conquistadors* in the Americas reveal the grim reality of a life nasty, brutish, and short. First Nations peoples (outside the three major Mesoamerican cities) mostly starved and certainly did not have access to widescale food production or advanced medicines and associated technologies. People-stealing ran rampant. Having been stranded in the Americas for eight years, Spanish explorer Álvar Núñez Cabeza de Vaca paints a picture of poor, unfed peoples who, during famines, relied on picking out the nuts from their own shit, grinding them up, and eating them—that is, if there wasn't a child available to cannibalize. De Vaca starved as well. One by one, each of 600 explorers died due to malnutrition, disease, thirst, or slaughter by a local. As de Vaca records, "Since a third of the men were quite sick and with every passing hour more were succumbing to illness, we were certain that we would all get sick and die."[30] We often forget that the Columbian Exchange was a two-way street. Both First Nations Peoples and Europeans killed each other with diseases neither knew anything about. As one example, syphilis, which plagued early modern Europe, came over the Atlantic from the Americas.[31]

30. Favata and Fernández (1993), p. 46.
31. Peera Hemarajata, "Revisiting the Great Imitator: The Origin and History of Syphilis," *American Society for Microbiology* (June 17, 2019).

Lack of nutrition and swapping exotic diseases aside, war was a constant way of life throughout the Americas. "[P]eople do not travel or trade much in that land because of the continuous warfare that goes on," remarked de Vaca.[32] Among some peoples it was the elder women of the tribe who urged men to war. The combat was so constant, in fact, that it evolved some truly odd forms of paranoid cultural behaviors. De Vaca writes of the customs of the Marimens and the Yguaces in this wise:

> When their daughters are born they cast them to the dogs, which eat them. The reason for doing this, according to them, is that all the people of that land are their enemies . . . and if their enemies were to marry their daughters, they would multiply so much that they would conquer them and take them as slaves. We asked them why they did not just marry their daughters to their own men, and they replied that they considered it an unseemly thing to marry them to their relatives and that it was better to kill them.

As for how these tribes survived without any women, they would "buy the children of strangers" to marry the men.[33]

Other peoples like the Coahuiltecans[34] also practiced a similar female infanticide, believing that it was better to kill the child than to have her marry into an enemy tribe. Though, it wasn't just baby girls that could have their lives cut short. Babies born slightly deleterious or with mild to severe retardation (of either sex), and/or one member from a set of twins, were buried alive. If a mother died during childbirth, the infant was slaughtered as well.[35]

De Vaca was not the only one to mention the "cruel, inhuman[,] and ferocious" ways the natives conducted themselves in war. Reflecting on the Karankawa, Fray Gaspar José De Solis, a mid-eighteenth-century Spanish chronicler, records: "When one nation makes war on another, the one that conquers puts all the old men and old women to the knife and carries off the little children as food to eat along the way." Older

32. Favata and Fernández (1993), pp. 64–5.
33. Favata and Fernández (1993), pp. 70–1.
34. Like the Pueblo, Coahuiltecan is not a single tribe, but rather an umbrella term which includes a variety of different peoples with similar languages and customs.
35. W.W. Newcomb, *The Indians of Texas: From Prehistoric to Modern Times* (TX: University of Texas, 1980), pp. 47–8.

children were sold as slaves. Still older youths and all the women would be kept as slaves for the tribe "with the exception of some of whom they reserve to sacrifice in the dance before their gods and saints."[36]

Most—perhaps *all*—First Nations societies practiced slavery. It was not uncommon for these slaves to eventually be sacrificed, eaten, or both. The Cherokee were especially harsh in their treatment of slaves and even acted as slave-catchers. They weren't hired very often, as they usually didn't bring the runaways back alive.[37] After the Civil War ended institutional bondage in the United States in 1865, First Nations peoples refused to give up their slaves until finely coerced by the government in 1866. For that brief moment in history, white Americans did not own a single slave, but indigenous peoples did. Odd as it might strike us, European colonization put an end to both the nonstop war and slavery amongst First Nations peoples.[38]

The worse angels of human nature know no ethnic bounds, no matter how long we sat in Man Maker's oven. First Nations peoples were not the holier than thou archetypes of moral and spiritual perfection so often depicted in popular culture, and especially in the psychedelic Renaissance. Neither were they the fragile, almost childlike, innocents who shared all their possessions, as postcolonialists paint them. They were humans. Each adapted to her own challenges, environment, and otherwise. And it is highly likely that without the intervention of Westernism, the slaughter might still be going on today.

The very idea of sinless, environmentally conscious indigeneity—the noble savage—is a product of the Western imagination. Postcolonialists are merely following the proscription already set out by those like John Collier (1884–1968), Commissioner of Indian Affairs during the Great Depression. Collier claimed that before colonization indigenous peoples existed in "perfect ecological balance with the forest, the plain, the waters, and animal life." Other writers have noted that, before the arrival of Europeans, the diverse indigenous populations of the Americas lived in

36. Quoted in Newcomb (1980), p. 77.

37. D'Souza (1995), pp. 75–6.

38. Vincenzo Petrullo, *The Diabolic Root: A Study of Peyotism, The New Indian Religion Among the Delawares* (PA: University of Pennsylvania Press: The University Museum, 1934), p. 26.

"balanced and fruitful harmony."[39]

But the real thrust of the noble savage myth came during the 1970s when Greenpeace founder Bob Hunter decided to exploit indigenous cultures like the Cree. During the psychedelic 60s, a Cree myth circulated about the Rainbow Warriors—those who would rise up to fight pollution. The legend came in poetic verse: "When the earth is sick, the animals will begin to disappear. When that happens, The Warriors of the Rainbow will come to save them."[40] It is a beautiful message that no doubt gives hope to anyone who cares about the environment. Only the legend of the Rainbow Warriors is not a Cree myth, but rather white American in origin. It derives from two evangelical Christians named William Willoya and Vinson Brown, who published a book titled *Warriors of the Rainbow* in 1962. They hoped that a Christian perspective would "evangelize . . . the Native American community."[41] The "indigenous environmentalist" was little more than a mascot later promoted by Hunter as an advertising campaign for Greenpeace.

Indigenous Traditions

Postcolonial Theorists tell us that it is necessary to preserve indigenous traditions. But rarely do they speak about what some of those traditions entail. We must accept them on their indigeneity alone, otherwise we disrupt the delicate disguise of noble savagery. While the postcolonial Theorist cries foul anytime a cultural custom is called into question, perhaps it behooves us to see what exactly some of these indigenous traditions looked like.

We begin with the explorers of the Paraguayan interior who encountered the Aché people, a hunter-gatherer tribe that practiced some rather interesting indigenous customs. Highlights include the following: should a woman grow weak, sick, or elderly to the point that she became a "burden" to the tribe, a young man would sneak up behind her with an axe and smash her skull in with it, killing her with that single hit; a child

39. Paul F. Boller, *Not So! Popular Myths about America from Columbus to Clinton* (UK: Oxford University Press, 1996) p. 8.
40. Quoted in Jeff Fynn-Paul, *Not Stolen: The Truth about European Colonialism in the New World* (Bombardier Books, 2023), p. 157.
41. John Tarleton, "Interview with Michael Niman" (July 1999).

who did not meet Aché beauty standards was buried alive; and when a "valued member" of the tribe died, the survivors would slaughter a little girl and bury her alongside the deceased.[42] This last practice was also popular among the Mayan Civilization;[43] perhaps the Aché appropriated it from there?

Moving north to the continental United States, the Comanche, located in the South Plains areas of Oklahoma and north central Texas, also practiced traditions worth exploring. Like most First Nations groups, the Comanche adhered to a level of misogyny unparalleled in Western Civilization—and that's saying quite a lot! Comanche women were not free agents of their lives, often passed between men (specifically brothers) for sexual favors. It was far more important to the Comanche that familial ties not be disturbed over sexual jealousy than it was to allow women bodily autonomy.

Women, however, could be punished for adultery. The penalty was carried out by the offended husband, who would right this wrong in one of two ways. If he was feeling charitable, he would only cut off the tip of her nose. Since women were viewed "as a sort of chattel," the defacement would lower her market value should she be sold to another man. Feeling less charitable, the offended husband might just kill the adulterous ex-wife. Failure to do so—showing any mercy on his wife whatsoever—would result in outpourings of emasculating mockery from the tribe. Should the wife die by her husband's hands or some other misfortune, he inherited her sisters to do with as he wished.[44]

The man with whom the wife had cheated had to make restitution to the husband in the form of guns, clothing, and horses or other beasts of burden. But this was only the case if the guilty man was poor and the offended man wealthy. One anthropologist tells us, "If a famous warrior confronted a weak, unknown man, the damages would be severe; on the other hand, a man lacking in military ability had a difficult time collecting any sort of payment from a powerful, aggressive adulterer."[45]

Although, the Comanche can still be seen as somewhat progressive.

---

42. Yuval Noah Harari, *Sapiens: A Brief History of Humankind* (London: Vintage Books, 2015), 59–60.
43. Sowell (1999), p. 267.
44. Newcomb (1980), pp. 170–71.
45. Newcomb (1980), pp. 176–77.

When a male member of the Shoshone—the tribe out of which the Comanche split—died, his widow was brought to his grave and slain—an eerie echo of the Southeast Asian practice of *suttee* (only there, the widow is burned alive alongside her husband's corpse). If the deceased had horses or cattle, these animals would be slaughtered alongside the widow. The Comanche opted for a less severe tradition—the widow would not be killed; she would just have her hair and a finger chopped off.[46] A Comanche woman *could* eventually obtain prestige in the tribe as a healer, but only after menopause. And only if her husband allowed it.[47]

The Comanche had hostile and deadly relationships with nearby tribes like the Kiowa, Apache, and Tonkawa, among others. This last group, the militarily-weak Tonkawa, often joined forces with *conquistadors* to fend off the Comanche and other tribes invading their land. The Comanche enslaved Mexicans, other neighboring peoples (like those mentioned above), and white Americans as well. The very term "Comanche" is a Ute word that means "enemy."[48] Thievery of crops ran rampant, as the Comanche both wanted corn and tobacco but lacked the desire to work producing them.

Similar to their European counterparts, First Nations peoples were quite superstitious. A contemporary of de Vaca, Andrés Dorantes de Carranza (c. 1500–1550), spent four years living among the Quevenes (of the larger Karankawa), and had witnessed around a dozen young boys who were buried alive or otherwise slaughtered due to a bad premonition in someone's dream.[49] The Comanche practiced a similar custom, as did some of the Coahuiltecans.[50]

Like Europeans of the time, one truly unforgivable transgression among First Nations peoples was practicing harmful sorcery or witchcraft. While Europeans often bear the historical brunt of this horrific social justice, First Nations peoples also believed that malevolent oper-

46. Newcomb (1980), p. 173.
47. Newcomb (1980), p. 187.
48. Newcomb (1980), p. 157.
49. Favata and Fernández (trans), (1993), p. 312.
50. Newcomb (1980), pp. 49 and 179.

ators caused storms and diseases by magical rituals.[51] All over Europe, innocent people could and would be executed for seemingly producing these kinds of natural phenomena through supernatural means—just like in the Americas. But such a parallel comes to a screeching halt in Europe by the early 1700s, when scientific advances in biology and meteorology had all but negated the need to burn innocent people for imaginary crimes. Whereas even by the mid-20th century, some First Nations peoples still believed in the efficacy of witches and their ability to cause diseases.[52] Not but a few innocent women were punished for it.

What does all of this say about cultural relativism? Are cultures that abstain from ritually murdering innocent women and children just the same as those that partake? Then why, if given the choice, would everyone you know avoid becoming a member of such a harsh culture? I do not intend to excuse certain brutalities that came with European colonization. I mention these indigenous traditions to put history into more proportionate context and remind the critical social justice ideologue that *all* our ancestors behaved in ways that we today find lamentable. We cannot reach a common understanding if we can't at least acknowledge that.

Giving the Land Back

At most any psychedelic event—conference, integration circle, fundraiser party, or otherwise in the United States and Canada—the host will inevitably open the proceedings by "acknowledging the land." This means she will tell us all that we are assembled on "stolen land," followed by a list of the various indigenous communities that once occupied the area. The subtext to the statement is that white Canadians and Americans should "give the land back" to the First Nations peoples who once inhabited any given area. To my knowledge, not a single one of these land-acknowledging (mostly white Canadian and American) people has

51. Clyde Kluckhohn and Dorothea Leighton, *The Navaho* (MA: Harvard University Press, 1974), pp. 192–93.
52. See Kluckhohn and Leighton (1974).

sought to rectify this problem by giving her house, car, and savings over to an indigenous family and moving back to her own ancestral land. Until that day comes, her land acknowledgments remain mere expressions of self-centered meaninglessness.

Let's play along anyway. Admittedly, I'm a little curious as to whom the United States returns the land. As one of many examples, the US government could give the land back to the last indigenous tribe to occupy the northwestern area of Texas, the Comanche. But then what do the US government land-returners say to the Apache, from whom the Comanche invaded, murdered, enslaved, and colonized the land? Does the land go back to the Comanche or the Apache? Some might say that it should go to the Apache as the original heirs to the land. But there's a hiccup. The Apache invaded, murdered, enslaved, and stole the land from the Pueblo People, who had earlier stolen it from the Plainview People, who earlier stole it from the Folsom People. Other, grander tribal conquests are also worth mention. Towards the end of the 18th century, the Iroquois Confederacy had stolen land "the equivalent of at least six times their original territory, all from neighboring tribes. . . . [T]hey had emptied much of Pennsylvania, West Virginia, Ohio, Indiana, and much of southern Ontario of its former inhabitants . . . despite the efforts of the French and English to protect many of the Iroquois' victims."[53]

Such progressions of intertribal warfare and colonization can be found all over the Americas. As one renowned anthropologist remarked, "A dominant Uto-Aztekan or Athapaskan culture may have supplanted an ancestral Hokan-Coahuiltecan culture, in much the same way that Americans replaced and relegated American Indians to marginal and generally unfavorable regions."[54] If the United States government was to return the land, exactly which invading, murdering, enslaving, colonizing indigenous groups should receive any given plot?

Acknowledging land grabs from Europeans and white Americans is okay, and you will no doubt be browbeaten about it at the next large psychedelic event you attend. On the other paw, the landgrabs committed by First Nations peoples against other First Nations peoples will go unmentioned.

---

53. Fynn-Paul (2023), p. 187.
54. Newcomb (1980), p. 33.

It's easy for postcolonial Theorists to criticize Western Civilization because they get to live in the comfortable confines of Western Civilization. They don't realize that their very ability to chant "give the land back" is only possible because the United States guarantees free speech and the right to assemble in protest. A Comanche youth telling a Comanche elder to "give the land back" to the Apache would have been ignored, beaten, or slaughtered.

Such an exercise of decolonization raises not only coarse truths but also pressing questions. If we decolonize the land does that mean we also uproot all those highways that now connect the farthest reaches of the plains, making long distance travel safer and more convenient? And what of the restaurants, hospitals, libraries, food storage facilities, Planned Parenthoods, farms, homeless shelters, cell phone towers, plumbing and sewer systems, air conditioning, central heating, food banks, toilet paper, pharmacies shelved with modern medicines, grocery stores, and other symbols of white supremacy? Surely, they must all be taken down—*deconstructed!*—in order to not insult whatever colonizing, murdering, enslaving First Nations group to which the United States returns the land. Surely, we can't say that all those things represent colonization *and* leave them all standing. They must be burned to the ground.

Just like the racist library near my house.

This chapter outlined only a small portion of the First Nations realities that postcolonial Theorists ignore. One could easily fill a book with more examples. None of this is meant to excuse the terrible ways some indigenous peoples were treated first by some Europeans and then by some Americans. I am sharing these harsh truths not to provoke, but rather to point to the subject of unity lost on DEI advocates like Ibram Henry Rogers (now known as Ibram X. Kendi), who (rather infamously) remarked: "The only remedy to past discrimination is present discrimination. The only remedy for present discrimination is future discrimination."[55] I'm not sure how psychopathic statements like that can possibly lead to a better world. Perhaps instead of cooking up clever ways to create injustice today, we reflect on the history of human evils and see the

55. Ibram X. Kendi, *How to Be an Antiracist* (NY: One World, August 13, 2019), p. 19.

horrible commonality of it all. How exactly does discriminating against people today retroactively fix the past? And does it not also ensure discrimination in the future? That doesn't sound like a sustainable plan for human progress to me.

And is that what we want our psychedelic Renaissance to be?

5

Psychedelia: A Brief History of the Western Traditions

Yes—clearly jealous of their lacking cultural contributions in the sphere of recreational drugs, white folks decided to just outright culturally appropriate one.

—Staff Writer at afru.com, "Psychedelic Privilege"

Something Awe-Inspiring

A common narrative in the psychedelic Renaissance today holds that Western peoples had no historical knowledge of plant medicines until sailing to the Americas. This perspective stems from the larger Decolonization Narrative we have already explored, which sees all things European as inherently evil and all things non-European as inherently benevolent. Since psychedelic postcolonial Theorists see psychedelics as *good,* such medicines must have been absent from Western civilization (which is *bad!*) until Europeans and white Americans alike stole them and the idea of psychedelic healing from indigenous peoples.

Chacruna Institute pushes the Decolonize Narrative with an impressive vigor. Drs. Bia Labate (co-founder of that organization) and

Monnica Williams (board member) write that the "healing properties of plant medicines and their derivatives were originally brought to Western consciousness by indigenous cultures around the world."[1]

But it isn't just those at Chacruna Institute who believe this narrative. The psychedelic critical social justice crowd, somewhat ironically, is often joined in chorus by conservatives who tend to feel uneasy about historical drug use in the West,[2] especially the plant medicine traditions found in the Abrahamic religions. Indeed, there is evidence to suggest that both Jews and Christians, from time to time, employed some kind of mind-altering substantia in their understanding of their respective faiths. This chapter will address the historically untenable position, whether coming from a postcolonialist psychedelic SJW or a conservative, which holds that Western civilization did not have any psychedelic traditions of which to speak until colonizers appropriated them from First Nations peoples.

But first, let's make sure we are all speaking the same language.

Defining Psychedelic

What does it mean to have a "psychedelic" experience? Some argue from a cultural perspective. Ecology professor and author Andy Letcher believes that during the late 1960s, "psychedelic" was "bound up with notions of authenticity, freedom, individualism, bohemianism, and rebellion."[3] Others argue from neurochemistry, claiming the determining factor for what makes something psychedelic depends on whether or not a drug interacts with the 5-HT_{2A} (serotonin) receptors. These scientists speak of the "classical serotenergic psychedelics (or CSPs)," limiting the family to LSD, ayahuasca, psilocybin mushrooms, DMT, 5-MeO-DMT, and mescaline.[4] I have a different way of understanding the term.

1. Monnica T. Williams and Beatriz Labate, "Diversity, Equity, and Access in Psychedelic Medicine," *Journal of Psychedelic Studies*, 4, 1 (2020), p. 1.
2. David Hillman, *The Chemical Muse: Drug Use and the Roots of Western Civilization* (Thomas Dunne Books, 2014), p. 2.
3. Andy Letcher, *Shroom: A Cultural History of the Magic Mushroom* (NY: HarperCollins, 2007), p. 97.
4. Valerie van Mulukom, Ruairi E. Patterson, Michiel van Elk "Broadening Your Mind to Include Others: The Relationship between Serotonergic Psychedelic Experiences and Maladaptive Narcissism," in *Psychopharmacology (Berl)*, May 2020: 2725–2737.

I believe that "psychedelic" has far more to do with a kind of numinous or otherworldly *experience* than it has to do with the way different substantia interact with this or that neuroreceptor.

I rest my understanding on the historical circumstances that birthed the word psychedelic in the first place: the correspondence between literary craftsman Aldous Huxley (1894–1963) and Canadian psychiatrist Humphry Osmond (1917–2004). In 1953, Osmond gave Huxley his first dose of mescaline in the latter's home in the Hollywood Hills. Huxley would end up penning arguably the most famous essay about the psychedelic experience in history, *The Doors of Perception* (1954), shortly thereafter. Osmond and Huxley carried on a lifelong friendship and wrote extensively to each other over the years. Reading their letters, it's clear that Osmond, who coined "psychedelic," was looking for something beyond brain chemistry to describe the experience. And he had precedent: the common medical term of the time for substantia like LSD and mescaline was "psychotomimetic," meaning "mimicker of madness."

Even the term "hallucinogen," coined earlier by Osmond, was now frowned upon by none other than Osmond himself.[5] Osmond wanted to move away from the madness model—away from clinical definitions. Huxley sought a word that meant "makes this trivial world sublime," settling on the word *phanerothyme*, a mingling of two Greek words meaning "to make the soul visible." (Note that we are in the realm of spirituality here, not neuroscience.) Osmond liked it and responded with a handful of possibilities, among them *psychelytic* ("mind-releasing") and *psychedelic* (mind-manifesting). When Huxley complained that he couldn't read Osmond's handwriting—had he written psychedelic or psychodetic?—Osmond replied with his now famous verse:

To sink in hell or soar angelic
Just take a pinch of psychedelic.[6]

The phrase specifically points to the extremes of otherworldly places: heaven and hell.[7] At no point did brain receptor agonism play any role

5. Max Rinkel, "Experimentally Induced Psychosis in Man," in Harold Abramson (ed.), *Neuropharmacology: Transactions of the 2nd Conference* (May 25–27, 1955), p. 240.
6. Quoted in Horowitz and Palmer (1999), p. 107.
7. Incidentally, Huxley would go on to title his second long essay about mescaline *Heav-*

in the coining of the term. Psychedelic was meant to define a specific experience. Osmond and Huxley might have agreed with some of the descriptors laid out by Andy Letcher (authenticity, freedom, and individualism) but would have scoffed at others (bohemianism and rebellion). And yet, Letcher is correct. In the late 1960s, a good decade after Osmond coined "psychedelic" to address the more numinous qualities of the experience, it did take on new meaning, including subversive attitudes. That again has changed recently with studies showing that psychedelics foster "prosocial behaviours" and help "address non-clinical but problematic interpersonal styles and behaviours."[8]

For many involved in the psychedelic sciences, the definition of psychedelic drifted further away from Osmond and Huxley's original intention and into the realms of neuroscience. Only Osmond and Huxley were not referring to brain receptor agonism as they wrestled for a new term, but were instead fixated on unlocking the deepest potential of the human mind (including psychic powers), access to usually uncharted realms of the unconscious, creative and artistic genius, mysticism, far out philosophies, epistemology, the next big leap in human evolution, and a taste of the sacred.[9] *That* is the context that forged the word "psychedelic."

And as it turns out, Western peoples have been using plant medicines for just such purposes throughout history.

Athens

Let's travel back 5,000 years to the Minoan Civilization where in the city of Gazi, archeologists' unearthed statuettes of women raising their arms, elbows kinked, palms open. These women could represent goddesses or human women like a priestess and/or a physician. Each of them sports

---

en and Hell, his follow-up to the more famous *The Doors of Perception.*

8. Mulukoma et al., (May 2020).

9. This is not to suggest that Osmond and Huxley didn't reference neurology and psychology from time to time in their letters. They certainly did. But that does not seem to have led them to determine that a new name was needed to replace "psychotomimetic." Osmond specifically stated that he wanted a word "uncontaminated by other associations." Horowitz and Palmer (1999), p. 107, and Grover Smith (ed.), *Letters of Aldous Huxley* (NY: Harper and Row, 1969); see letters 623, 631, 643, 655, 658, 668, 670, 671, 679, 681, 687, and 691.

an elegant crown. One crown features birds flying around the top of the rim; another shows the horn of consecration (or the horns of the sacred bull). But the crown that arrests our attention is the one that features three opium bulbs. While we do not know the full significance of these figurines, there can be no doubt that whoever made them had a high opinion of opium. There is a reverence about the statuettes that speaks through the ages. The stoic looks on the women's faces. The way their hands are raised in a pose of serenity.

The statuette featuring the opium crown was found beside a "tubular vase" used for inhaling burning opium. Sadly, we will never fully know what it all meant. It could be the remains of a medical prescription, opium having value as a pain-relieving drug. Or it could have been something closer to what we would call entheogenic. We must also recognize that our progenitors had very different ideas about medicine, magic, and religion than we do today, seeing them as interrelated. An opium ritual would have been no exception. Indeed, there is every chance that whoever inhaled that burning opium in the cavern with her statuette was performing a medical *and* entheogenic ritual. Either way, the archeologists concluded that "[t]he use of opium, for religious purposes at least, was known in Crete in the same period."[10] Thus we are granted a primitive example of Western entheogenism, thousands of years in the past, at a time when not a single Minoan civilian had ever heard of First Nations peoples.

It was this practice—inhaling opium under watch of a goddess or priestess as represented by the statuette—that I believe slowly crept north from Gazi to Athens forming the basis of the most popular ritual of the ancient world, the Rites of Eleusis. These rites were unique in the ancient Grecian world, as we have a text that accompanies them, the *Hymn to Demeter*, ascribed to Homer (c. 8th century BCE). This founding myth behind the Rites of Eleusis tells the story of Persephone, daughter of the grain Goddess Demeter, strolling through the plains of Nysa. At some point, she finds a flower called *narcissus* (from where we get our word "narcotic"[11]) and plucks it from the ground, prompting Hades, the Lord

10. P.G. Kritikos and S.P. Papadaki, "The History of the Poppy and of Opium and their Expansion in Antiquity in the Eastern Mediterranean Area," *United Nations Office on Drugs and Crime* (January 1, 1967).
11. Carl A. P. Ruck, "The Wild and the Cultivated: Wine in Euripides' Bacchae," *Jour-*

of the Underworld, to bring her into his subterranean domain.

Scholars remain unsure as to the nature of the rites. But we can make some educated guesses. The idea behind the Eleusinian Mysteries might have been to take initiates through Persephone's journey into the Underworld, the ceremony offering them a simulacrum of her experience. The ritual featured a moment when the initiates would imbibe a ceremonial drink, *kykeon*, which some scholars believe delivered some kind of entheogen.[12] After all, subsequent to drinking the *kykeon*, they would see a vision of Persephone rising from the Underworld. Even a blind man, Eukrates, claimed to have seen Her.[13] While popular psychedelic consensus holds that ergot—the fungal precursor for synthetic LSD—was most likely the active ingredient in the *kykeon*, there is surprisingly zero evidence to support such a claim.[14] Most likely, these ancient Grecians were drinking an opium-laced concoction.[15]

Interestingly, thousands of miles away, a satellite of the Eleusinian Mysteries uncovered in Catalonia, Spain, does show evidence of sacred ergot usage. Archaeobotanist Jordi Juan-Tresserras disinterred both skeletal remains and a ceremonial drinking vessel from the archaeological site, Mas Castellar de Pontós. Both the drinking vessel and the teeth of the skull tested positive for ergot.[16]

The ancient Greco-Roman world did not have laws against dispensing psychoactive plant material until just before the Common Era. Using these substances in temples in sacred ways was one thing, but in 81 BCE, the Roman general Sulla issued a decree punishing those who

---

nal of Ethnopharmacology, 5 (1982), p. 235.

12. See Carl A.P. Ruck et al., *The Road to Eleusis: Unveiling the Secret of the Mysteries* (CA: North Atlantic Books, 2008).

13. Carl A.P. Ruck, *Sacred Mushrooms of the Goddess: Secrets of Eleusis* (CA: Ronin Publishing, 2006), p. 17.

14. The latest book on the topic has been Brian C. Muraresku, *The Immortality Key: The Secret History of the Religion with No Name* (NY: St. Martin's Press, 2020). While Muraresku makes an excellent case for entheogenic use in the ancient world, he presents no solid evidence for ergot use at Eleusis.

15. For my full thoughts on opium at Eleusis, see Hatsis (2018), p. 54 *ff.*

16. See Jordi Juan-Tresserras, "La Arqueología de las Drogas en la Península Ibérica: una síntesis de las Recientes Investigaciones Arqueobotánicas," *Complutum*, 11 (2000); for an excellent breakdown of Juan-Tresseras' work, see Muraresku (2020).

"sold evil drugs to the public or who keeps them for killing." Among the drugs mentioned are mandrake, hemlock, and Spanish fly.[17] The Roman jurist, Julius Paulus Prudentissimus (3rd century CE), opined against drug-taking for abortions and magic. A later Germanic law specifically references "Magic Philters or Poisoned Potions."[18]

Condemnations of drug use also existed outside legal bodies. The common term for a recreational drug in the Roman world was *pocula amatoria* (or "love philter"; *philtron* in Greek). Plutarch believed that such love philters resulted in the takers becoming "dull-witted, degenerate fools."[19] Christian authors were not far behind. St. Basil (c. 330–c. 379), warned that women employed magic ritual and drugs to "dull . . . intelligence."[20] Boethius (d. 524 CE), a former pagan turned Christian, also poopooed the effects of mind-altering substances: "This terrible drug is so strong that it cuts to the core of a person's being. The drug enters the inner-essence of the self. Those pharmaka that destroy the body are not nearly as powerful as those that corrupt the mind."[21] The very condemnation of intoxication by church leaders is ample proof that Christians were sampling psychoactive potions. And some of the higher-ups were themselves entertained by this or that substantia. One Syrian bishop, Theodorat, rather enjoyed taking opium to shut out all the noises of the world so that he could contemplate Bible passages.[22] Even Ambrose of Milan noted that certain members of the cloth were using opium "almost daily" due to digestive issues.[23] His tone seems to indicate that the digestion issues were nothing more an excuse to enjoy opium.

17. Daniel Ogden, *Magic, Witchcraft, and Ghosts in the Greek and Roman Worlds* (UK: Oxford University Press, 2009), p. 280.

18. Katherine F. Drew (trans. and ed.), *The Laws of the Salic Franks* (Philadelphia: University of Pennsylvania Press, 1991), p. 83–4. Note: Poison (*vene*—from which we get our word "venom"), depending on context, can be translated four ways: as a medicine; as a poison (the way we think of poison as harmful or deadly); as a recreational drug; as an entheogen.

19. Plutarch, *Conjugalia Praecepta*, sec. 5.

20. St. Basil of Caesarea, *Letters*, 188.8.

21. Boethius, *Consolatio philosophiae*, 4.3; *"Haec venena potentius, detrahunt hominem sibi, dira quae penitus meant, nec nocentia corpori mentis uulnere saeuiunt."*

22. Richard Littledale, *Commentary on the Song of Songs* (London: J. Masters, 1869), p. 339.

23. Quoted in Theodorate of Cyrus, *On Divine Province* (NJ: Paulis Press, 1988), p. 193, n. 52.

Like many First Nations' practices, there were some aspects of ancient Western psychedelia that were inhumane from a modern perspective. Worship of Hecate, the Greek goddess of crossroads, involved entheogens and animal sacrifice (specifically black dogs).[24] Grecian oracles, notably those who operated in the Temple of Apollo at Delphi, sat on a tripod over a fault line in the earth. From this tear in Gaia's bosom, psychoactive vapors (said to be the God Apollo himself) would rise into the chamber, lulling the oracle into an entheogenic trance. We know the vapor was powerful, as Plutarch—who was a priest of the Temple of Apollo—records that he once witnessed an oracle become so overwhelmed by the fumes that she had a panic attack, or what we today might call a "bummer."[25] Still, these women were not free agents, but instead the property of the temples, wholly controlled by the priests.

Jerusalem

Like the ancient pagans, the ancient Hebrews were well aware of the intoxicating effects of psychoactive plants like mandrake, which appears twice in the Old Testament, specifically for its magical aphrodisiac qualities. First, in the story of Rachel's infertility (*Gen* 30:14), wherein she had become so desperate to conceive that she traded a night with her husband Jacob to her sister Leah in exchange for some of her nephew's mandrakes. The plant as well finds favorable mention in the *Song of Songs* (*Cant.* 7:13) for its prized aphrodisiac affects.

The Old Testament also mentions another plant, *kaneh bosm*,[26] the meaning of which remains the subject of debate today. Our modern Bibles translate *kaneh bosm* as the "fragrant cane"; conservative scholars usually consider this cane to be calamus, a marshy reed. That was until a Polish anthropologist, Sula Benet (1903–1982), traced the etymology of *kaneh bosm* and compared it with surrounding dialects like Sanskrit (*cana*), As-

24. Manolis Sergis, "Dog Sacrifice in Ancient and Modern Greece: From the Sacrifice Ritual to Dog Torture," *Folklore*, 45 (2010), p. 69. For entheogenic use *vis-à-vis* Hekate sacrifices, see Hatsis (2018), p. 92.
25. Plutarch, *De defectu oraculorum*, 51.
26. Exodus 30:23; Song of Songs 4:14; Isaiah 43:24; Jeremiah 6:20; and Ezekiel 27:19.

syrian (*qunnabu*), and Greek (*kannabis*), among others. There is a clear etymological link that would suggest *kaneh bosm* was the ancient Hebrew word for cannabis.[27]

Still, conservative scholars wouldn't budge.

However, new evidence has put a lot of weight behind Benet's assertion. About fifty miles south of Jerusalem, the remains of a small temple—the Temple of Arad—was recently unearthed. The temple features two incense pillars which have tested positive for frankincense and cannabis.[28] There's very little wiggle room here. Whichever rabbi was worshipping in that space was inhaling cannabis as he prayed. What's more, ancient writers attest to highly psychoactive varieties of frankincense that are unknown to us today. The poet Virgil, physician Dioscorides, and the Christian theologian Tatian, all acknowledged that powerfully psychoactive forms of frankincense existed in the ancient world.[29] The cannabis additive seems to have entered the temple through the worship of Asherah, Yahweh's original (though mostly forgotten), wife. Ancient semitic peoples linked Asherah with cannabis and such traditions seem displayed at Arad.[30] As the patriarchs took power, they tore Asherah, and the cannabis used in her worship, from their divine status.

Psychedelic Christianity

When we call attention to the foundations of Western Civilization originating in Athens and Jerusalem, we really mean "Judeo-Christianity" when referring to the latter. While Christianity today has a somewhat puritanical bent on the subject of drugs, ancient and medieval Christians weren't as anal. Like today, Christianity in the ancient world took on a variety of forms and doctrines. Many of those Christian groups, which some modern scholars' herd under the umbrella term "gnostic,"[31] em-

---

27. Chris Bennett, *Cannabis and the Soma Solution* (OR: Trine Day, 2010), p. 353.
28. Alex Fox, "Archaeologists Identify Traces of Burnt Cannabis in Ancient Jewish Shrine," *Smithsonian Magazine*, June 4, 2020.
29. Hatsis (2018), p. 93.
30. See Chris Bennett, *Cannabis: Lost Sacrament of the Ancient World* (OR: Trine Day, 2023).
31. I agree with other scholars who feel that the term "gnostic" is too broad to be of much use. While I find that "Neo-Platonism" is a more apt term, I retain "gnostic" here because of common usage.

ployed mind-altering potions in their rituals. Church Fathers indicate that both Carpocrates (from Alexandria) and the infamous Simon Magus (from Samaria) concocted these kinds of potions and drugged their respective congregations with them, presumably to some kind of mystical effect.[32] We know of one Valentinian gnostic named Marcus who several Church Fathers charged with using substantia in his religious rituals. A common drug found in such potions throughout the Roman empire was mandrake.[33]

Medieval alternative-Christian offshoots, condemned by the Church as heresies, continued the alleged practices of the Carpocratians, Simon Magus, and Marcus—that is, dosing their congregations to demonstrate the divinity of the groups' leaders. Delegates attending the Council of Paris in 819 CE warned of such magicians who drugged the food of their constituents to convince them of their power.[34] Another Christian writer spoke of one heretical leader putting "drugs in food" (*applicando incentive in cibriis*) to help sway the new recruit's mind.[35]

Perhaps our best evidence for medieval Christian psychedelia comes from France in 1022 CE. A knight named Aréfast was dispatched to Orléans to root out a group of heretics. While disguised as a curious potential candidate seeking information about the sect, Aréfast was told by the leaders that new initiates must first feast on "heavenly food" (*caelestri cibo*) that generated "angelic visions . . . and sated by that comfort [he] will be able to go where [he] will at [his] leisure"[36] After Aréfast ratted

32. For Carpocrates, see Irenaeus, *Against the Heresies*, 1.25.3; for Simon Magus, see Epiphanius, "Contra Haereses," 2.2 in G.R.S. Mead, *Simon Magus: Essays on the Founder of Simonism Based on Ancient Sources* (Leipzig, Germany: edidit G. Dindorfius, 1859).

33. Dioscorides, *Pharmacorum simpilicium*, p. 238; *". . . huius radicem ad amorem dant."*

34. Nigel Glendinning (*trans.*), Julio Caro Baroja, *The World of the Witches* (UK: Pheonix Press, 2001), p. 56.

35. "Recollectio," in Joseph Hansen (ed.), *Quellen und untersuchungen* (Bonn, Germany: Carl Georgi, 1901), p. 161; *"et applicando incentive in cibariis, aut per superius tactos provocancia partem sensitivam."*

36. Quoted in Martin Bouquet et al., "Acts of the Council in Orlans," *Recueil des historiens,* (Poitiers: Imprimerie de H. Oudin Frères, 1878), p. 537–38; "*Deinde caelestri cibo pastus, interna satietate recreates, videbis persaepe nobiscum visiones angelicas, quarem solatio sultus, cum eis quovis locorum sine mora vel difficultate, cum volueris, ire poteris; nihilque tibi decerit . . .* " For a more detailed analysis of this incident, see

them out, this particular group of heretics was rounded up and locked in a cottage, which was then set ablaze. All burned alive.

Later, when orthodox Christianity rose into an institutional Goliath, mandrake still found favor among Christians as an entheogen. The author of the anonymous Trudperter Hohelied (c. 1160), worked the intoxicating effects of mandrake into her own mystical understanding of the Trinity when she wrote:

> The bark of the mandrake root brings stupefaction. This root denotes God, the image of whom was Christ. On earth he was a man. For us he is a medicine and a security for eternal life. He is the root. . . . The root's bark is the Holy Ghost, this means the numbing vapor which makes all lovers of holy Christ sleep.[37]

I believe this author was referring to achieving a *somnitheogenic* experience—that is, "generating divinity in dreams."[38] Mandrake doesn't just cause visions and horniness while awake, but also produces dreams so vivid and lucid that one feels like they have stepped into an alternate reality, every bit as real as waking life.

Witches

Some of the best evidence we have for Western psychedelia comes in the form of the popularly called witches' "flying ointment" of the early modern period. Women would use these ointments to fall into a deep, lucid dream state where they would feel that they were flying to mountaintops to join others in worshiping a goddess (i.e., a *somnitheogenic* experience). The Latin word for this kind of spirit flight is *transvection* (or "carried across"). This practice of having religious experiences outside a Christian framework added fodder to the Church's larger mission of eradicating the many local goddesses in which common people still believed. Stories of interactions with these goddesses abound in the source literature.

Hatsis (2015), pp. 64–8.

37. Quoted in H. Klug (trans.), Van Arsdall et al., "The Mandrake Plant and its Legend: A New Perspective," *Old Names—New Growth: Proceedings of the 2nd ASPNS Conference, University of Graz, Austria* (6–10 June 2007), p. 316.

38. See Hatsis (2018), p. 9.

Dominican theologian Johannes Nider (1380–1438) and the Bishop of Ávila, Spain, Alonso Tostado (1410–1455), were sober and clear when they wrote of wise-women rubbing their bodies with medical ointments and believing that they are *transvecting* to witch dances.

Nider tells us that during his travels in southern Germany he encountered a worshiper of the fertility Goddess Hulda (*unholdan*), who recited magical words as she oiled up her body with a magical ointment. She seems to have believed that the ointment would allow her to *transvect* to the Heuberg, a mountaintop in southern Germany, to join the ceremonies that took place there.[39] The soporific unguent caused her not to lift off but to lie down; she eventually fell into a deep sleep. Nider's message is clear: this woman had deluded herself with a drugged ointment. But that was just his theological opinion; to the *unholdan*, the experience was likely very real—something she might have called "somnitheogenic" had the word existed at the time.

Likewise, while commenting on the book of *Genesis*, Alonso Tostado digresses to briefly discuss the way some people used mind-manifesting medical drugs to enjoy otherworldly experiences: "There are certain women that we [theologians] call 'witches' who claim to use these . . . medical ointments in conjunction with magical words to transport whenever they desire to diverse places to meet with other women and men. There, they will indulge in all sorts of foods and pleasures."[40] Tostado is clearly speaking of an experience that we today would call "psychedelic" (i.e., taking substantia to have a specific kind of ethereal experience), even though the word did not exist in his day.

French doctor Jean de Nynauld (c. 1550–c. 1650) demonstrates that by the Renaissance Era, magicians and witches were well-acquainted with psychedelic mushrooms. He even differentiates between the famous, red-topped white spotted *Amanita muscaria* (or "sleepy mushroom") and the *psilocybe* (or "maddening mushroom"). Nynauld says that these mushrooms are used by magicians to "show the shadows of the

39. Johannes Nider in Hansen (1901), p. 437; *"und salb machent und enweg farent . . . vulgo Herberg dictum."*

40. Alonso Tostado in Hansen (1901), p. 109; *Sunt enim mulieres quaedum, quas maleficas vocamus, quae profitentur facta quondam unction cum certis verborum observationibus ire, quando voluptatum generibus, tam in cibis quam in complexibus perfruantur."*

underworld."[41] Earlier, another physician named Girolamo Cardano had even distinguished between what we today might call a "good trip" (e.g., visions of "pleasure-gardens, banquets, beautiful ornaments and clothing, handsome young men, kings, [and] magistrates") from a "bad trip" (e.g., "demons, ravens, prisons, desert wastes, and torments").[42]

In the 20th century, researchers became curious about the powers of these ointments. Basing his recipe on one from the mid-1500s, German folklorist Will-Erich Peukert (1895–1969) concocted his very own flying ointment sometime in the 1950s. Peukert "dreamed of wild rides, frenzied dancing, and other weird adventures . . . connected with medieval orgies."[43] A centuries' old Western psychedelic tradition rediscovered in the modern world!

Raising Demons

Like wise-women, ceremonial magicians of the medieval and early modern Western world also ingested entheogenic plants in their magical rites from time to time. Ceremonial magic isn't like the stage magic we see today in figures like David Copperfield and Chris Angel. It is highly complicated procedure filled with any or all of the following elements: astrological calculations, cleansing rituals, daemonic and angelic invocations in Hebrew and/or Latin, drawing sacred geometric symbols, lengthy prayers, and, on occasion, substantia.

The founding text of medieval Western ceremonial magic, *Picatrix* (mid-13th century), mixed magical lore from Persia, India, Greece, Assyria, Egypt, and Chaldea, and includes mind-manifesting uses of substantia. One spell to invoke the "servant of the Moon" requires mixing a staggering amount of cannabis resin (1–1.5 lbs.!) with plane tree resin while the "Sun is in Virgo." Another, ghastlier, spell requires cooking a

---

41. Jean de Nynauld, *De la Lycanthropie, Transformation et Extase des Sorciers* (Paris: Chez Jean Millot, 1615); reprint of the original edition Éditions Frénésie, Paris, France (1990), p. 49; *"morelle furieuse* [reading *"furieux"*] . . . *morelle endormāte"; "desquels le Diable se sert pour troubler les sens de ses esclaues."* (Marie Phillips, trans).

42. Cardano, *De subtilitate*, p. 592; *"Sed tamen dormire creduntur dum haec vident, videt autem theatra, viridaria, coenas, orantus, vestes, formosos iuuenes, Reges, magitratus, item daemonas, coruos, carceres, soliditudinem, tormeta."*

43. Quoted in Michael Harner, *Hallucinogens and Shamanism* (UK: Oxford University Press, 1973), p. 139.

severed head in eight ounces of opium (!) mixed with equal parts human blood and sesame oil, which allows a person to see "whatever [she] wants to see." A similar spell involving opium requires not a severed head but a penis.[44]

Other grimoires like the *Sworn Book of Honorus* (c. late 14th century) incorporated psychedelic spells as well. Heinrich Cornelius Agrippa von Nettesheim (1486–1535) carried these ideas from the medieval era into the Renaissance.[45] His *Three Books of Occult Philosophy* (1531) features fumigation mixes of henbane and opium that when inhaled, would "makes spirits forthwith appear in the air or elsewhere," a clear reference to the visionary properties of the ingredients.[46] Elsewhere, he notes the use of mandrake as a sex-enhancing drug.[47] *Three Books of Occult Philosophy* was one of the most widely circulated grimoires of his day, meaning there is no telling how many ritual magicians used plant medicines to invoke spirits. These traditions survived into the 20th century in the form of ceremonial magicians like Aleister Crowley (1875–1947) and Allen Bennett (1872–1923).[48]

(Incidentally, they have also been carried into the 21st century among certain folks I know personally.)

Exploring Inner Space

Physicians and magicians continued to concoct psychedelic brews up to and throughout the Industrial Revolution. Poets and writers were enthralled by cannabis, no doubt to access the plant's creativity enhancing effects. Most famous among these new inner-explorers

44. Quoted in Chris Bennett, *Liber 420 . . .* (2018), p. 182.
45. Jake Barlett Winchester, *Necromantic Shamanism in 19th Century London* (Wedfty Media Division, 2020), p. 8.
46. James Freake (trans.), Donald Tyson (ed.), Cornelius Agrippa von Nettesheim, *Three Books of Occult Philosophy* (St. Paul, Minn.: Llewellyn Publications, 1992), p. 133.
47. Catherine M. Dunn (ed.), Henry Cornelius Agrippa of Nettesheim, *Of the Vanitie and Uncertaintie of Artes and Sciences* (Northridge: California State University Foundation, 1974), p. 203.
48. See Patrick Everitt, "The Cactus and the Beast: Investigating the Role of Peyote (Mescaline) in the Magick of Aleister Crowley," M.A. Western Esotericism Thesis, University of Amsterdam (2016), p. 13.

was undoubtedly Fitz Hugh Ludlow (1836–1870), who took readers through the highs (and lows) of his hashish experiments. The pages of his book *The Hashish Eater* (1857) contain numerous passages testifying to the psychedelic nature of high doses of hash. Consider the following: "Though far from believing that my own ecstasy has claim to such inspiration as an apostle's[,] the states are still analogues in this respect—they both share the nature of disembodiment, and the soul, in both, beholds realities of greater or lesser significance, such as may never be apprehended again out of the light of eternity."[49] There is very little that isn't *psychedelic* about that sentiment. And he wasn't alone. Poets, philosophers, seers, and artists were also experimenting with high doses of cannabis—and soon, peyote—to explore the creative inner workings of their minds.

Contemporaries like the Rosicrucian Paschal Beverly Randolph (1825–1875) found much use for entheogenic ointments and potions in his search for a deeper spirituality. Traveling to Europe in early 1855, Randolph fell in with secret societies who experimented with hashish. He was charmed by a certain Dr. Jaques-Joseph Moreau de Tours (1804–1884), a member of the Club de Hashischins in Paris, who believed that proper cannabis use could reveal the reality of the soul. Randolph borrowed this line and incorporated psychedelics into sex magic. His mind-manifesting ointments included an astonishing amount of substantia; the ingredients of one are as follows: 50 grams of henbane, 20 grams of belladonna,[50] 250 grams of opium (!), and 300 grams of hash (!!). Both partners were to dose themselves with it and work to make sure they orgasmed at the same time. Only then would "the mystic doors of the soul open to the spaces."[51]

49. Quoted in Donald P. Dulchinos, *Pioneer of Innerspace: The Life of Fitz Hugh Ludlow, Hasheesh Easter* (Autonomedia, 1998), p. 81.
50. Henbane and belladonna are members of the Solanaceae family of plants. They have similar mind-altering potentials as mandrake.
51. Quoted in John Patrick Deveny, *Paschal Beverly Randolph: A Nineteenth Century Black American Spiritualist, Rosicrucian, and Sex Magician* (NY: State University of New York Press, 1996), p. 71.

The 1800s also saw the first concerted efforts by Western peoples to use plant medicines as aids in psychology—as new ways to explore their own minds. The first person (for which we have reliable information) to consider this new paradigm was the British chemist Humphry Davy (1778–1829). Somewhat ironically, the first modern psychedelic experiments did not involve plants or mushrooms at all.[52]

It wasn't weird that Davy conducted his first psychedelic experiment on April 17, 1799. He was right on time. Davy lived on the cusp of a new scientific enlightenment. In nine months the clocks would reach midnight, turning the 18th century into the 1800s, the century that brought us the battery, the locomotive, the camera, electromagnets, fiber optics, spectroscopes, braille, toilet paper (*yes!*), the first electric light, and the first modern trip report—those latter two contributions coming from Davy himself. He lived at the dawn of the modern world, and dutifully contributed to its unfolding. His insatiable thirst for experiment and knowledge would not go unnoticed; he eventually joined the Royal Institution to teach chemistry.

Inventions and accolades aside, Davy was a rarity in early psychedelic research—a person willing to take a new drug to see how it affected him. He straddles the historical line that bridges those like Paracelsus (1493–1541), the 16th century alchemist-magician who mixed concoctions of cannabis, opium, mandrake and often drank them himself, and Shasha Shulgin (1925–2014), the "Godfather of Ecstasy," who designed, synthesized, or otherwise sampled a variety of research chemicals like MDMA and 2CE in his laboratory in Northern California. For Davy, the drug was nitrous oxide, first discovered by Joseph Priestley (1733 –1804) in 1772. He recorded his self-experiments and those of others in his book *Researches, Chemical, and Philosophical, Chiefly Concerning Nitrous Oxide* (1800). Therein, Davy describes the effects of Apollo's vapors, updated for the modern day. One paralytic patient to whom he gave nitrous oxide remarked that she "felt like the sound of a harp;"[53] another experimenter, a Mr. J.W. Tobin, was "elevated to a

52. Mike Jay, *Emperors of Dreams: Drugs in the Nineteenth Century* (UK: Dedalus, 2005), p. 14.

53. Quoted in Sir Humphrey Davy, *Researches, Chemical and Philosophical* (London: J. Johnson, 1800), p. 496.

most sublime height."[54] As so often happens with psychedelic experimentation, conscious expansion gave way to spiritual revelation. Born a generation after Davy's nitrous oxide tests commenced, the American poet, philosopher, and mystic Benjamin Paul Blood (1832–1919) discovered nitrous oxide while having dental work performed. His take on the gas, which he likened to a "revelation," could "Initi[ate] . . . Man into the Immemorable Mystery of the Open Secret of Being, revealed as the Inevitable Vortex of Continuity."[55]

This consciousness-expansion approach to drug use filtered into the *hoi polloi.* Around the same time (the 1840s), mind-altering experiments, both mystical and psychological, were taking place in Paris under the direction of Dr. Moreau de Tours at the Club de Hashischins, where Paschal Beverly Randolph was first turned on to hash. Though, he was far from the only eccentric to take kindly to the drug. Dr. Moreau de Tours, influenced from a high dose session of hashish, believed that the drug ferried the user to the realm of madness, and safely returned her back to sanity once the effects had waned. He was mostly interested in what he referred to as the "hallucinations" caused by hashish. Such hallucinations, he felt, were "the most frequent symptom and the fundamental fact of delirium, mental illness, and madness."[56] He took his theory to les Hôspital Universitaire la Pitié-Salpêtrière, publishing the findings in his book, *Hashish and Mental Illness* (1845). This, not any indigenous psychedelic practice, represents the beginning of psychedelic psychotherapy in the West, i.e., doctors ingesting a drug to better understand the minds of their more compromised patients. And it was in this tradition of self-experimentation with research chemicals, natural and synthetic, that carried into the 20th century and led to one of the greatest psychedelic discoveries in history.

54. Quoted in Davy (1800), p. 501.
55. Quoted in William James, *The Varieties of Religious Experience* (New York: Signet Classics, 2003), p. 328.
56. Gordon J. Barnett (trans.), Jacques-Joseph Moreau, *Hashish and Mental Illness* (NY: Raven Press, 1973), p. 165.

Wunderkind

On 16 April 1943, the Swiss chemist Albert Hofmann (1906–2008) took a break from his work at Sandoz Pharmaceuticals. He had been trying to develop a migraine medicine from ergot, a fungus that grows on rye grains, but started to feel dizzy and decided to leave for home. Once arrived, he experienced a "dreamlike condition," while a "stream of fantastic pictures" flooded his mind. The phenomena eventually waned, leaving Hofmann not but a little confused as to what had caused such bizarre sensations. He reckoned he had accidentally absorbed one of the chemicals in his lab. Since it was Friday, he would have to wait a couple of days to find out. Returning to work the following Monday, anxious to follow the thread of formulae that may have caused his ordeal, he inhaled a chloroform-like substance he had used while preparing his ergot derivative. The effects were trivial. He then decided the culprit must have been the only other chemical he handled back on Friday—the 25th synthesis of his experiments with ergot—called "LSD-25." Little over an hour after taking what he believed to be a small dose of LSD—250 millionths of a gram—Hofmann once again felt odd and decided to head home. As it turns out, 250 millionths of a gram is a *gigantic* dose of LSD, throwing Hofmann into a spiral of fear as he reached his front door. His wife and children were visiting in France, so his neighbor, Mrs. R, came to his aid with a bucket of milk hoping it would relieve him of his symptoms. It did not. Hofmann's fear intensified to the point that he thought he was dying.

After a while he relaxed and started to enjoy the experience. He eventually went to sleep; he describes waking up the next morning: "I had the feeling that I saw the earth and the beauty of nature as it had been when it was created . . . it was a beautiful experience! I was reborn, seeing nature in quite a new light."[57]

The therapeutic possibilities for LSD were recognized almost immediately. Werner Stoll (1915–1955), son of Hofmann's boss Arthur Stoll (1887–1971), brought the strange new chemical to Burghölzli Hospital for further experimentation. In his first published article on LSD,

57. Stan Grof, "Stan Grof Interviews Dr. Albert Hofmann, Esalen Institute, Big Sur California 1984," *MAPS Bulletin* 11 no. 2 (2001), p. 25.

Stoll admits that it can be used to "support a therapeutic effect."[58] Moreover, in a private letter to the director of Burghölzli, Stoll confided, "It transports the subject into a magical world" and "gifts him supernatural powers and overwhelming experiences inaccessible to his mundane surroundings."[59] But the real excitement came from doctors believing they finally had a way inside the minds of their mentally disturbed patients—exactly the reason for which Dr. Moreau de Tours employed cannabis.

Though the possibilities didn't end there. Early LSD experimenters also noticed that the drug caused abreaction, or the sudden remembering of a long-forgotten memory. When Sandoz sent samples of LSD to the United States and elsewhere, the shipment included a pamphlet outlining what these early researchers believed to be the medicine's greatest attributes: first, to "elicit release of repressed material," and second, for doctors "to gain insight in the world and ideas and sensations of mental patients."[60] Once Sandoz started to ship internationally in the early 1950s, psychedelic psychotherapy enjoyed an evolutionary boom in the West. Following in the line of Moreau de Tours and, later, Werner Stoll, Dr. Charles Savage (1918–2007) began his LSD experiments in 1952. Dr. Savage had earlier worked with mescaline and was familiar with the psychedelic terrain. He soon took note of the euphoria caused by LSD and wondered "if such a euphoria might be of value in the treatment of depression."[61]

During this first wave of LSD experimentation, doctors began to develop the protocols that are still largely in place today, notably the adage of "dose, set, and setting." Briefly, dose refers to the amount of medicine a person ingests; set refers to a person's mindset; and setting refers to

58. W. Stoll, "Ein Neues in sehr Kleinin Mengen Wirksames Phantastikum" *Schweizer Archiv fur Neurologie und Psychiatric*, 64, p. 483; *" . . . therapeutischen Effekt vermuten konnte"*; (trans., Peter Conolly-Smith.)

59. Quoted in Erika Dyck and Chris Elcock, *Expanding Mindscapes: A Global History of Psychedelics* (MA: MIT Press, 2024), p. 144–45.

60. Albert Hofmann, *LSD, My Problem Child: Reflections on Scared Drugs, Mysticism, and Science* (FL: MAPS), p. 73.

61. Charles Savage, "The Resolution and Subsequent Remobilization of Resistance by LSD in Psychotherapy," from the Round Table "Psychodynamic and Therapeutic Aspects of Mescaline and Lysergic Acid Diethylamide," held at the annual meeting of the American Psychiatric Association, May 3, 1956. Transcripts reprinted in *Journal of Nervous and Mental Diseases* 125, no. 1 (January– March 1957). 434–35.

the environment in which a person takes the medicine. One of the first doctors to receive a supply of LSD was Ronald Sandison (1916–2010), the Deputy Medical Superintendent of Powick Hospital in Worchester, England. He quickly established an LSD Block and transformed that corner of the drab hospital into a livelier environment, complete with musical instruments, toys, a record player, and a small petting zoo.[62] One white American doctor, Juliana Day (1919–2013), adopted a hands-off approach to facilitating LSD. She wouldn't interrupt her patients when they started speaking of cosmic insights, but rather gave them the space to be seen and heard.[63]

If Dr. Moreau de Tours' experiments with cannabis birthed modern psychedelic psychotherapy in the mid-1800s, this new therapeutic model came of age with LSD during the 1950s, when scores of psychiatrists, chemists, allergists, and spies sampled it, mescaline, and psilocybin mushrooms trying to unlock the hidden powers of the mind.

One of those doctors was Los Angeles based psychotherapist, Oscar Janiger (1918–2001). He not only facilitated LSD sessions, including to noteworthy authors like Anaïs Nin (1903–1977) and Aldous Huxley, but also hosted psychedelic gatherings at his house. The purpose of these gatherings, as mystic-philosopher and regular attendee Alan Watts (1915–1973) recalls, was to find the " 'essential' or 'active' ingredients of the mystical experience."[64] Janiger looked to the West when designing these gatherings. Indeed, he made no secret about his wish to replicate "the ritual created by the Greeks at Eleusis."[65]

In those days, any accredited doctor could write a letter to Sandoz that explained her research interests and, if approved, receive a supply of LSD for experimentation. Only Janiger couldn't write to Sandoz speaking of ancient Grecian mystery religions and mystical experiences. And he was too honorable a man to scam Sandoz by coming up with a bogus

---

62. Antonio Melechi, "Drugs of Liberation: From Psychiatry to Psychedelia," *Psychedelia Britannica: Hallucinogenic Drugs in Britain* (London: Turnaround, 1997), p. 38–39.
63. Juliana Day, "The Role and Reaction of the Psychiatrist in LSD Therapy," *Journal of Nervous and Mental Diseases* 125, no. 1 (Jan–March 1957), pp. 437–38
64. Alan Watts, "Psychedelics and Religious Experience," *California Law Review* 56, no. 1 (1968), p. 75.
65. Oscar Janiger, "Personal Statement by Oscar Janiger," *Bulletin of the Multidisciplinary Association for Psychedelic Studies*, 9, no. 1 (Spring 1999), p. 6.

experiment he never intended to conduct. Instead, he got his LSD from a former spy for the US government, the legendary Captain Alfred Matthew Hubbard (1901–1982).

Psychedelic Conservatism

Captain Al Hubbard is much celebrated in the psychedelic Renaissance for his cavalier, jovial, good-ole-boy approach to medicine-work. Hubbard's life is complicated by the tales he spun about it. Not one to shy from telling a good story, teasing fact from fiction about Hubbard's biography remains a Sisyphean task. We do know that at some point he joined the Office of Strategic Servies (OSS), forerunner to the CIA. In 1947 he took position as director of scientific research at Limited, a uranium corporation based in British Columbia.

As for psychedelic facilitation, Hubbard was Catholic, and incorporated Christian art in his psychedelic sessions, regardless of a person's religious bent. Myron Stolaroff (1920–2013), a Jewish engineer turned psychedelic pioneer, felt the brunt of Hubbard's methods on his first trip in April 1956. Stolaroff swallowed 60 micrograms of LSD; then, Hubbard's friend Father J.E. Brown, a priest of the Cathedral of the Holy Rosary, blessed him. As the LSD began to open Stolaroff's eyes to both the wonders of the cosmos and the infinite in every grain of sand, Hubbard bombarded him with pictures of Jesus![66] Stolaroff would later act as psychedelic missionary by bringing LSD to the Sequoia Seminar, a Bible-study group located in Palo Alto.

Father Brown also took warmly to LSD, seeing it as a spiritual technology for Christians to embrace. In a mailer he sent out to his congregation, he included the following thoughts:

> We ... approach the study of psychodelics [*sic*] and their influence in the mind of man anxious to discover whatever attributes they possess, respectfully evaluating their proper place in the Divine Economy. We humbly ask Our Heavenly Mother the Virgin Mary, help of all who call upon Her, to aid us to know and understand the true qualities of

66. Myron Stolaroff, *Thanatos to Eros: 35 Years of Psychedelic Exploration* (Berlin: VWB, 1994), pp. 23–4.

> these psychedelics ... according to God's laws to use them for the benefit of [hu]mankind here and in eternity.[67]

Father Brown was not alone in wanting to use LSD to strengthen the Catholic faith. In one of Aldous Huxley's many letters to Humphry Osmond, he mentions someone who was using LSD "as an instrument for validating Catholic doctrine."[68] Huxley was likely referring to Hubbard.

Maria Huxley (1898–1955), an early psychedelics explorer, was conservative—famously fretting over whether Canadian psychiatrist, Humphry Osmond, who visited the Huxleys in Los Angeles back in the mid-1950s, would have a beard.[69] Maria took part in many of the early psychedelic experiments with Aldous and his friend, author Gerald Heard (1889–1971), along with their supplier, Al Hubbard. It was Maria, in fact, who influenced her husband to write the most famous essay in psychedelic history, *The Doors of Perception*.[70] And it was Maria, in fact, who typed up the manuscript (Aldous was legally blind). Had she lived to see the psychedelic 60s it's unlikely she would have approved of the hippie counterculture. For Maria, the sacredness—the *mystery*—of the psychedelic experience mattered most.

The public face of mid-century conservatism, Clare Boothe Luce (1903–1987), and husband Henry (1898–1967), founder of *Time-Life Magazine*, published articles favorable to LSD and mescaline in their periodical. For the Luces, there was nothing rebellious or anti-conformist about psychedelics at all. In fact, Henry desired to use the deep insights of the LSD space to become "the spokesman for the conventional values of Middle America," specifically, "country, church, capitalism, and party."[71] Like Al Hubbard, the Luces preferred to have a priest, Father

67. Quoted in Jay Stevens, *Storming Heaven: LSD and the American Dream* (Grove Press, 1986), p. 71.
68. Smith (1969), p. 843.
69. Horowitz and Palmer (1999), p. 33
70. See Hatsis (2021), p. 143.
71. Robert E. Herzstein, *Henry R. Luce, Time, and the American Crusade in Asia* (Cambridge, United Kingdom: Cambridge University Press, 2005), p. 240.

John Murray (1904–1967), around whenever they took LSD. Father Murray was with Henry on his first LSD trip. Other times he would council Claire while she was on LSD, especially during her very public divorce from Henry.

It was only in the late 1960s that psychedelics became truly politicized. While psychedelic explorers of the 1950s were inclined towards a more conservative approach to these medicines, hippies of the late 1960s preferred anything but. Public figures like Timothy Leary (1920–1996) and Ken Kesey (1935–2001) freely dosing unsuspecting people with LSD, while not the sole reason psychedelics became illegal, did not lend credibility to the movement. While the psychedelic Renaissance tends to highlight the outliers in psychedelic history that contributed to creating visionary culture, the majority of unnamed scientists and governmental authorities viewed LSD, mescaline, and mushrooms as psychotomimetics, drugs that make you insane. From their perspective, a crazy-making drug found use recreationally by scores of young people. When we look back a decade prior to the 1960s, we see a far more conservative approach to handling plant medicines. We only think the 1960s was emblematic of Western psychedelia because popular culture typically presents that decade as the beginning and end of Western psychedelia.

Whether one places the origins of psychedelia in the West at the dawn of civilization with cannabis and opium (as I do) or feels that only CSPs count as "psychedelic" doesn't matter to our larger inquiry. Neither the ancient traditions in Europe nor the modern clinical approaches to psychedelia in the West—what Chacruna affiliates refer to as the "White-dominant medical framework"—borrowed much from First Nations peoples.[72] The characterization of global medicine as "white-dominant" is little more than an echo of CSJ psychedelia's oppressor-oppressed narrative. Advances in medicine are not "white";

72. See Jamilah R. George et al., "The Psychedelic Renaissance and the Limitations of White-Dominant Medical Framework: A Call for Indigenous and Ethnic Minority Inclusion," *Journal of Psychedelic Studies*," Vol. 4, 1 (2020): 4–15.

they are universal, the result of physicians and chemists from all over the world basing new experiments on older research.

Entering altered states of consciousness through substantia goes back to the days of the Minoan Civilization, Greece, Catalonia, pagan Rome, fringe Judaism, Christian Europe, and is later found among medieval witches and magicians, alchemists, poets, other assorted seekers, and is still with us today. Western Civilization has a far richer psychedelic history than perhaps many conservatives and postcolonialists are ready to admit.

May they find common bond in their error.

6

Decolonizing Psychedelia: A Brief History of First Nations' Medicine Work

The scientific progress and clinical progress
of the modern psychedelic medicine movement owes
much of its success to the history of indigenous healing practices.
—Jamilah R. George, "The Psychedelic Renaissance"

A Dark and Shameful Chapter

I sat in attendance at the 2022 Spirit Plant Medicine Conference as Francine Douglas of Sacred Circle, an indigenous health and wellness organization, took the stage. Her speech was quite moving at times. I didn't know much about the history of Canadian-indigenous relations and was touched as Douglas mentioned the Anti-Potlatch Laws enacted against her people, the Stol:lo, in 1885. The legislation effectively outlawed her tribal culture and language until cooler heads realized just how terribly wrong it all was and lifted the ban in 1951. Douglas herself was luckily never alive to see those days, so her speech mostly focused on a common theme found in psychedelia as of late: centering the psychedelic Renaissance around First Nations voices. The idea is that First

Nations peoples have some kind of "ancestral knowledge of psychedelics [that] roots back to their origins," which Westerners do not possess—an erroneous framework we have already addressed in the last chapter.[1] At one point during her presentation, Douglas played a movie trailer that featured renowned psychiatrist Dr. Gabor Maté repeating the noble savage stereotype as he sat with a group of First Nations elders. "It's necessary that we as a culture turn to you for the healing," says Dr. Maté, "because the healing principles embedded in your traditions and your culture are so much wiser, so much more connected."[2] Dr. Maté is a fine psychiatrist; but as we will see, a historian he is not.

Douglas's talk also featured a truly ghastly segment, when she referenced "215 indigenous children [that] were unearthed in unmarked graves" at a Christian-run indigenous school in Kamloops, British Columbia. The subplot was that the Church authorities at the school had heartlessly murdered the children through neglect and shamefully tossed their bodies into a common grave, telling no one of their foul deed. "I had my first medicine journey with Sacred Circle about a week after the announcement of the 215 children," Douglas announced from the stage. The mushrooms she consumed on that journey told her that the "children found [under Kamloops] have been waiting. Waiting for their families to find their connection . . . waiting for you, our allies, our neighbors, our friends, our community, to be ready to witness our pain. To cry for us and to cry with us."[3]

It's a heart-wrenching story, one that should cool the heels of any bigot. But there's just one problem with the mushroom's message to Douglas: *not a single child has been unearthed from the Kamloops Indian Residential School campus.*

Unfortunately, Douglas (or the mushroom) was merely parroting a then unconfirmed news report that had broken a year earlier in July 2021, when Chief Rosanne Casimir of the Tk'emlups te Secwepemc First Na-

1. Touleimat (2022).
2. "Medicine: St'elmexw."
3. Francine Douglas, "Swoxwiyam and Sqwelqwel: The Power of Indigenous Knowledge and Cultural Ceremonies for All with Francine Douglas," Spirit Plant Medicine Conference, 2022.

tion claimed that ground-penetrating radar had exposed the bodies of children buried near the Kamloops Indian Residential School, which opened in 1890. "It's a harsh reality and it's our truth, it's our history," she told the press.[4] The idea is that children were kidnapped or otherwise forced into these schools where they were neglected and abused by the staff. Eventually dying, the staff callously dumped the corpses in a mass grave near the campus. Rumors had circulated about the bodies for years, but no hard evidence was ever presented.

Prime Minister Justin Trudeau announced this "dark and shameful chapter" in Canada's history.[5] News of the discovery reached all the way to the Vatican, followed by an apology from Pope Francis for this grave injustice, which, of course, stoked the flames of retaliation. Across Canada, churches—many of them built by First Nations peoples—were burned to the ground. The Canadian government quickly allocated $27 million to efforts of identifying the deceased and transporting their remains back to their families.

We are still waiting for a single name to be released.

In fairness to Douglas, many First Nations children in those schools toiled under conditions that we today would call neglectful and abusive. But they hardly suffered in a vacuum. Lots of children of various ethnicities endured harsh environments in dilapidated schools. In fact, the indigenous child mortality rate "was comparable to the Canadian average."[6] It's sad on all fronts, and I am reluctant to consider that white or black Canadian children's lives are somehow worth less than any other child's life—indigenous or otherwise.

It all started when an anthropologist at the University of the Fraser Valley, Dr. Sarah Beaulieu, determined to find those long-rumored bodies of indigenous children by using ground-penetrating radar around the Kamloops Indian Residential School. She was the first to claim that 215 corpses of indigenous children were found on the grounds. But as the

4. Ian Austen, "'Horrible History': Mass Grave of Indigenous Children Reported in Canada," *NY Times* (May 28, 2021).
5. Quoted in Jacques Rouillard, "In Kamloops, Not One Body Has Been Found," *The Dorchester Review* (January 11, 2022).
6. Rouillard, "In Kamloops, . . ." (2022).

story heated up, Beaulieu walked back her initial claims about finding actual bodies. Now the ground-scanning imagery showed that they were "*probable* burials." She then walked back her statements a little more, claiming to have "barely scratched the surface," and only finding "disturbances in the ground such as tree roots, metal and stones."[7] So, *no bodies.* On Dr. Beaulieu's faculty page for the University of Fraser Valley, we find that while she might spend her time hunting for "residential school burial sites," there is no indication that she has found any to date.[8]

There is a sad irony to it all. Kamloops sits on indigenous territory and was founded by an indigenous elder, Shuswap Chief Louis Clexlixqen (1830–1915). Furthermore, the school is a mere stone's throw from the Kamloops Reserve Cemetery. Are we to believe that indigenous schoolmasters buried indigenous children under an indigenous school when there is an indigenous cemetery not far away?

All this raises questions about the mushroom journey Douglas took a week after this bogus story hit the press. If the mushroom voice truly came from some spiritual realm outside Douglas's own mind, how did it not know that the news reports were mistaken? For those who believe that even psychedelic experiences are subject to reductionist materialism, this certainly seems to confirm that position. In this case, the message Douglas received was not from "out there," but instead from inside her own mind.

Though we might entertain a different possibility. Sure, the voices Douglas heard were generated by her, not some outside spiritual entity; but does that mean that *all* visions and voices encountered in psychedelic spaces are the product of the mind? Oaxacan *curandera* (or "medicine woman") María Sabina (1894–1985) would claim otherwise. For María Sabina, not all people were suitable vessels for the mushroom's secrets. Those who were worthy (like herself) entered "the world where everything is known" where they could sample the nectar of divine wisdom.[9] Such chosen people have access to knowledge that transcends culture,

7. Quoted in Rouillard, "In Kamloops, . . ." (2022).
8. See University of the Fraser Valley, "Faculty: Sarah Beaulieu."
9. Halifax, *Shamanic Voices: A Survey of Visionary Narratives* (NY: Penguin Press, 1991), p. 132.

space, and time. Others, like María Sabina's own sister, Anna María, could not enter this sacred realm. The true voice of the mushrooms did not speak to her. She was not worthy.[10] Maybe such spaces are real (i.e., generated outside the mind), and Douglas simply doesn't yet know how to access them. Perhaps it requires more training than merely citing indigenous status?

At the time of this writing, no bodies have been found at Kamloops, despite Douglas's insistence that they were "unearthed." Every spiritual psychenaut must ask herself if the mushrooms were wrong or if Francine Douglas was wrong. Or, as an atheist might contend, the mushrooms were wrong because Francine Douglas was wrong. Can Douglas really enter the world where everything is known, like María Sabina, due to nothing more than her indigeneity, or is she barred from admission like Anna María, likewise indigenous?

One of the more solipsistic aspects of the Decolonialize Narrative, as Douglas herself articulated at the conference, is the belief that since the US and Canadian governments undoubtedly wronged First Nations peoples, the latter knows more about psychedelics than most everybody else. The plea is, of course, a non-sequitur; but there is a deeper issue. If historical wrongs are our standard for psychedelic knowledge, then does not *every* person on earth have the right to make a similar appeal? Exactly whose ancestors have not been subjugated by another's sometime in history? And how is the pain always so specifically caused by Westerners? Some of the gifts exchanged at the Stol:lo Potlatch were slaves, whose progeny would surely know nothing of their original tribal customs. Does the pain Douglas feels from having her grandparent's customs erased by the Canadian government (which were reinstated before Douglas was born) recognize the pain the Stol:lo caused by erasing other peoples' cultures (which today have not been recovered) through enslavement? These aren't easy questions. Perhaps misreporting facts about serious issues and citing one's indigeneity as evidence is not the most accurate way to answer them.

10. Halifax (1991), p. 133.

While I question the current Decolonize Psychedelia Narrative, I hold a deep respect for First Nations peoples and their extraordinary techniques with plant medicines. Today's ceremonies are truly beautiful, inspirational, and medically valuable, and I consider myself thoroughly improved for having participated in them. The question is whether or not the therapeutic value of indigenous ceremonies goes as far back as does their use of the plants and mushrooms themselves.

In the last chapter we dispelled the first psychedelic postcolonial myth, which holds that Western Civilization had no psychedelic traditions until the 20th century. But there exists a second part to this baseless claim; namely, that since Western peoples had no psychedelic traditions, modern protocols employed by Western doctors were stolen from indigenous peoples, who, as Gabor Maté contends, practiced much wiser, more connected traditions than did Europeans.

Let's find out.

Indigenous Psychedelic Traditions

Psychedelic Theorists like Jamileh George have promoted a meme of cultural appropriation, reinforcing an oppressor-oppressed narrative within psychedelia, claiming that while "the White-dominant culture borrows from the cultural practices and ceremonial expression of often marginalized and disenfranchised indigenous groups, members of these groups end up alienated from the practices informed by their own cultural traditions."[11] But George never indicates how those indigenous cultural traditions were practiced historically or how this "white-dominant" medical framework utilizes them currently. She merely asserts the claim while withholding any convincing evidence to support it. Since Chacruna's Theorists and other psychedelic postcolonial thinkers have apparently not checked the historical record to see what indigenous psychedelic traditions looked like, it is up to us to do so here. Only then can we determine whether these indigenous psychedelic traditions represent, as psychedelic postcolonialist Belinda Eriacho calls them, "common belief systems shared by Native American cultures," and if

11. Jamilah R. George et al., "The Psychedelic Renaissance . . ." (2020), p. 5.

Western doctors smuggled such techniques into their own practices.[12]

Beginning in Peru, we find the Nazca, famous for their giant geoglyphs depicting a humanoid figure and animals like a monkey, a spider, and a bird, among others. Recently, scientists also discovered that the Nazca not only engaged in human sacrifice of both adults and children but also kept the heads as trophies of a sort. These "trophy heads" have allowed ethnobiologists to run tests on the kinds of foods the sacrificees consumed before the big show. They discovered a psychedelic pharmacopeia that appears to have been fed to the victims beforehand, among them San Pedro cactus, coca leaf, and a possible ayahuasca analog.[13]

Other Mesoamerican psychedelic traditions were quite ruthless and imperially pompous, filled with gratuitous grandeur for the entertainment of the privileged male elite—women and commoners were forbidden from partaking. One contemporary, ethnically mixed Dominican friar, Diego Durán (1537–1588), notes the coronation ceremony of the Aztec emperor Tizoc (d. 1486), who took office in 1481. Tizoc and the local "priests . . . mayors . . . and tax collectors" ate the mushrooms in preparation for a four day ceremony, which included dancing, distribution of lavish gifts to the local gentry, and terminating with the prisoners of Metztitlan marching to the Stone of the Sun (i.e., "altar of sacrifice'), who would be executed for Tizoc and his guests' pleasure.[14] The king's name means, after all, "The one who makes sacrifice" (*el que hace sacrificio*).[15]

The ninth emperor of the Aztec Empire, Moctezuma II (c. 1460–1520), is perhaps most famous for the revenge he takes against gringos who haphazardly drink unfiltered water in Central America. Though, I reckon most would prefer praying to the Porcelain God for a few days over how Moctezuma II treated residents of surrounding cities like Tlax-

12. Eriacho, "Considerations . . .," in Labate and Cavnar (2021), p. 58.
13. Jennifer Nalewicki, "Before Being Ritually Sacrificed, This Nazca Child was Drugged with Psychedelics," *Science Alert* (Nov 1, 2022).
14. See Jose F. Ramirez, *Historia de las Indias de Nueva-Espana, y Islas de Tierre Firme por El Padre Fray Diego Durán* (Mexico: Imprenta de J. M. Andrande y F. Escalante,1807).
15. Enrique Vela, Mexican Archaeology, "Tízoc, 'He Who Makes Sacrifice' (1481–1486)," reproduced in *Arqueología Mexicana* (2023).

cala, Huexotzinco, Cholula, Atlixco, Tecoac, and Tliliuhquitepec. Moctezuma II had no real enemies from these areas but found war to be a form of recreation for the ruling class. He was a tyrant who wielded tremendous power, unleashing a wave of terror on the surrounding peoples whenever he was bored. He also greatly desired the taste of human flesh, and the residents of those cities were always on the menu. Diego Durán had earlier witnessed Moctezuma II's coronation and is not sparing in detail when describing how the Aztec nobility incorporated psychedelic mushrooms into their sacred rites:

> The sacrifice finished, and the steps of the temple and court remaining bathed in human blood, they all went off to eat raw mushrooms, on which food they lost all their senses and ended up in a state worse than if they had drunk much wine; so drunk and senseless were they that many of them took their own lives, and by dint of those mushrooms, they saw visions and the future was revealed to them, the Devil speaking to them in that drunken state.[16]

The nature of these visions is anyone's guess. But the likelihood that the Aztec elites were all working through their traumas in a supportive, therapeutic environment—i.e., the approach created by Western doctors during the 1940s and 1950s—remains quite low.

Durán tells us that some of Moctezuma II's political rivals—princes from the Tlascalan—had attended his coronation.[17] At some point the Tlascalan nobles were made. Moctezuma II chose not to execute them, but rather to show them with great spectacle just how regal and extravagant he could be. He fed them psychedelic mushrooms and enjoyed a four-day party complete with dancing, feasting, and human sacrifices. We don't really know how many people were sacrificed by the bemushroomed priests as they looked upon human hearts pulled from the chests of their slaves and offered to the sun. The Aztec wall made of sacri-

---

16. Quoted in Valentina Pavlovna Wasson and R. Gordon Wasson, *Mushrooms, Russia, and History* (NY: Pantheon Books Inc., 1957), p. 218.
17. It is possible that the Tlascalan ate peyote (much as their neighbors did), but concrete evidence is lacking. See *Omar Stweart, Peyote Religion: A History* (OK: University of Oklahoma Press, 1994), p. 18.

ficed skulls (*tzompantli*) numbers in the tens of thosuands.[18] And perhaps Moctezuma II was not as charitable as he seemed. The mushrooms fed to the Tlascalan princes caused such disturbance and confusion that "many of them took their own lives."[19]

The great Aztec emperor also employed priests to consume mushrooms for other reasons like prognosis. The priests' visions were supposed to foretell the outcomes of battles, the Aztecs being quite fond of war. Priests who predicted defeat of Moctezuma II were promptly executed, despite their visions actually proving fatidic.[20] It would seem that mushrooms did not lead the Aztec nobility to peace and love. Instead, the ruling class enjoyed a certain brutality and cocksureness as a complement to the mushroom experience. One eyewitness to the regal spectacles, Franciscan friar Toribio de Benavente (1482–1569), noted how the mushrooms "sharpened [the Aztecs'] cruelty."[21]

Wholly absent from Aztec mushroom traditions is any sense of equality, empathy, humility, healing, or even basic human rights—those things one will find in a modern, Western clinical setting. And they don't seem to have been too concerned with the principles of JEDI. Nor was the Aztec gentry working through their trauma. When we speak of "colonization" in this instance—specifically the famous humanitarian disagreements between Moctezuma II and Hernán Cortés—we are talking about eradicating genocide, human sacrifice, and cannibalism.

Not all indigenous mushroom ceremonies involved such divine gore. Equally interesting within the annals of psychedelic history are the stories of some indigenous peoples who would eat mushrooms and have glorious visions of owning a lot of slaves. Others saw visions of taking captives in war (or falling captive themselves). Still others saw wealth in their future.[22] These experiences were no mere flights of fancy to the people having them, but rather prophetic visions of things to come. Even here, there isn't much of what we would call "medicine work" among these

18. Fynn-Paul (2023), pp. 144–5.
19. Quoted in Wasson and Wasson (1957), p. 218.
20. Letcher (2007), p. 75.
21. Quoted in Wasson and Wasson (1957), p. 219.
22. Wasson and Wasson (1957), p. 224.

early First Nations psychedelic traditions. It was all rather self-centered and violent.

And while postcolonial Theorists never seem to mention it, First Nations healers did expect payment for their services. Cherokee healers accepted compensation of "a coat, a quantity of cloth, or a sum of money."[23] Other healers could be as ruthless as Big Pharma. In what Álvar Núñez Cabeza de Vaca dubbed the Village of Misfortune (Coahuiltecan tribe), a cured individual gave all her possessions (and even some of her family's) to the healer. Paying the healer impoverished her. Although, that's not to say that a patient had no recourse. One medicine-worker who failed in his task to heal was murdered by the patient's family.[24]

THE CHRISTIAN SHAMAN SLAVE

Powerful healers also had to worry about being kidnapped by neighboring tribes due to their notoriety. Four unlikely candidates, de Vaca, and his three surviving companions—Estebanico (arguably the first black Muslim explorer in North America), Andrés Dorantes Carranza, and Alonso del Castillo Maldonado—became just such healer-slaves. Their owners, a tribe of the Coahuiltecan, believed that these foreign men had supernatural powers based on, well . . . *their skin color*. While the former three (de Vaca, Estebanico, and Carranza) were captives of the Coahuiltecan, they were urged by the locals to heal them using tribal techniques: e.g., blowing on sick people and/or waving away their illnesses with their hands. After scoffing at the idea (de Vaca was, after all, a *conquistador*, not a man of the cloth), he decided to give it a try (mostly because the Coahuiltecan promised to starve him should he refuse). De Vaca was in luck. Christians held a similar medical superstition involving hand gestures—one still seen today in megachurches. That is, making the sign of the cross over a sickly person as a remedy. A group of ailing Coahuiltecans were brought before de Vaca and his companions, who proceeded to make the sign of the cross over them, blow on them, say the Our Father and Hail Mary, and then prayed to the Christian God

23. James Mooney, *Cherokee Shamanism* (Simplicissimus Book Farm, 2015), p. 9.
24. Newcomb (1980), p. 52

"to heal them and inspire them to treat us well."[25] One by one, the natives claimed to be cured by the foreigners. The sign of the cross was the first symbol of Western occultism the Coahuiltecans had ever seen. It blew their minds.

Sometime later, after parting with the Anagados, de Vaca and company found themselves among the Avavares (another Coahuiltecan tribe), with whom their companion, Alonso del Castillo Maldonado, had been held. Word of the foreigners' remarkable healing abilities had spread to various tribes who now asked for such treatment. A few Avavares approached Maldonado and asked him to heal the pain in their heads. Maldonado had always been a little hesitant to play the healer, constantly wondering if his many sins would prevent him from performing a successful treatment.[26] Nonetheless, he made the sign of the cross over them and "commended them to God," which seems to have cured their headaches.[27]

But here we meet several curiosities that make postcolonialism tricky for the psychedelic Theorist: what are we to make of the fact that, without any threat of force from the foreigners whatsoever, these various tribes adopted Christianity for what they believed to be its remarkable healing powers? Additionally, de Vaca tells us that after every treatment, the Avavares would be overjoyed and celebrate with an *areítos*, a three-day ceremony in which peyote was sometimes ingested (depending on local custom). Let's suppose for a moment the Avavares used peyote in their *areítos*. At what point does Christianity become part of their indigenous psychedelic tradition? This Christianity was not riveted onto the locals with any aggressive imposition by de Vaca and company; indeed, at that time they were not grandiose conquerors of an exotic land, but instead abject slaves of the Coahuiltecans. Truly the locals found value in Christianity and, in the case of the Avavares, incorporated the sign of the cross into their *areítos*, quite possibly representing the first Christianized psychedelic ceremony in the Americas.

And it all happened without a whisper of violent force.

25. Favata and Fernández (1993), p. 62.
26. Otherwise known as Donatism, a Christian philosophy that holds living a moral life as essential to healing.
27. Favata and Fernández (1993), p. 77.

After escaping one of his terms as a slave-healer, de Vaca became a trader. One of the main items he traded were "seashells which they use to cut a certain fruit that looks like a bean, used by [the locals] for medicinal purposes and for dances and festivals."[28] De Vaca was most probably speaking of the mescal bean, a powerful psychedelic and purgative that grows in the pods of the mountain laurel tree.

We know from later sources that tribes like the Iowa would drink a mescal bean decoction that would keep them stimulated and dancing all night. By sunrise the effect of the mescal bean and the dancing would cause the revelers to vomit in prayerful crescendo. This cleansed them of evil spirits.[29] Perhaps that, or something like it, is the medicinal effect to which de Vaca refers? To be sure, those *areítos* might have only involved innocuous social activities that we can all get behind: dancing, drumming, chanting, and (at times) psychedelic substantia.[30]

Other indigenous traditions are a little less praiseworthy. Recall the Quevenes, who buried children alive based on ominous dreams. They also, among other tribes of the area, practiced a violently misogynist plant ritual. The men—Quevenes women were barred from participation—would brew a stimulating tea from the *ilex vomitoria*, a species of holly, and yell "who wants to drink?" At that moment, all the women of the tribe would have to freeze in place "even if they [we]re carrying a heavy load," while the men partook in the ceremony. Should a woman move out of place the men would spill out their cups and beat her senseless.[31]

If we accept the former tradition—spiritual cleansing through dance, ceremony, and ingestion of the mescal bean—into modern psychedelia based solely on its indigeneity then what argument can we make for eschewing the latter, where women were ritually beaten, based solely on indigeneity? There has to be something more than an indigenous-dominant medical framework on which to base modern psychedelia.

---

28. Favata and Fernández (1993), p. 65.
29. James H. Howard, "The Mescal Bean Cult of the Central and Southern Plains: An Ancestor of the Peyote Cult?" *American Anthropologist*, Vol. 59, No. 1 (February 1957), p. 78.
30. Fynn-Paul (2023), p. 63.
31. Favata and Fernández (1993), p. 89.

Still, I find some psychedelic postcolonialists are correct that overlooked perspectives from contemporary indigenous communities should have a seat at the scientific psychedelic table—though, not for worth of their indigeneity, but rather for the merits of the ideas themselves. I have personally seen the healing power of indigenous technologies in psychedelic spaces and believe they should be explored, not shunned, by the scientific arm of the psychedelic Renaissance. One truly remarkable practice by the Wichita of Kansas that probably involved the psychedelic mescal bean was witnessed by an anthropologist in 1904, who records:

> Thus, in the ceremony of the medicine men, after the novitiate has been placed in a trance, he usually holds speech with some fierce wild animal, who visits him and instructs him—should he prove brave and not become scared. Thus[,] he obtains power that he uses in doctoring, and in his songs, sung during the medicine-men's ceremony, he tells of his experience with the animal.[32]

This is fascinating. Truly there is something here to be explored from the perspective of natural philosophy—a kinship with wild nature, achieved through an indigenous form of psychedelia that transcends species.

Sign me up for *that* workshop!

But cultural respect must be a two-way street. Modern Westerners look for value beyond heritage—a most necessary correction to historical discrimination when far too many people in the Americas were shut out of important conversations due to their immutable characteristics.

Big Moon

Another myth of the psychedelic postcolonialist holds that First Nations psychedelic use was universal and unchanging.[33] Nowhere is that idea less true than with the spread of peyote across the continental United States. Peyote is a small cactus that grows in eastern Texas and northern Mexico and has a deep, centuries-old relationship with the few groups who knew of its existence for medication, ceremonial dances, and as a

32. Quoted in Rudolph C. Troike, "The Origins of Plains Mescalism," *American Anthropologist*, 64 (1962), p. 950.

33. Eriacho, "Considerations . . .," in Labate and Cavnar (2021), p. 50.

recreational inebriant. Its journey from a small, isolated region along the Texas-Mexican border to as far north as Canada tells a story not of a peaceful, universal, and sacred indigenous tradition, as psychedelic postcolonialists might imagine, but rather a shifting and unfolding variety of cultures drenched in intertribal warfare, misogyny, and various evolving practices and perspectives pertaining to peyote.

Peyote enters the historical record by name in the late 1570s when Spanish missionary Bernardino de Sahagún (c. 1499–1590) noted its use among the Chichimec[34] peoples in his *Historia General de las Cosas Nueva España.*[35] Undoubtedly, the Chichimec groups were one of few peoples that had been consuming the cactus well before it ever made its way to ink and parchment. De Sahagún records nothing of healing or what we might call therapeutic use. Instead, the Chichimec preferred to enjoy peyote as a recreational inebriant or to induce stamina and fearlessness in war. Though we might consider that group ceremony, in and of itself, is a form of medicine in certain respects. But so far as using peyote for ways we might call psychedelic-therapy, the Chichimec still come up short.

The Coahuiltecan groups, who we met earlier, also consumed their substantia of choice, peyote, in a manner that I imagine would be unpalatable to plucky psychedelic postcolonial Theorists today. Both captives and fellow tribesmen would be roasted and consumed, along with peyote, in psychedelic ceremony. However, eating the flesh of a fellow tribesman was considered taboo. Therefore, the men—Coahuiltecan women were barred from participation—would grind the bones of the deceased into powder and flavor the cactus with it.[36]

More insightful accounts come from a Norwegian ethnographer, Carl Lumholtz (1851–1922), who in 1890 explored areas of what he called “unknown Mexico.” During the expedition to regions that were

34. Like the Pueblos and the Coahuiltecans, “Chichimec” is a catchall term for a variety of peoples that share limited to noticeable linguistic and cultural traits, while still remaining distinctive.
35. Richard Evans Shultes and Albert Hofmann, *Plant of the Gods: Their Sacred, Healing, and Hallucinogenic Powers* (VT: Healing Arts Press, 1992), p. 48
36. Newcomb (1980), p. 132.

"foreign even to most Mexicans," Lumholtz's team discovered various unidentified (at least in a zoological sense) plants, animals, and even cave dwellers.[37] One such people they encountered was the Tarahumara, a tribe not wholly untouched by Western influence as evidenced by their knowledge of Christianity. But what really struck Lumholtz was the Tarahumara deification of a certain cactus.

Only shamans—for lack of a better word—who took on the dual role of physician and priest to the tribe, could handle the cactus, called *Hikuli*, which after it was eaten, "cause[d] a state of ecstasy."[38] Most Tarahumara had several shamans living in their village. The *Hikuli* was used less as a cure for illness and more as preventative medicine.[39] The Tarahumara believed that sickness itself derived from the spirit world and therefore used the cactus to drive sorcery from their villages. Some shamans also used the plant for more practical matters such as healing physical ailments like snakebites, rheumatism, and other wounds. Lumholtz records that the primary "effect of the plant is so much enjoyed by the Tarahumares that they attribute to it power to give health and long life and to purify body and soul."[40]

Hikuli also had magical properties. Carrying *Hikuli* would stave off bear attacks, and deer wouldn't run away during hunting season. The Apache supposedly would not fire their guns at a *Hikuli*-carrying Tarahumara. Spellcasting enemies of the Tarahumara wouldn't stand a chance of harming anyone in the village via sorcery after a peyote ceremony. It was also said to aid sportsmen in a variety of games—no doubt due to its stimulating properties. Christian Tarahumara crossed themselves when in close proximity to the cactus and explained the nausea that accompanies eating it as the devil fleeing from their stomachs.

The Huichol, who lived several hundreds of miles away, also incorporated peyote into their culture. Lumholtz was astonished to discover that despite the vast terrain between the two groups, which "are neither related to nor connected with each other. . . . show many points of resem-

37. Carl Lumholtz, *Unknown Mexico: A Record of Five Years' Exploration Among the Tribes of the Western Sierra Madre* (NY: Charles Scribner's Sons, 1902), p. xvi.
38. Lumholtz (1902), p. 357.
39. Lumholtz (1902), p. 311.
40. Lumholtz (1902), p. 359.

blance" including the deified name of the cactus itself.[41] The Huichol employed *Hikuli* as a somatic medicine, "for anything from a minor ache to a major wound."[42] Uncommon for the majority of peyote-using peoples of Mexico, women were allowed to participate in the Huichol rites, though we only have modern accounts of their inclusion.[43]

It wasn't until the 1890s that peyote spread throughout the continental United States *en masse*, riding off the dissipating trails of the Ghost Dance, a spiritual ceremony that was supposed to rid the land of white Americans. Its prophetic and visionary capabilities synergized with the ongoing skirmishes that erupted across the plains in those days. For the Comanche, peyote allowed warriors to hear an advancing enemy.[44] Comanche women's traditional position in peyote rituals was "a subordinate one," although they later had more active roles.[45] For the Tonkawa, peyote was to be used "only in wartime."[46] One indigenous elder remarked that tribes of the plains "played war like [white Americans] play baseball."[47]

Off the battlefield, we find very little evidence of a "universal" tradition for peyote use (despite some similarities here and there). Due to cultural needs and specific environments and challenges, peyotism "necessarily existed in a variable form . . . which led to the creation of new rituals and sometimes even somewhat antagonistic doctrines."[48] The cactus passed through many hands of many people, creating an ethnographic nightmare for anyone trying to trace the spread of peyote from sea to shining sea. Two men, Quanah Parker and John Wilson (Wokova or "Moonhead")—both half Comanche, half white American—played a major role in disseminating peyote across the US.

41. Lumholtz (1902), p. 357.
42. Weston Le Barre, *The Peyote Cult* (OK: University of Oklahoma Press, 1989), p. 28.
43. Le Barre (1989), p. 32.
44. Le Barre (1989), p. 27.
45. Perhaps influenced by the first wave of feminism which hit the United States in the late 1840s. Alice Marriott and Carol K. Rachlin, *Peyote: An Account of the Origins and Growth of the Peyote Religion* (NY: Thomas Y. Crowell Company, 1971), p. 30.
46. Quoted in La Barre (1989), p. 119.
47. Quoted in Marriot and Rachlin (1971), p. 11.
48. Petrullo (1934), p. 31.

Wokova (a Delaware by birth) lived among the Caddo of Oklahoma, but at some point traveled to Arizona and New Mexico where he learned of peyote. Returning to the Caddo, Wokova announced that peyote had given him a new vision, one applicable to the Delaware. His rite was called the "Big Moon" ceremony, named after the large crescent moon altar around which the participants sat. He took the name "Moonhead," declaring that only he and his closest followers could perform the ceremony, creating a peyote service monopoly on the plains. He also expected (as all healers did) to be paid for his efforts, which included accepting women as a fee. Some Christians even participated in Big Moon ceremonies. In fact, Wokova believed himself to be "the forerunner of Christ," while his disciples believed him to be the Nazarene himself.[49]

Wokova was what we today would term a "ladies' man," whose appetites included borrowing married women, who he would "discard ... when their appeal for him was gone." Wilson's womanizing ways did not endear him to everyone. Often the subject of much debate, Wokova was defended by those like white American ethnographer James Mooney (1861–1921), who described him as "smart" with "a keen sense of humor,"[50] while a Kiowa man, Ahpeatone (or "Wooden Lance"), proclaimed, "There is no truth in [Wokova]. If we must change our beliefs, let us believe the missionaries. At least they are kind and generous."[51]

The nature of peyote visions also changed depending on tribal doctrine. For the Comanche and other war-mongering groups across the plains, the peyote visions were necessary for prophesying the enemy's advances. Among the Delaware, all visions—warlike or otherwise—were shunned. "Peyote should not be eaten for visions," said Delaware tribesman Joe Washington. "Many Indians eat it to get visions and hear things. ... But that is a wrong way to use it. ... A man who gets visions doesn't learn anything from peyote. ... By giving you these visions Peyote tells you that you have no business in the meeting."[52]

49. Petrullo (1934), p. 46.
50. Quoted in Mrs. Andy Welliver, "Wokova," *Nevada Historical Society Quarterly*, Vol. XI, No, 2 (Summer, 1968), p. 14.
51. Quoted in Mariott and Rachlin (1971), p. 22.
52. Quoted in Petrullo (1934), p. 66.

A Sacred Medicine

By the 1880s we see evidence of peyote's use to treat mental health issues, but only in highly localized ways. One Delaware chief, Elk Hair (d. c. 20th century), was suicidal and the "herb doctors" could not cure him.[53] An Anadarko friend of his, Johnson Bob, who learned of peyote by way of the Comanche, tried to convince Elk Hair to give it a try. Elk Hair at first refused, wanting nothing to do with the cactus (despite his indigeneity). But after reflecting on the poor state in which he'd leave his family, he sampled peyote as a last effort. It worked. So astounded by peyote's remarkable healing abilities, Elk Hair gave some to his ailing sister, who was also cured as if miraculously.

By the time peyotism spread across North America, many First Nations peoples had already adopted Christianity by force or by desire, causing obvious disagreements among them. Some embraced Christianity as a part of peyotism, while others scorned the wedding. Wokova believed in a Christianized peyote rite, which caused him to lock horns with those like Elk Hair who did not. Joe Washington, Elk Hair's, nephew, objected that Wokova "was mixing . . . Christianity and Peyote. That was bad. The Christian way of worshiping is good and Peyote is good, but the two should not be mixed."[54] Others found that peyotism was "among the innumerable variants of Christianity."[55] One Kickapoo peyotist attested, "We use the peyote in our religious ceremonies and it means the same to us as the reading of the Bible in the religious meetings of the white people—we use it in the worship of Our Father."[56]

And what of the psychedelic postcolonialist's insistence that Europeans and white Americans learn from the centuries of peyote use among the First Nations? Historically, it gets tricky because in some cases, Euro-

53. Petrullo (1934), p. 41.
54. Quoted in Petrullo (1934), p. 43.
55. James S. Slotkin, *The Peyote Religion: A Story in Indian-White Relations* (Il: University of Chicago, 1956), p. 65.
56. Quoted in Slotkin (1956), p. 139.

peans and white Americans were familiar with peyote *before* many First Nations peoples. As one example, the Diné only discovered peyote in 1901,[57] which comes *after* physicians like John Raleigh Briggs (1851–1907), Weir Mitchell (1829–1914), and Havelock Ellis (1859–1939), and natural philosophers like William James (1842–1910), had already sampled it.

In 1887, Briggs published the first known personal account of a peyote experience in two journals, *The Medical Register* and *The Druggists' Bulletin*.[58] The latter was read by the general manager of pharmaceutical company Parke-Davis and Co., George S. Davis (1847–1914). By 1889, Parke-Davis was producing peyote tinctures. By the early 20th century, peyote-chocolates were available.[59] Arthur Hefter would synthesize mescaline from peyote in 1897. And it all came before the Diné, the Kickapoo, the Potawatomi, the Cherokee, and many other tribes had ever heard of peyote. And of those tribes of the continental US who discovered peyote before white Americans like the Comanche, the Ute, and others? Their use only goes back to the 1870s and 1880s. In fact, the earliest image and description of the cactus appears in an 1846 edition of *Curtis's Botanical Magazine*, courtesy of W. J. Hooker—three decades before even the Comanche employed it.[60] Where are the deep, centuries-old, psychedelic psychotherapy peyote traditions we are told existed among these various peoples?

And what of the claim with which we opened this chapter—that Westerns doctors stole indigenous psychedelic practices and now bankroll on them without acknowledging their indigenous origin? Exactly which aspects of these indigenous psychedelic practices are we talking about? Collecting trophy heads like the Nazca? The human sacrifices and ornate parties of the Aztec elites? The human bone-infused peyote rites of the Coahuiltecans? The near total exclusion of women from

57. Marriott and Rachlin (1971), p 39.
58. We know Briggs was not the first American to sample peyote. Reports of soldiers trying the "dry mule" exist; however, I know of no known accounts from the partakers.
59. Everitt (2014–2016), p. 50.
60. Sir William Jackson Hooker, "Echinocactus Williamsii," in *Curtis's Botanical Magazine* (London: Reeve, Benham and Reeve, King William Street, Strand, 1847), Vol. III, Third Series, Tab 4296.

psychedelic spaces? The complete absence of JEDI from First Nations psychedelia?

Psychedelic postcolonial Theorists never tell us.

In the CSJ anthology *Psychedelic Justice*, Belinda Eriacho tries to bridge the gap between First Nations and global medical practices. While I support her initiative, Eriacho overlooks many historical truths we have already covered in this section, creating a false narrative that sees Western doctors as simply hopeless when it comes to understanding psychedelia without instruction from indigenous peoples. And while I agree with Eriacho that much can be learned from allowing a variety of perspectives, she seems unaware of the historical realities that have shaped her stance. As we saw earlier, Western doctors were quite familiar with psychedelics without any First Nations input whatsoever.

Eriacho's points may be well-meaning, but they also invite glaring contradictions. She tells us that "there are 573 federally-recognized tribes in the United States, and each is distinct with their own culture and language."[61] But she also speaks of the "Native American's World View" and the need for Westerners to have "a basic understanding of the philosophical and social contexts of Native American society."[62] I'm confused. I thought each of these groups had its own culture and language. Do all 573 tribes share a similar world view or not? Furthermore, if tribal *individuality* is what the psychedelic postcolonial Theorists seek, then each indigenous groups' understanding of best psychedelic practices must be dealt with on a case-by-case analysis—not based on any claim to the land or heritage.

No one can deny that First Nations peoples saw many horrors as the American expansion pushed westward. The slavery, the landgrabs, the murder, the broken treaties, the empty promises—all serve to blight the United States' historical integrity. But Eriacho seems unaware that these unjust brutalities littered the Americas before any Europeans ever

61. Eriacho, "Considerations . . .," in Labate and Cavnar (2021), p. 50.
62. Eriacho, "Considerations . . .," in Labate and Cavnar (2021), p. 55.

stepped on the Atlantic shoreline. The colonization and slaughter of Eriacho's people, the Diné, by the Pueblo Peoples is rather infamous. The Pueblo—the only indigenous peoples to successfully oust the Spanish—also readily appropriated from them, acting "as intermediaries in the transmission of various European technologies," to the Diné. Weaving, painted pottery, animal domestication, and equestrian goods like saddles and bridles entered Diné culture by way of their conquerors, the Pueblo, who took these crafts and ideas from their earlier enemies, those dashing Spaniards.[63] And perhaps most scandalous: the Diné, who migrated south from Canada, had earlier stolen the land from the Pueblo! The Diné also had dustups with the Comanche, Pawnee, Ute, and Apache over territory, horses, slaves, and women. And yet, Eriacho tells us, "Native Americans as the original people of this country believe that all beings in the universe are sacred: from the tiniest insects ... to fellow human beings."[64] I'm sure the slaves sacrificed for Moctezuma II's grotesque pleasure would fully agree. Perhaps Eriacho believes in the sacredness of all living beings. But historically, that was not a Diné cultural trait.

And Eriacho knows it. Until just a few years ago, "[a] lot [of Diné] women have gone missing or [were] murdered," she admits. Abduction of women in the Southwest ran rampant amongst First Nations tribes into the 20th century—even Eriacho's own great-great grandmother was kidnapped by Mescalero Apaches.[65] Recently, the Diné was given hope by President Donald Trump, whose *Executive Order 13898*, signed 26 November 2019, focused on "addressing the crisis of missing and murdered Native Americans and Alaska Natives."[66] All that at a time when we were badgered to abolish the police.

63. Kluckhohn and Leighton (1974), p. 37.
64. Eriacho, "Considerations ...," in Labate and Cavnar (2021), p. 55.
65. María Mocerino, "This is Not Native American History, This is US History with Belinda Eriacho" (October 2, 2020).
66. Press Release, "Presidential Task Force on Missing and Murdered American Indians and Alaska Natives Release Status Report," *Office of Public Affairs, US Department of Justice* (December 10, 2020).

Indigenous Reciprocity

Because psychedelic postcolonialists believe that white Americans and Europeans stole psychedelia from First Nations peoples, they berate the former to "center" the latter. "You need to let the indigenous lead," said a young woman (who has been involved in psychedelia for all of five minutes) as she protested Rick Doblin (who has been involved in psychedelia for over thirty years) at the Multidisciplinary Association for Psychedelic Studies (MAPS) Psychedelic Sciences 2023 conference.[67]

At Chacruna Institute, indigenous reciprocity is a hot topic. Notwithstanding several affiliates publishing articles about it, cofounder Dr. Bia Labate insists that "even if you only like psilocybin or synthetic mescaline or LSD or MDMA, and you think 'what I'm doing here has nothing to do with indigenous people and therefore I owe nothing,' you're wrong. All of us owe something. . . . Because we just studied [indigenous] practices and got the idea that these substances heal—such as famous researchers in Canada that participated in Native American teepees, and by observing how Native Americans used peyote to treat alcoholism, started to propose a similar study with LSD."[68]

The Canadian researchers to whom Dr. Labate refers were Drs. Humphry Osmond and Abram Hoffer (1917–2009), who sat in a peyote ceremony hosted by the Red Pheasant Band in October 1956. However, their witness to the ritual had nothing to do with learning how to use peyote to treat alcoholism or any other malady. Osmond and Hoffer's participation proved a more noble reason. The Minister at the House of Commons in Ottawa, after applying zero effort to investigate the issue, had determined that peyote was just as much a danger and social vice as alcohol. Osmond and Hoffer called bullshit and wanted to show the Canadian government that peyote was not dangerous at all and, in fact, much safer than alcohol by consuming it.[69] They had no plans of learning indigenous therapeutic practices with peyote that night.

Dr. Labate has taken the meeting out of historical context in order to make a case for indigenous reciprocity. That isn't scholarship, it's ide-

67. BobCool7, "Protesters Interrupt Rick Doblin at MAPS Psychedelic Science 2023 Closing Ceremony" (June 23, 2023).
68. Rebel Wisdom, "Psychedelic Capitalism and the Sacred" (2021).
69. Only Osmond ingested the peyote.

ology. As we saw in the previous chapter, the therapeutic potential of LSD was first recognized in Switzerland in the early 1940s by psychiatrists who knew nothing of First Nations peoples' uses of peyote.

Additionally, the idea of employing LSD to treat alcoholism on a widescale did not come from First Nations peoples, but rather from Alcoholics Anonymous founder Bill Wilson (1895–1971) during a vision he had when he was in the throes of another mind-manifesting plant with a rich European history, belladonna, which was sometimes found as an ingredient to the flying ointments we explored in the previous chapter.[70] The idea wasn't new. The Winnebago had been using peyote to treat alcoholism since the early 1900s, giving some weight to Dr. Labate's stance. Though, like Delaware use of peyote to combat suicidal depression, treating alcoholism was localized to the Winnebago. However, Wilson did not know this when the belladonna vision came to him. Is it so impossible to believe that two different people (a Winnebago healer and Bill Wilson) could have had the same idea?

Turns out, that's exactly what happened.

Correct as Dr. Labate may be that the Winnebago use of peyote to treat alcoholism predated Bill Wilson's revelation, she misses a deeper truth as she opts for identity politics: that two culturally separable peoples determined that psychedelics could treat alcoholism without conferring with each other is strong evidence that psychedelics are quite useful in treating alcoholism. That's more interesting than identity politics. And anyway, treating alcoholism with peyote wasn't an *indigenous* thing, it was a *Winnebago* thing; just as treating alcoholism with LSD wasn't a *white American* thing, it was a *Bill Wilson* thing.

Science and Spirits

One of the haughtier assertions made by some psychedelic postcolonialists is that ideas can be scientifically valid even if they aren't validated scientifically. We are told that such ideas are merely a "different way of knowing." But to call something that is factually incorrect "a different

70. Howard Markel, "An Alcoholic's Savior: God, Belladonna or Both?" *New York Times*, April 9, 2010. For belladonna (nightshade) as an additive in flying ointments, see Hatsis (2015), p. 189.

way of knowing" is quite unscientific. We have to be able to speak the same language.

Consider ayahuasca, the visionary brew of the Amazon, which contains only two ingredients: the banisteriopsis caapi (b. caapi for short) vine and the chacruna leaf. Indigenous Peruvian traditions would have us believe that the b. caapi vine (translated roughly as "vine of the soul") curries the psychedelic goodies into the mind; however, it's actually the chacruna leaf—not the vine—that possesses the active DMT. The b. caapi vine, while necessary for the brew, is a monoamine oxidase inhibitor (MAOI), which stops the breakdown of DMT by MAO enzymes in the stomach, permitting the body to admit the medicine. As regards phytochemistry, the indigenous elders, in this case, are wrong. Perhaps there is some kind of as-yet-undiscovered approach to phytochemistry that will one day demonstrate that the b. caapi vine contains the active DMT—I'm open to it. But until that day, we can scientifically say that it does not.

And there is more. The claim that ayahuasca is some ancient medicine that has been used by Peruvians since before written history is similarly erroneous. While the locals might enjoy spinning yarn of that type for tourists, anthropological and linguistic evidence shows that cooking and drinking ayahuasca is probably closer to three centuries old. Nonetheless, that is still an impressive passage of time to carry a torch. Anthropologist Bernd Brabec de Mori tells us, "It's a romantic image that Indigenous people have been using everything they do for thousands of years. . . . If we change the picture, it's kind of unromantic, and it seems that people like romanticism."[71]

Still, while ayahuasca is certainly old, it isn't ancient.

Errors like this matter little to someone like me, who simply wants to enjoy the inarguable benefits of drinking ayahuasca. I am very open about my religious beliefs and the role entheogens play in them, so at the end of the day, I side with non-scientific modalities on a very deep, personal level. All my most meaningful healing has come from sitting with the medicine in fantastically *non*-clinical settings. However, when we are talking *science* (and in this case we are), these differences matter.

71. Manvir Singh, "Psychedelics Weren't as Common in Ancient Cultures as we Think," *Vice* (December 10, 2020).

I use substantia almost exclusively for religious purposes, and yet there is nothing about sitting with Gaia in the womb of the infinite, which I have done many times under high doses of mushrooms (and fewer times with ayahuasca), that has prepared me for a career in the STEM fields. My ideas on neurochemistry are not of equal validity to those of a neuroscientist—no matter my cultural heritage.[72]

I feel similar about Western mistakes in medical science. In the 13th century, German theologian Albertus Magnus (c. 1200–1280) discussed the medical properties of the *Amanita muscaria*, the famous red-topped, white-spotted mushroom, popular in fairy tales and buildings in Smurfland. The mushroom is also highly psychoactive and has been used as an entheogen in various places and times in history. However, Albertus positioned the mushroom within the context of the four humors theory, an ancient and outdated way of understanding medical science.[73] According to that theory, the body was composed of four humors: yellow bile, black bile, blood, and phlegm. When these humors were balanced (i.e., there was the right amount in the body), a person was healthy. When the humors were unbalanced (e.g., an excess of blood and/or a depletion of yellow bile in the body, etc.) a person was sick. The remedy for unbalanced humors was bloodletting—physicians and barbers would draw blood from a person to realign the humoral levels. Many people died from this kind of operation, including George Washington (1732–1799).

Since the four humors theory is today a totally discredited way of understanding medical science, almost everything Albertus claims about the *Amanita muscaria* is incorrect. For that reason, I find it best to avoid citing my European heritage in a Hail Mary attempt to give Albertus's mistaken ideas about mushrooms and medical science any weight in a modern scientific psychedelic discussion.

72. By that logic, I have more knowledge of, say, opium due to my Greek ancestors' use of it for medicine, recreation, and religion than does a First Nations physician who specializes in addiction treatment. I simply don't believe that.

73. Albertus Magnus, *De Vegetabilibus Libri VII. Historiae Naturalis Pars XVIII* (Berolini: Typis Et Impensis Georgii Reimeri, 1867), p. 136.

All our ancestors knew very little about the measurable natural world. They knew some things, for sure, but we know a lot more today. To snub one's nose at the years of trials and torments, failed experiments, imprisonments, and executions of scientists as they slowly and painstakingly brought Europe out of rampant and crippling superstition and into an Enlightenment, I believe, can only be done in poor taste. All of our ancestors prayed for the kinds of medicines, technologies, and conveniences brought to the world by Western Civilization that we all take for granted on a daily basis. To dismiss that is profoundly ungrateful. To say that indigenous peoples have *nothing* to learn from science is profoundly anti-scientific and reeks of the very arrogance we are told only exists in Western models.[74] In fairness, there are many First Nations psychedelic thought leaders who welcome the wedding of their traditions with those of the West, agreeing that there is much to be shared from both hemispheres.[75]

That's the trip I'm on too.

It gets exciting when we consider that maybe psychedelic experiences represent something beyond any current scientific understanding. Francine Douglas's faux pas aside, I have seen enough evidence to question for myself whether or not entheogenic experiences are all in our head. Science can only measure the natural world. If the psychedelic experience truly is something super . . . or rather—*adjacent* natural—then scientific method as we presently understand it has no jurisdiction. Perhaps psychedelic spaces are a part of the natural world that we do not as of yet have much understanding. Or perhaps psychedelics are so wondrously revolutionary that there is room for both a scientific and spiritual understanding of them waiting to be discovered. If a specific indigenous practice can be shown to work repeatedly it immediately becomes science. It becomes part of the natural world that we used to misunderstand. For *that* reason, not any claims to heritage or grievance, indigenous technologies deserve a seat at the scientific table.

---

74. Murray (2022), p. 57.

75. Lara Jakowski and Patrick Belem, "Eskawata Kayawai: The Spirit of Transformation" (2023).

But until we spiritual and religious people—whether First Nation, European, or otherwise—can create tests for measuring our claims, perhaps it's best if we have our own conversation elsewhere. Science has nothing to do with your, my, or anyone else's religious beliefs. Perhaps one day they will all interlace like a beautiful, tie-dyed embroidery, but all available contemporary data suggests that spiritual belief and scientific inquiry are, as Stephen Jay Gould noted, "nonoverlapping magisteria."[76] At the time of this writing, the possibility of wedding science and spirituality is exciting, but distant—even if psychedelics seem to point some people (this author included) in that direction. The facts just aren't there yet. So I welcome First Nations peoples to see if they can conduct falsifiable tests that demonstrate whether their immaterial philosophies fit in with material science. But if they don't, it's probably not because science is racist. Indeed, there is no scientific validity to my entheogenic mythopoetics either. It is more probable that we are dealing with nonoverlapping magisteria that neither indigenous psychedelic beliefs nor my own beliefs can, at this time, reconcile.

The extreme end of psychedelic decolonization ideology tells people what medicines they are and are not allowed to use based on heritage.[77] If ancestry matters for using various psychedelic substances, how much does it matter? We saw that the early 17th century French physician Jean De Nynauld was well familiar with magicians who used *Amanita muscaria* and *psilocybe* mushrooms. Is four centuries a long enough time span? Can French and French-Canadian people now use psychedelic mushrooms without hassle from psychedelic postcolonialists? After all, their cultural use dates to around the time ayahuasca was first discovered, and is at least three centuries *older* than many contemporary First Nations peoples' peyote practices. Furthermore, does their French lineage include this new category of "white," opening the door for anyone living in the Americas with European roots to partake? If so, at what point do all these people transform from Irish, French, German, Italian, Spanish,

76. See Stephen Jay Gould, "Nonoverlapping Magisteria," *Natural History*, Vol. 106, No. 2 (January 1997).
77. Arfu Staff, "Psychedelic Privilege . . .," (undated . . . because dates are "oppressive"?).

Polish (etc.) into "white?" And what if our French-Canadian friend isn't interested in ritual magic, but instead focused on healing trauma? Or exploring her subconscious mind to produce more profound art? Is she allowed to eat mushrooms to those ends without first receiving instruction from a First Nations elder? Must she only use them for visionary magic, as her French predecessors did, or can she apply them to other endeavors like healing trauma?

And what if I, of Greco-Roman heritage, do not prefer the substantia of my ancestors, who found divine revelation in opium? There isn't any hope for finding ayahuasca, which I like *way more* than opioids, anywhere in my bloodline, as the b. caapi vine and chacruna leaf are not native to Europe. Moreover, what do I do about my use of the *Amanita muscaria* mushroom? While that mushroom appears nowhere in my Greek ancestry, it does appear in my Italian ancestry.[78] Which part of me is allowed to consume the mushroom from a psychedelic postcolonial perspective—the Greek part or the Italian part? How do I split the difference? Since I already eat *Amanita muscaria* mushrooms in ceremony today, does that mean in a few centuries or so my Greek descendants will be able to do so without hassle? Will my Greco-Roman "ancestorness" validate their future use?

Denying a person the kinds of medicine that might heal her deepest psychic wounds based on her heritage cuts against the principles of the psychedelic Renaissance. If *Amanita muscaria* mushrooms are a healthy medical alternative to, say, sedatives like benzodiazepines (or "benzos") for some people, why not allow them to use the former over the latter? I have a friend and colleague who used that mushroom for exactly that purpose.[79] It saved her life. And the Italian part of my heritage couldn't care less if *Amanita muscaria* mushrooms appear in her cultural lineage. Psychedelic medicines are far too powerful to be approached with such shallow prejudice, such cynicism.

To reiterate, none of this is meant to disparage First Nations peoples in any way. I have sat with peyote and ayahuasca and absolutely feel deep reverence and respect for the indigenous facilitators, the medicines, and

---

78. Batista Grassi, "Il Nostro Agarico Moscario Sperimentato come Aliment Nervoso," *Gazzetta degli Ospitali Milano*, Vol. 1 (188), pp. 961–972.

79. Amanita Dreamer, *Dosing Amanita Muscaria and What to Expect* (GA: Amanita Dreamer Publishing, 2023), p. 19.

the ceremonies. I have watched *ayahuasqueras* pull harmful spirits (for lack of a better description) from the souls of the distressed. I stand in awe of their remarkable healing abilities. Western medicine has as much to learn from these traditions of the western hemisphere as First Nations peoples have to learn from the eastern hemisphere. Imagine for a moment that psychedelics may very well serve as a bridge between science and spirituality. I remain cautiously optimistic.

I merely refuse to accept that spiritual wisdom remains the sole domain of First Nations peoples. There is psychedelic insight to be found all over the world by countless peoples of any ethnicity—from places and medicines as distant and different as Africa and iboga, Siberia and *Amanita muscaria*, Catalonia and ergot, India and Soma, and many more that your friendly, neighborhood psychedelic nerd can name. It is one of the things that many civilizations have in common—we can all marvel at the wondrous effects of these extraordinary medicines. Psychedelics aren't a Western thing or an indigenous thing. They are a *human* thing.

Like the Hekate puppy sacrifices and the near-enslavement of Delphic oracles courtesy of my Greek forbearers, we must come to terms with the fact that not everything our ancestors did while working with substantia should be emulated by us today. Why bring past cultural divisiveness into current psychedelia? What purpose, besides browbeating those who look different, does it serve? Is that truly what these awe-inspiring visions are telling us? Perhaps instead of using the bloodshed of history to demonize each other in the present we use it to grow towards mutual understanding and a deeper strengthening of the human bond. We could transmute the universal traumas of the past, perpetrated by all of our ancestors, into gold.

7

Memeing María Sabina: How Social Media Whitewashes Culture

I am wise even from within the womb of my mother.
I am the woman of the winds, of the water, of the paths,
because I am known in heaven, because I am a doctor woman.[1]

—María Sabina Magdalena García

Cultural Erasure

I have always had a penchant for the odd byways of culture, the outrageous, the weird—all that polite company finds offensive. The thought of losing a single precious inch of some exotic cultural paradigm—even one reduced to a barroom factoid—can bring a somber ripple to the edge of my eye. I find myself shouting expletives into the stagnant air of gridlocked highways over the loss of the library of Alexandria. I clutch the

This chapter first appeared in an abridged form as an article on psanctum.org, written by Eden Woodruff and the author.

1. Quoted in Henry Munn (*trans.*), Álvaro Estrada, *María Sabina: Her Life and Chants* (CA: Ross-Erikson, 1981), p. 56.

steering wheel in despair accepting that I will never know what a Neanderthal twenty-something-year-old ever dreamed about. And seriously . . . what were the Minoans doing with their Poppy Goddess statuettes and opium-smoking vases? Did it have anything to do with what happened later at Eleusis?

I think of the cultural traditions and languages that have disappeared every bit as much as brachiosauruses and dodo birds, shout more expletives into the traffic-jammed air, then suddenly stop, return to reality, and wonder what kind of nutjob I must look like to my fellow motorists.

Cultural erasure takes many forms. There is no doubt that first Europeans and then white Americans outlawed a rich medley of both benign and brutal indigenous practices in the Americas. But not all these traditions fell to sword and Bible. As we saw earlier, a fair amount of religious syncretism could take place in the Americas without any force by *conquistadors* at all (*à la* de Vaca, the Christian shaman slave). Should the Christianity that the locals freely adopted be decolonized from any surviving rites? If so, how is that honoring the ancestors who chose a Christian way of life voluntarily?

Still, we can recognize that for many First Nations peoples, the banning of their languages, religions, and other cultural affinities was a harsh and demoralizing blow that no doubt created a kind of cultural trauma passed down generationally, which perhaps contributes to many of the social problems found on reservations today.

But cultural erasure wasn't the strict province of Europeans coming to the Americas. Some indigenous practices ended for other reasons. Some peoples of the Americas simply didn't prefer their cultural inheritances and opted for modernity instead. An overlooked, but nonetheless important reason indigenous traditions did not survive in some cases was that First Nations youths were losing interest in the old ways, opting for the comfort and convenience of Western Civilization instead. The tribal elders recognized this apathy among the younger generations but could do very little about it. Clyde Kluckhohn and Dorothea Leighton write of the "[Diné] girl who has been to boarding school for many years usually has no desire to live in a hogan [i.e., a Diné home built of dirt and logs] when she marries. But to have a house with a wooden floor, running water, and other conveniences to which she has become accustomed."[2]

Conquistadors aside, cultural erasure was almost a sport among First Nations peoples, all the way up to the 20th century. We might note the colonization of the Hopi by the Diné. As late as the 1940s:

> The Navajo Tribal Council . . . posted a sign warning off all trespassers, including Hopis, from the Great Inscription Rock on which for centuries all Hopi initiates . . . have inscribed their clan signatures. Similar signs have been erected on sites of Hopi ruins. Today Navajos are trespassing at every Hopi spring, at every Hopi shrine, in every Hopi field, and are swarming into every Hopi village to steal every article left unguarded in Hopi homes.[3]

That certainly sounds like cultural erasure and colonization to me! How will psychedelic postcolonialists explain those worse angels of the Diné nature? Further, how will they explain that the only thing that stopped the slaughter of the Hopi by the Diné was an intervention by the US government? Finally, if the United States returns the land to the Diné, will the Diné then give the portions of the land they stole from the Hopi back to them?

Furthermore, what are we to make of the fact that not every indigenous person approved of using psychedelic medicines like peyote? In some instances, intertribal feuding erupted over the demarcation line between those who saw value in the cactus and those who did not. Writes anthropologists Alice Marriott and Carol Rachlin, "the fellow tribesmen of the peyotists, learning of a [peyote] meeting, would tear down or burn the ceremonial tipi, stamp out the sacred fire, and spill the sacred water on the ground."[4] Are we to honor the anti-psychedelic indigenous voice or the pro-psychedelic indigenous voice? Either way, we erase someone's cultural identity.

Sometimes cultural erasure occurs in far more subtle forms than youth-

2. Kluckhohn and Leighton (1974), p. 168.
3. Frank Waters, *Book of the Hopi: The First Revelation of the Hopi's Historical and Religious World-View of Life* (NY: Ballantine Books, 1971), p. 402.
4. Marriot and Rachlin (1971), p. 47.

ful indifference to the old ways, indigenous anti-peyote agitators, or by way of sword and Bible. Sometimes we don't even mean to do it. Sometimes our own need to show how progressive we can be does the erasure for us. In the late summer of 2020, a Facebook post sharing some very sweet and inspiring advice in the form of a poem, coupled with a photo of an elderly woman, went viral. It wasn't controversial; instead, it recommended a way of living that's a strong departure from how most of us with access to social media live today. It asked us to embrace simple pleasures, enliven our senses, tend to our needs, and restore ourselves by immersing our body, mind, and soul in the sensual embrace of nature.

The poem reads:

> Heal yourself with the light of the sun and the rays of the moon. With the sound of the river and the waterfall. With the swaying of the sea and the fluttering of birds. Heal yourself with mint, neem, and eucalyptus. Sweeten with lavender, rosemary, and chamomile. Hug yourself with the cocoa bean and a hint of cinnamon. Put love in tea instead of sugar and drink it looking at the stars. Heal yourself with the kisses that the wind gives you and the hugs of the rain. Stand strong with your bare feet on the ground and with everything that comes from it. Be smarter every day by listening to your intuition, looking at the world with your forehead. Jump, dance, sing, so that you live happier. Heal yourself, with beautiful love, and always remember . . . you are the medicine.

The message is truly lovely, and it ends on a really beautiful and empowering note. But we think it was the message in combination with the photo and name of the author that truly resonated with people. The photo shows the weathered face of a woman of advanced age—the kind of face one rarely sees in the virtual public square. "Advice from María Sabina, Mexican healer and poet," the post promises us.[5]

Ah yes, *María Sabina.*

She who can enter the world where everything is known.

Psychedelic researchers and those with a general interest in the area have been familiar with the Mazatec *curandera* (or "medicine woman")

5. See Rythmia's Facebook post from September 1, 2020, as just one of many social media pages to share it.

for over half a century since she became the first known indigenous Mexican to allow four white Americans to take part in a psilocybin mushroom ceremony (or *velada*) in 1955. When two of the participants, married couple Valentina Pavlovna Wasson (1901–1958) and Robert Gordon Wasson (1898–1986), published articles of their experience in the spring of 1957, this remote woman and her mystical practices were suddenly thrust into a strange new world.[6] The world of mid-20th century America. Unbeknownst to her at the time, María Sabina became somewhat of a celebrity in the United States and beyond.

And now with this meme, María Sabina's life once again became available to thousands of people who'd otherwise never have heard of her.

Only María Sabina almost certainly didn't write that poem.

In fact, it sounds nothing like her.

We reason that the poem went viral because it speaks to a deep longing we hold for nurturing grandmotherly wisdom. As many are aware (but still can't seem to escape) social media thrives by keeping people engaged in divisive, often hostile, exchanges. We suppose it's no wonder that a poem allegedly written by a wise elder offering gentle advice, free of any political ideology, would be such a hit. But in the process—as is often the case these days—we had merely reshaped an exotic culture into our own likeness and image, turning María Sabina into our indigenous "fairy godmother."

The fairy godmother reaches across every aisle.

Psychenauts tend to have a very modern view of what medicine people were like in history, often truncating their cultural and regional differences into a few basic patterns (recall Belinda Eriacho's insistence that there exists some nebulous "Native American worldview"). The poem paints María Sabina as a sort of Pocahontas character *à la* Disney's 1995 film. For example, while Pocahontas sings about "paint[ing] with all the colors of the wind" in the movie, the poem asks that you "Heal yourself with the kisses that the wind gives you and the hugs of the rain." We tend

6. See Valentina P. Wasson, "The Sacred Mushroom," *This Week* (May 19, 1957) and Robert Gordon Wasson, "Seeking the Magic Mushroom: A New York Banker Goes to Mexico's Mountains to Participate in the Age-old Rituals of Indians who Chew Strange Growths that Produce Visions," *Life* (May 13, 1957).

to view indigenous peoples as perfect beings in tune with nature and timeless truths—the noble savage trope is above reproach. But María Sabina, gifted healer as she was, also had a lot of pride in her abilities. "Ego death," so often taken as a truism of the psychedelic experience, did not exist for María Sabina.[7]

She was very much a gatekeeper of the healing potential of the mushroom; it would be quite out of character for Sabina to have uttered anything like "you are the medicine," as the poem reads. Her livelihood was based on taking the mushroom medicine *herself*, exploring the world where everything is known, and relaying whatever prescriptions obtained while there to her patients.[8] We tend to think that she often dished out mushrooms to her clients willy-nilly because she shared them with the Wassons after only knowing them for a few hours. But that was hardly typical (her family and inner circle notwithstanding—they often ate the mushrooms with her); outsiders coming to Sabina to be healed rarely, if ever, ate the mushrooms themselves (another departure from Western therapy practices wherein the client, not the facilitator, consumes the medicine). Sabina believed that she had a unique gift that allowed her to heal with mushrooms. Even her own sister, Anna María, who ate the mushroom often, was not worthy of its healing knowledge. "The mushroom is similar to your soul. . . . And not all souls are the same. . . . Ana María, my sister . . . talked to the mushrooms, but the mushrooms did not reveal all their secrets," said Sabina.[9] This is hardly the kind of person who would say, "you are the medicine."

She, María Sabina—along with her mushrooms—was the medicine.

Not even her own sister was worthy.

The redefining of María Sabina began with Valentina and Robert Gordon Wasson. In their published accounts of their adventures in Oaxaca, the Wassons painted *la curandera* as more primitive than she actually was

7. "Ego death" is the belief held by some psychenauts that a person can reach such a deep and profound psychedelic state that the ego simply dissolves or "dies," and a person experiences a feeling of pure oneness with all of creation. We will explore this more in chapter 14.

8. Estrada (1981), p. 47.

9. Quoted in Halifax (1991), p. 133.

to further their own preconceived biases of an unbroken Ur-mushroom religion originating thousands of years ago. Their very thesis depended upon it.[10]

As it turns out, modern women do not possess the requisite pixie dust of the best fairy godmothers—or so thought the Wassons. Sabina's television watching, beer drinking, and tobacco smoking disrupted the picture the Wassons were trying to frame—so they left María Sabina's *all too human* habits out of their stories.[11] Although she wasn't as primitive as the Wassons reworked her, the poem still holds very *modern* ideas of which María Sabina had likely never heard.

Take as an example the poem's nod to the Third Eye, which is how we interpret the line that implores us to look "at the world with your forehead." But the Eastern idea of the Third Eye only enters the Western Hemisphere in the 1956 novel by Cyril Henry Hoskin, *The Third Eye*; there is zero evidence that this Eastern concept penetrated María Sabina's village, Huautla de Jiménez, a remote area of Oaxaca, by 1985, the year she passed on. Nonetheless, the math, it seems, works like this: the Third Eye is a *spiritual* concept + María Sabina was a *spiritual* woman = María Sabina must have known about the Third Eye.

Modern psychenauts tend to associate the Third Eye with other tropes of modern, holistic psychedelic spirituality. In order for María Sabina to be worthy of the title "medicine woman" (and more importantly, act as our indigenous fairy godmother), she must have been familiar with everything your friendly SoCal neighborhood crystal-gazer knows: quantum theory, Chinese medicine, astrology, *The Secret*, pineal glands, sacred geometry, Jungian shadow work, the deep esoteric Spiritual Theory of Everything that ties it all together . . .. and of course, the Third Eye. This is less a deduction to evidence and more a whitewashing of various spiritual traditions, totally unrelated to each other, that evolved on opposite corners of the globe, joined together by our SoCal crystal-gazer who wishes to paint spiritual women like María Sabina into *her own* likeness and image. In this way, our crystal-gazer can both elevate María Sabina as a divinity and then join her in the heavens. *We've* heard about these things (Chinese medicine, quantum theory, Carl Jung, etc.)

10. Letcher (2007), p. 110.
11. Letcher (2007), pp. 107–08.

because Western Civilization (specifically the United States) is a melting pot of diverse cultures and ideas. But it strains credulity to imagine someone living in the nearly impenetrable mountain village of Huautla de Jiménez in the mid- (and even late) 20th century would have heard of Jung, quantum theory, sacred geometry, or the Third Eye. In fact, the first Buddhist temple in the area, Casa Tibet México Sede Oaxaca, was founded in 1998—over a decade after María Sabina left us to dance on the stars.

We hypothesize that since María Sabina has become a respected "elder" among psychenauts, said psychenauts cannot imagine her as ignorant of the kinds of notions we have come to believe about spirituality today. Whoever cited María Sabina as the author of the poem, perhaps unconsciously, riveted our modern ideas onto the famed *curandera*; however, in doing so she negated the fascinating amalgam of Sabina's practice.

We only have one source (published in two places) for María Sabina's poems and lyrics. They are first found on a record made by Robert Gordon Wasson in 1956 titled *Mushroom Ceremony of the Mazatec Indians of Mexico*; secondly, English versions of her poems (all sung in Mazatec on the record) appear in Henry Munn's *María Sabina: Her Life and Chants* (1981). Munn also preserves for us the lyrics to another of María Sabina's *veladas*, which took place in 1970, as recorded by Julia and Celerino Cerqueda. The viral poem is not included in this collection, meaning it could not have come from Sabina. If you're still not convinced, please compare the following excerpts.

From the Poem:

> Put love in tea instead of sugar and drink it looking at the stars. Heal yourself with the kisses that the wind gives you and the hugs of the rain.

From *María Sabina: Her Life and Chants:*

> ha ha ha

so so so
so so so
so so so
Whirling woman of colors
Whirling woman of colors
Woman of the network of lights
Woman of the network of lights
Clock woman
Clock woman
ha ha ha
so so so
so so so
so so so . . .[12]

Do you really believe the same woman wrote both those verses?

Another fact about María Sabina overlooked to paint her as our indigenous fairy godmother is that she was a devout Christian. The number of times she refers to Jesus, Mary, the Christian God, and other Christian saints in her actual poems is staggering. The viral poem contains 12 lines. Not a single one touches upon Sabina's two favorite topics found carpet bombed throughout her lyrics: first, Jesus; second, her relationship with him. Again, let's go to Sabina's own lyrics. Here are the words she chose when she allowed Julia and Celerino Cerqueda to record her *velada* in July 1970:

Father Jesus Christ
God the Son and God the Holy Spirit
Lord Saint Peter
Lord Saint Paul
Saint, saint, saint,
Holy saint Father, says,
Father Jesus Christ, says
God and Son, says
God the Holy Spirit, says
Saint Peter
Saint Paul
Saint, saint . . .

12. Estrada (1981), p. 114.

. . . you get the idea.

Can this really be the same woman who wrote "Be smarter every day by listening to your intuition, looking at the world with your forehead"?

Of course not.

We often struggle to hold two opposing truths: María Sabina the *Christian* and María Sabina the *curandera* seem antithetical to us.

And yet, María Sabina was a devoutly Christian indigenous medicine-worker. From her perspective, the psychedelic mushrooms she ate were "the blood of Christ."[13] To tear her religion from her is to tear an important piece of her cultural identity from her.

The Unread Library Effect

The "Unread Library Effect" results from having access to knowledge sources (books, libraries, databases, archives, Google), and believing that a person's proximity to information means she understands complex issues. "The shallows of explanation," Robert Anton Wilson deemed it.[14] Psychenauts are not immune. Because psychedelics can inflate the ego,[15] psychenauts can at times unwittingly rewrite historical incidents and personages in their own likeness and image, even if they do not intend to. Their justification, whether they realize it or not, rests in the collision of ego-inflation and the Unread Library Effect.

The nature of the Internet (more specifically social media) expedites this process. One can easily be in touch with thousands of people who share the same erroneous belief, actively reinforcing it in each other. And then mob mentality takes over. Simply join any social media forum of flat-Earth believers, tell them Earth is spherical, and await the pile on. Or rather, join any social media forum about psychedelics, state that María Sabina did not write that poem, and watch the "peace and love" crowd go absolutely apeshit.

In this case, one large organization that shared the poem was the Chapel of Sacred Mirrors, Allison & Alex Grey's psychedelic art church

13. Estrada (1981), p. 40.

14. Quoted in Peter Boghossian and James Lindsay, *How to Have Impossible Conversations: A Very Practical Guide* (NY: Go Hatchette Books, 2019), p. 36.

15. Charles Savage, "LSD, Alcoholism, and Transcendence," *The Journal of Nervous and Mental* Diseases, Vol. 135 (November 1962), p. 433.

with over 190,000 followers. At the time of this writing the post has over one thousand likes and over eight hundred shares. MAPS, the largest psychedelic organization on the planet, posted a portion of the poem, which has 1,400 likes and over 300 shares. But the misinformation didn't stop with arguably the most famous entheogenic artists and largest psychedelic organization of our day. A Facebook group called Folklore, Customs, Legends, and Mythology shared the meme as well; it has 19,000 likes and 17,000 shares. The group has over 900,000 members. At this point, millions of people have seen this misattribution. "Truth" is no longer created by, well, *truth*, but rather created by "influencers." And I don't see it getting much better with A.I. I hope I'm wrong.

Like most misattributions haphazardly believed in the Internet Age, the viral nature of the poem includes both positives and negatives. The positives: more people inside and outside of psychedelia now know about this extraordinary woman. The negatives: the poem tears Sabina from her culture and places her into a more easily digestible paradigm for the "cannabis and yoga" demographic of the 21st century American public.

To talk about the realities of María Sabina's life is not to denigrate her (as we have been accused of doing in the past). It's to bring the full context of this woman's life into public awareness. María Sabina and the misattributed poem merely scratch the surface of a much deeper problem: namely, Googling info, while a good start, is not "doing research." Google should be a *starting* point; but for far too many folks it's an *ending* point. Moreover, our desire for social media "likes" and "reactions" far outweighs our need to tell a more complicated story about an extraordinary woman. Make the post, get the likes, feel the dopamine rush, move on to the next historical or philosophical butchering. It might behoove us to remember that Internet algorithms are designed to show us what we want to see, not what is accurate or true.

We are, in a soft way, *hypnotizing ourselves*.

In chapter 2 I mentioned how I did not necessarily disagree with all the premises of Karl Marx and Friedrich Engles and would address it later. I'd like to make good on that promise now. In 1893, Engels floated the idea of "false consciousness," which held that people living good lives in prosperous societies were not truly happy (much as they may believe themselves to be) but were instead slaves that could not see their bondage. Their contentment rested in a *false* consciousness (i.e., they weren't really happy); all one needed to do was realize it and break free from the mental chains. And while I find no merit in Marx and Engel's fantasy of utopian communism, I sometimes have difficulty determining whether or not we *do* somewhat live in a false consciousness today—only it's one caused by an invention that Engels could not have predicted: the Internet—specifically social media. While unquestionably a revolutionary—dare I say *miraculous*—tool that puts all the world's knowledge in anyone's hands, the Internet also comes with airbrushed selfies, cascades of baseless claims, and shameless self-aggrandizement in a never-ending quest to have strangers validate our existence. We believe almost anything we read on our social media troughs so long as it jives with our confirmation biases. Algorithms ensure that we will only see that with which we are likely to purchase or agree, creating a false consciousness and obliviousness about the world around us. And that's to say nothing of the rampant censorship of ideas and perspectives coming from Big Tech.[16]

This is the problem with the social media age—we *think* we know people. We get drips and drabs of their lives without realizing that photos from Hawaii and birthday selfies only represent a tiny fraction of the whole. We get quotations besides images with "ancient wisdom" that isn't much older than my cat, believing it gives us a window into something or someone who otherwise would be unreachable. It is a sad testament for far too many otherwise good people who get caught up in a shaky mix of myopic thinking, tractability, and a deep longing for meaning in this life.

María Sabína serves as only *one* example of this phenomenon.

16. See Ramaswamy (2021). See also "Michael Shellenberger's Guide to Escaping the Woke Matrix," University of Austin (June 26, 2023).

PART III

THE RACIST NARRATIVE

8

Locoweed: The Racist Origins of Anti-Cannabis Laws

In the history of drug prohibition, concern about health, racism, and xenophobia were thus born as siblings.

—Thiago Rodrigues and Biatriz Labate, "Prohibition and the War on Drugs in the Americas"

Before [drug prohibition], marijuana was only the word for a sacred and medicinal herb.

—Nidia Olvera-Hernández, "We Must Continue Calling the Cannabis Plant 'Marijuana'"

The Little Star That Follows

In both the psychedelic Renaissance and the larger American society, it is taken as a given that the War on Drugs, specifically laws banning cannabis—the "peoples' psychedelic"[1]—began as a racist undertaking to keep first Mexican Americans, and then black Americans, under a

1. To borrow from author and facilitator Stephen Gray.

white supremacist boot. University of Pennsylvania law professor Michael Vitiello claims, "At the start of the twentieth century, states began criminalizing marijuana based on unquestionably racist grounds."[2] Toni Smith-Thompson and Yusuf Abdul-Qadir[3] of the New York Civil Liberties Union (NYCLU) write, "As early as the turn of the 20th century, marijuana was framed by the dominant culture as dangerous and associated with Black and Brown people."[4] They are followed by a host of popular articles making similar claims.[5] And, of course, such ideas are found among Chacruna Institute affiliates.[6] If the war against cannabis began as a war against black and Mexican Americans then we will find evidence for this fact on the local level, when state lawmakers started to draft the first anti-cannabis regulations. We need to see where, when, and why legislators started implementing such unholy laws. Only then can we determine if racism provided a driving force for the policies.

While the use of cannabis by Europeans for medical and occult reasons goes back centuries into the past, Americans started using it regularly for artistic, spiritual, and recreational pursuits *en masse* in the mid-1800s. This cannabis did not come from Mexico, but rather was obtained in either of two ways: a person could purchase hash from local pharmacies who themselves had it shipped all the way from India by way of British cargo vessels; or they could grow the plant personally.

There were no laws. As we saw in our last section, cannabis had a stellar reputation among poets and writers especially, producing works like Fitz Hugh Ludlow's *The Hasheesh Eater*, Rosetta Howard's *If You're a*

---

2. Michael Vitiello, "The War on Drugs: Moral Panic and Excessive Sentences," *Cleveland State Law Review*, Vol. 26, Issue 2 (2021), p. 448
3. Assistant Director and Senior Racial Justice Strategist of NYCLU, respectively.
4. Toni Smith-Thompson and Yusuf Abdul-Qadir, "How Legalizing Cannabis Makes the Case for Reparations" (April 9, 2021).
5. Nick Wing, "Marijuana Prohibition was Racist from the Start. Not Much has Changed," *HuffPost* (Jan 14, 2014); Chris S. Duvall "Decriminalization Doesn't Address Marijuana's Standing as a Drug of the Poor," *The Conversation* (June 30, 2015); "Racism, Weed & Jazz: The True Origins of the War on Drugs," *News Beat* (August 25, 2017); Laura Smith, "How a Racist Hate-Monger Masterminded America's War on Drugs," *Timeline* (Feb 27, 2018)—to name a few.
6. Wendy Chapkis, "What Psychedelic Researchers and Activists can Learn from Medical Marijuana Legalization" (April 21, 2017).

Viper,[7] and many more. Their symphonic odes to the flights of cannabis, specifically hash, still delight readers and listeners to this day.[8]

Like most peoples familiar with cannabis, the average American used the plant as a medication for a variety of afflictions like pain management, menstrual cramping, appetite stimulation, and to ease depressive episodes. In 1889, cannabis was even recommended for alleviating opium addiction by no less an authority than *The Lancet*![9] A slight change occurred in medical- and governmental- protocols in 1906 with the passing of the Pure Food and Drug Act, the first legislative document to mention cannabis. In short, any intoxicating ingredients found in medications had to be listed clearly on the prescription label. This idea was already old news. Back in 1866 the editors of the *Boston Medical Services Journal* had deemed, "If the manufacture of this [cannabis] candy cannot be prohibited or its sale restricted in this country by law, the public should at all events be made acquainted with its dangerous character."[10] An ominous byproduct of the law meant that, for the first time, government authorities became "the watchdog over all drugs and medications that Americans took to feel better."[11] The next step came with the passing of the Harrison Act in 1914, which exerted federal regulations to include nonmedical uses of substantia. This was the first time in US history that a distinction was drawn between recreational and medical uses of intoxicants. Still, we are not yet in the age of aggressive police raids and long prison stretches.

Writers tend to begin the story of racist anti-cannabis legislation with the infamous Marihuana Tax Act of 1937.[12] We will deal with the Tax

---

7. Cynthia Palmer and Michael Horowitz (eds.), *Sisters of the Extreme: Women Writing on the Drug Experience* (VT: Park Street Press, 2000), p. 92.
8. See Gwyllm Llwydd, *The Hasheesh Eater And Other Writings: Illustrations by Gwyllm Llwydd* (CreateSpace, 2018).
9. Amanda Reiman et al., "Cannabis as a Substitute for Opioid-Based Pain Medication: Patient Self-Report," *Cannabis and Cannabinoid Research*, 2, 1 (2017): 160–166.
10. Quoted in Dale H. Gieringer, "The Origins of Cannabis Prohibition in California," *Schaffer Library of Drug Policy*, Vol. 26, No. 2 (June 2006), p. 6, n. 17.
11. Martin A. Lee, *Smoke Signals: A Social History of Marijuana* (NY: Scribner, 2012), p. 41.
12. Laura Smith (2018); News Beat (2017); Carl Hart, *Drug Use for Grown-Ups:*

Act in the next chapter. For now, we will unravel the real story, which begins not in the 1930s but rather in 1889 when the state of Missouri issued a revision of its statutes. The new law held that "every person who shall maintain any house, room or place for the purpose of smoking opium, hasheesh or any other deadly drug, shall be guilty of a misdemeanor."[13] Here is our first anti-cannabis law in the United States and it says nothing about race. The penalty amounted to a misdemeanor and didn't even technically outlaw smoking cannabis—it only targeted the parlors where cannabis and other drugs were consumed. We must then look elsewhere for the racist origins of anti-cannabis legislation.

And so we find ourselves in merry New England, specifically Massachusetts. The Bay State is important to our story. Legislators there would set the vanguard for anti-cannabis regulations in the United States. Let's dig deep into history and unearth that dastardly racism that must have been prominent among the Plymouth colonizers.

New England

Our tale begins when the indefatigable sex-moralist Anthony Comstock (1844–1915) came to Boston from New York and held a meeting before a large crowd gathered at Park Street Church on 28 May 1878. The topic? The evils of pornography. Comstock had made a name for himself a few years earlier when he successfully outlawed sending smut and/or information about birth control through the mail.[14] And now, he was on a larger mission: to found an organization in Boston that would mirror his New York Society for the Suppression of Vice. And so, on that spring day in Boston, the meeting attendees birthed The New England Society for the Suppression of Vice (NES).

An early administrator of the NES was a man named Henry Chase. Taking position in 1882, he initiated an aggressive campaign resulting in the drafting of laws against "immodest and indecent" materials including books, pictures, and theater performances, the latter of which came with a hefty penalty: those recitals deemed lewd would result in a $500

Chasing Liberty in the Land of the Free (2021), p. 161.

13. Gieringer, "The Origins . . ." (2012), p. 7 n. 24.

14. George Fisher, "Racial Myths of the Cannabis War," *Boston University Law Review* Vol. 1, Issue 3 (2021), p. 953.

fine, a year imprisonment, or both.[15] Chase also fought a war against brothel keepers. But the Society did some good work too. For example, they investigated rape cases (among other injustices against women) and intervened on behalf of the victims.

Eventually, the New England chapter would grow apart from its New York roots, fully rechristening itself as the New England Watch and Ward Society (incorporated 1887). Their target? "[T]hose agencies which corrupt the morals of youth."[16] Race played no role when it came to protecting children. Watch and Ward mostly continued the fight against pornography, but strategies were about to change.

The laws banning cannabis in New England began with a single person—a relative of Henry Chase, a plucky social reformer named Jason Franklin Chase (or Frank as he preferred; 1872–1926), who became the head of the Watch and Ward Society in 1907. He immediately set about directing some of Watch and Ward's resources to the "suppression of habit-producing drugs." By 1910, they were regularly prosecuting cocaine users.[17] That same year, the state of Massachusetts successfully criminalized unprescribed opium and a variety of opiates and opioids. Cannabis had managed to slip the noose that time.

But the situation would soon change thanks to toxicologist Dr. William Boos, who erroneously believed that hashish was "1000 times more harmful than either morphine or opium." And Boos certainly had his prejudices when he spoke of "foreigners" bringing hashish into the United States. But as it turns out, he was not referring to Mexicans. No, the real threat according to Boos came from India, where hashish was, as he put it, "the favorite drug of murderers."[18] The age-old stereotype of intoxicated bandits in Southeast Asia, thousands of miles from any black or Mexican American, was the culprit. Those like Boos were not the first writers to draw a connection between the people of India and drugs used in criminal activity. Renaissance Era Dutch physician Johann Weyer (1515–1588) warned of certain people in India who put the

15. Fisher, "Racial Myths . . ." (2021), pp. 954–5
16. Quoted in Fisher, "Racial Myths . . ." (2021), p. 953.
17. Fisher, "Racial Myths . . ." (2021), p. 955.
18. Quoted in Fisher, "Racial Myths . . ." (2021), p. 958.

highly psychoactive datura flower and seed "into the food of those they intend to rob. And those who have partaken thereof appear disoriented . . . dissolved in laughter; with perfect nonchalance they allow the thieves to remove whatever they wish."[19] And, of course, Boos always had the legend of the "Order of Assassins," a Persian cannabis-smoking paramilitary order, on which to rest any prejudices.

This first law specifically banning the Lord's plant, ratified in Massachusetts in 1911, totally ignored both black and Mexican Americans, and focused exclusively on the hash coming from the East. Which makes sense because hash *did* come to the US from the East. Pointing out where hashish comes from is not racist, it's geographically accurate. When it came to pornography, Frank Chase had no problem citing a French, or Italian, or South American origin—most probably because that too was geographically accurate. And while he certainly traced the supply chain back to India, he never linked hash *use* with any particular ethnicity.[20]

According to Watch and Ward, the real threat came not from Southeast Asians, black or Mexican Americans but rather *white American* doctors who were seen as the scourge of New England, over-prescribing hash to their patients and "profiting by their misfortune." Furthermore, according to Watch and Ward, those people who used hash were not insane or rapists or part of some criminal underworld. They were *always* listed as "victims," not criminals.[21] The criminals were the *doctors*. During the initial furor caused by the Harrison Act, 25,000 doctors were arrested for prescribing such medications! About 3,000 of those doctors earned stretches in prison for their efforts and many more had their medical license annulled.[22] The overwhelming majority were white American. If such laws were drafted to oppress black and Mexican Americans, both

19. George Mora et al. (trans., eds.), Johannes Weyer, *Witches, Devils, and Doctors in the Renaissance* (Binghamton, N.Y.: Medieval and Renaissance Texts and Studies, 1991), p. 230.

20. Notwithstanding a couple of comments like "All the opium illegally sold in Boston . . . was sold by Chinese" and a reference to Southern cocaine use by black Americans, the overwhelming majority of Watch and Ward's collected documents says nothing about linking drug use with any specific race. Moreover, regarding ethnic stereotypes about cannabis and race, the source materials say nothing. See Fisher (2021), p. 961.

21. Fisher, "Racial Myths . . ." (2021), p. 961.

22. Lee (2012), p. 41.

Watch and Ward and the Harrison Act authorities totally forgot to use them to such ends.

But Chase wasn't done yet. Moving quickly, he drafted anti-cannabis laws for Maine, New Hampshire, and Vermont—hardly bastions of black and Mexican Americans. Census reports from 1910 turn up a total of twenty-nine Mexican people living in Massachusetts. Indeed, the legislative language spoke not of "marijuana" (the common Mexican word for that plant at the time[23]) but of "cannabis indica"—the medical term for what we today would call "hash."[24]

The Maine and Vermont laws were ratified in 1913 and 1915, respectively; the New Hampshire bill did not pass muster in that state at the time. As the pusher of these laws, Chase remained consistent: race didn't matter, addicts were victims, and white American doctors were to blame—those were the battle cries of the New England anti-cannabis crusaders. We are at the dawn of anti-cannabis legislation and arrests in the United States, and black and Mexican Americans are nowhere to be found.

We might also consider that the Massachusetts anti-cannabis and morality bills had precursors with other substances. Beginning with a decidedly ethnicity-less intoxicant, alcohol, which was prohibited in 1852; cocaine (without a prescription) in 1898; and in 1910, a year before Frank Chase set his eyes on hash, the Bay State had outlawed morphine, codeine, heroin, and opium.[25] The concerted war against cannabis did not begin in any border town or ghetto, as the Racist Narrative would have us believe. It began in New England (specifically Massachusetts) and was a mere extension of older morality drug-purveying laws that targeted white American doctors who overprescribed medicines. There simply wasn't anything racist about this.

And things do not look any more accurate regarding the racist-laws claim when we consider the order in which the following states ratified anti-cannabis legislation outside New England: Indiana, California, and Wyoming all outlawed cannabis in 1913—the same year as Massachusetts and Maine. Perhaps, due to its proximity to the Southern border,

23. *Mota* seems to have replaced "marijuana" as the popular term in Mexico these days.
24. Fisher, "Racial Myths . . ." (2021), pp. 950–51.
25. Fisher, "Racial Myths . . ." (2021), pp. 962–3.

we might find some anti-Mexican sentiment in the California legislation. *But Indiana and Wyoming*? Since California is often brought up as a citadel of anti-Mexican sentiments (in a way that, due to lack of Mexican and black American populations, both Wyoming and Indiana are not[26]), let's take a look and see what truth, if any, we can find to support the claim that anti-cannabis laws were tied to racism against Mexican Americans who emigrated to California.

The Sunshine State

Cannabis had entered California, specifically San Francisco, in the 1860s, creating what one writer of the time called a " 'Hasheesh' mania."[27] Some have credited Fitz Hugh Ludlow (of *The Hasheesh Eater* fame), who holidayed in the Bay Area around that time, with introducing the herb to the West Coast. Perhaps that's true. Regardless, soon hash would be regularly available at any corner pharmacy in San Francisco, like Richards & Co., which advertised "Hasheesh Candy." But Ludlow's most notable show of influence in the Bay Area was on the acclaimed author Mark Twain (1835–1910). Sometime after the two authors met, Twain was seen walking down Clay Street—the very street on which Richards & Co. was located—on 17 September 1865, high as a kite on hash. The event even made the local paper; *The San Francisco Dramatic Chronicle* (since redubbed *The Chronicle*), stated, "Yesterday, Mark Twain and the 'Mouse-Trap' man [i.e., Tremenheere Lanyon Johns (1839–1875)] were seen walking up Clay street [*sic*] under the influence of the drug, followed by a 'star' [i.e., a police officer], who was evidently laboring under a misapprehension as to what was the matter with them."[28] Amusing as the story is it also tells us something important for our purposes. The great Mexican migration that took place after the Mexican Revolution (1910–1920) would not commence for another several decades. The hash

26. California also had a very low black American population at the time, a total of 145 in the entire state; see "State of California in 1860," p. 5. By 1900, that number would climb to 3,721; see "A History of Black Americans in California." These numbers are not large enough to have influenced statewide legislation.
27. Quoted in Gieringer, "The Origins . . ." (2012), p. 5.
28. Ellen Komp, "Mark Twain's 'Hashish' Experience in San Francisco," *San Francisco Gate* (Oct. 2, 2011).

Twain ingested did not come from Mexico. In fact, the San Francisco drug wholesale firm Redington & Co. listed "Fluid extracts of *Indian hemp*, (foreign) *cannabis indica*," a "powerful narcotic," for $3 per pound."[29] It says nothing of "marijuana."

This wasn't Mexican grass.

This was Big Pharma stuff.

Few other local newspapers from the time mention cannabis use. Those that do leave ethnicity unmentioned, save one. In 1895, the *San Francisco Call* reported on a certain tobacco expert, Mr. Nahon, who was in the market to buy forty acres of land to grow his preferred plant. During his quest he happened upon "Arabs and Turks" who grew cannabis, using the seed for birdfeed and the flower to, well . . . *you know*. The article mentions nothing derogatory or racist about these gentlemen or their use of "kiff." Quite the contrary, Mr. Nahon wanted to go into business with them! For he had, in fact, already come into contact with hash while traveling overseas. After smoking, the "spirit [was] in a new realm—a paradise. . . . The air filled with melody . . . odorous with delicate perfumes." Finally, the smoker was "lulled into a peaceful sleep by the music of his imagination." One wonders if Mr. Nahon was retelling his own experience with hash. In any event, he decided to portion off some of those forty acres he would soon acquire to grow cannabis.[30]

Who can blame him?

Perhaps the most interesting story from that time deals with a group of Los Angeles spiritualists who believed that cannabis unlocked "Magic Powers." One incensed writer had this to say about the clique:

> [Hash] was introduced into this country through a demand of ignorant mediums and spiritualists for a stimulus upon their occult powers, it being claimed for the drug that it would assist the medium in materializing the spirits with which they wished to communicate. . . . By its use they claim ability to force the spirits of the dead to stalk forth and hold converse with their living loved ones.

The author worried that the people of Los Angeles were being driv-

29. Quoted in Gieringer, "The Origins . . ." (2012), p. 6; *italics* mine.
30. "Local Hash-Easters: Arabs Near Stockton Growing Indian Hemp and Making the Drug," in *San Fracisco Caller*, June 24 (1895), p. 7.

en insane by this melodious mix of magic and marijuana—one of the earliest American mentions that enjoying hash turned a person into a "raving maniac." Though, this madness was largely relegated to the user fighting imaginary enemies or committing suicide, not attacking other people. The hash came not from Mexico but was "distinctly Hindoo . . . imported from India."[31] But that was not the only thing imported from the East. The notion that cannabis drove a person mad probably came to the ports of Southern California from Arabian doctors in the Middle East,[32] which appears to be the origin point of the sterotype.[33]

Black and Mexican Americans were not yet in any legislator's racist crosshairs; Asian Americans[34] were. Californians' drug of choice at the time was opium coming from China, not cannabis coming from Mexico. One writer from the era, Harry Hubbell Kane, posited two reasons this was the case. First, comparing opium to cannabis, he wrote, "Here, as there [i.e., Eastern countries], the practice is not one of steady, daily intoxication with [cannabis], but it, more like alcohol, is resorted to at certain times, when the system seems especially to crave it, or the temptation is offered."[35] Kane next points to doctors as the reason cannabis wasn't very popular in California, remarking, "If physicians used [cannabis] as freely, as carelessly, and in large doses, as they are using opium, morphine and chloral, hashich [*sic*] takers would be more common."[36] That's why California lawmakers focused on opium, enacting the first prohibition in 1875, which outlawed opium-dens during a surge of anti-Chinese immigration sentiments. Black and Mexican Americans cannabis smokers couldn't have been further from the minds of California lawmakers of the time.

31. "Insanity Caused by Hindoo Drug," *Los Angeles Herald*, May 14 (1905), p. 3.
32. W.B. O'Shaughnessy, *The Bengal Dispensary and Companion to the Pharmacopeia* (London: W. H. Allen and Co., Leadenhall Street, 1842), p. 584.
33. Origin point at least for Southern California. As we shall see in a moment, this stereotype comes from other places too.
34. Meaning Chinese and Hindu.
35. H.H. Kane, *Drugs that Enslave: The Opium, Morphine, Chloral, and Hashisch Habit* (PA: Presley Blakiston, 1881), p. 206.
36. Kane (1881), p. 207. As we saw, this would change by the early 20th century in New England.

Not much changed as the nineteenth century gave way to the twentieth. A study conducted in the 1930s—one imbued with offenses committed by immigrant populations—measured criminality from 1910 to 1936 and did not list a single cannabis arrest or incident. Furthermore, ethnographer Paul Taylor decided to conduct a study on farm communities in California during the 1920s. During that time, he never once came into contact with cannabis and was wholly ignorant of it. And there is a good reason for this. Modern ethnographers have thoroughly examined the "borderlands and . . . Mexican immigrants in general," finding "that marijuana use was rare in Mexican immigrant communities during the early twentieth century."[37] Tempting as California might seem for a racist origin of anti-cannabis legislation, the historical record indicates that we will have to look elsewhere.

The Big Easy

Another possible city that might point to the racist beginnings of anti-cannabis law is New Orleans. The Crescent City was not only a hotbed of jazz clubs, speakeasies, gambling dens, and brothels, but also saw a surge of cannabis use in the 1920s. In a commendably researched study, Adam R. Rathge investigated 225 arrests made for cannabis use in New Orleans which "reveals a user population with characteristics different from those often described by contemporary commentary and subsequent historical studies."[38]

The first hint of cannabis as a social menace in New Orleans occurred in August 1920, nearly eight months after Prohibition became law on 17 January 1920. It came as a report to prohibition commissioner John F. Kremer from Louisiana Governor John M. Parker. "Two people were killed a few days ago by the smoking of this drug," wrote Governor Parker, "which seems to make them go crazy wild."[39] By 1923 the first city ordinance was passed banning cannabis in New Orleans alone; it would be followed by a statewide ban the following year, which targeted

37. Isaac Campos, "Mexicans and the Origins of Cannabis Prohibition in the United States: A Reassessment," *Social History of Alcohol and Drugs*, Vol. 32 (2018), p. 14.
38. Adam R. Rathge, "Mapping the Muggleheads: New Orleans and the Marijuana Menace, 1920–1930," *Southern Spaces* (Oct. 23, 2018).
39. Quoted in Rathge, "Mapping . . ." (2018).

transport, sale, possession, and use by all except those with a doctor's prescription.

The locals called cannabis "muggles," inspired by a Louis Armstrong (1901–1971) song of the same name. Armstrong himself often recorded and played live while high on cannabis, so it makes sense that such a jazz town like New Orleans would follow his beat.[40] NOLA police officers and journalists started referring to cannabis smokers as "muggleheads," a precursor to our current term, "potheads." Like in California, those muggles at first did not come from Mexico. A contemporary news report from the *Times-Picayune* referred to "Indian hemp, Cannabis indica." The author even suggested that the word "marijuana" came from the Eastern word "majoon," a term used in Calcutta for a mix of "sugar, butter, flower, milk, and *Sidhee* or *Bang* [i.e., hash]."[41] Majoon was written about by physicians in rather enticing terms, the ingestion of which caused "extatic happiness, a persuasion of high rank, a sensation of flying, voracious appetite, and intense aphrodisiac desire."[42] However, the authors of the article decided to ignore all that pleasantness and focus on the etymology of the word "hash," supposedly deriving from the term "assassin," stoking images of Southeast Asian outlaws who drugged their victims before violating them in some way. Though, *Times-Picayune* balanced their stance by also claiming, "Some individuals become pugnacious, while others fall into a state of reverie. After small doses there is a great tendency to causeless merriment."[43]

We can detect the first uttering of a Mexican connection to the popularity of cannabis in New Orleans in 1923, several years after other states had already banned it. One article from that year mentions "another victim of Mexican dope."[44] However, the real problem didn't revolve around Mexican or black Americans, who, of the 225 reports studied by Dr. Rathge amounted to a total of thirty-three, meaning 192—a sizable majority—of those arrested were white American. Of those former thirty-three, only eleven were identified as Mexican, and seven of the eleven were all arrested in a single bust. "The arrival of Mexican immigrants

40. Lee (2012), p. 11.
41. O'Shaughnessy (1842), p. 583.
42. O'Shaughnessy (1842), p. 584.
43. Quoted in Rathge, "Mapping . . ." (2018).
44. Quoted in Rathge, "Mapping . . ." (2018).

smoking marijuana did not capture the attention of civic groups and law enforcement," says Rathge,

> Neither was anti-Mexican or racist sentiment central to the discussion of the New Orleans city ordinance or state law prohibiting marijuana. . . . [T]he absence of blatant anti-Mexican sentiment and the limited number of arrests undermines the intense emphasis on Mexican immigrants found in many histories of marijuana prohibition.

Additionally, Rathge found "almost no references" to either black Americans in general or to jazz musicians specifically. Finalizing his tally, Rathge finds only six mentions of black Americans smoking cannabis. All available evidence "reveals little connection between these groups [i.e., black and Mexican Americans] and marijuana use. . . .[T]he available arrest evidence from the *Times-Picayune* suggests the most common marijuana user in the city was a white male in his early twenties."[45] With New England, California, and Louisiana proven dead-ends for the racist origins of cannabis laws, it's time to explore ground zero for evidence of such bigotry—the line separating Mexico and the United States.

Borderland

Around the turn of the 20th century, a new term began to creep into southern Texas news reports and police statements: "locoweed"—the plant that made a person crazy. It is unlikely that this stereotype traveled from our Los Angeles spiritualists and those who condemned them all the way to the southern border at this point in history. Additionally, that earlier typecast of the maddening hash in LA started with Middle Easter doctors, all far removed from Mexico. And harm caused by violent cannabis outbursts among Los Angeles mediums was usually inflicted upon the individual mugglehead, not an innocent target. But locoweed was different and far more concerning. Locoweed caused the smoker to commit violent acts against the public.

45. Rathge, "Mapping . . ." (2018).

In 1886, medical student Genaro Pérez interviewed Mexican soldiers for his thesis titled *La Marihuana.* As it turned out, sometimes soldiers would lace a newbie comrade's cigarette with cannabis, sit back, and watch the fireworks. Pérez did not think the jokes so funny. "Soldiers who smoke [cannabis] . . . *go crazy and run around doing lots of disordered things,*" he claimed. But Pérez was also somewhat balanced in his assessment, adding that those soldiers more accustomed to the effects of the smoke often "became happy and sing."[46]

Pérez was echoed a few years later by an American psychiatrist living in Mexico, Charles Pilgrim. Around the 1890s, Pilgrim had caught word from local authorities that the Mexican pharmacopeia included flora that drove a person to madness. The two plants brought to his attention were cannabis and datura (called *toloache* by the locals). And while Pilgrim made sure to include testimonies from Mexican doctors who scoffed at the idea that cannabis caused insanity, he was also careful to note how the stereotype was popular among common people.[47]

The buzz about this crazy-making locoweed eventually reached Washington, DC, no doubt due to the bizarre stories coming from the Southern border. On 15 September 1915, a *joint* recommendation between the Department of Agriculture and the Secretary of the Treasury issued T.D. 35719, which would outlaw "Drugs, dried flowering tops, pistillate plants of Cannabis sativa, linne, [and] importation . . . if intended for other than medical purposes."[48] This amendment effectively extended Section 11 of the Pure Food and Drug Act of 1906 to include cannabis. The Department of Agriculture had been spurred by a report coming from Ciudad Juárez, Mexico, concerning a Mexican man who apparently smoked marijuana and, with knife in hand, pursued two American tourists to slaughter. "Death to Protestants," he yelled. He would go on to stab a police officer and a horse before being taken out by a cue stick to the dome while in a billiard hall, courtesy of one of

46. Quoted in Isaac Campos, *Home Grown: Marijuana and the Origins of Mexico's War on Drugs* (NC: University of North Carolina Press, 2012), p. 166; *italics* in original.
47. Campos (2012), p. 163.
48. R.C. Smith, "Report of the Investigation in the State of Texas Particularly Along the Mexican Border," Department of Agriculture, Bureau of Chemistry (April 15, 1917), p. 7.

the pool sharks.[49]

The assistant to the chair of the Bureau of Chemistry at the Department of Agriculture, Reginald Smith, was sent to the local pharmacies of border towns like Eagle Pass, San Antonio, El Paso, Del Rio, and Brownsville to investigate how the change to the law was moving along. Had the local pharmacies curbed their cannabis sales? Did the druggists agree with the decision? How did the residents of these border towns respond? Did cannabis really cause crime and insanity? *Where did the idea of locoweed come from*?

It's difficult to tell for certain, but after reading various firsthand reports of cannabis use stemming from the Mexican-US border it seems that locoweed was not the regular cannabis grown in Mexico, but instead imported *hashish* from major pharmaceutical companies. My hypothesis is based on an incontrovertible fact about cannabis products: namely, pharmaceutical-grade *hash* is much, *much* stronger than wild grass. We see good evidence for this from border-town pharmacies like the International Drug Store in El Paso, which distinguished between "Marihuana [and] . . . 'Locoweed.'"[50] That the pharmacy was called "International" offers more clues—their supply came not just from local and domestic sources, but also foreign (probably British) companies.

More concrete evidence comes from a local Mexican owner of the V. R. Ramirez Drug Store (also in El Paso). Señior Ramirez himself regularly received packages of "Indian Hemp" from pharmaceutical giant Parke-Davis and Co. The local Mexican population "seemed to prefer it to their native grown Marihuana," he said. And Ramirez knew the reasons, "because it was stronger . . . and more uniform in strength," he claimed.[51] High-grade hashish had crossed the border into Mexico courtesy of other pharmaceutical companies like the Warner Drug Company. Interestingly, when E. M. Duggan, who represented Warner Drug Co. in Mexico, sold "Cannabis indica in herb form" (i.e., grass marijuana) no instances of "insanity" were reported. However, when Duggan sold the pharmaceutical-grade hash, he said it "dr[o]ve the person using it crazy and makes him irresponsible and absolutely fearless of any dan-

49. Campos (2018), p. 20.
50. Smith (1917), p. 46.
51. Quoted in Smith, "Report . . ." (1917), p. 42.

ger."[52] Another pharmacist from El Paso, a Mr. Pollard, knew why hash sales had increased: the Mexican War for Independence. Mexican soldiers fleeing north caused a "noticeable demand" for cannabis. "I believe," admitted Pollard, "that the difficulty in obtaining Mexican herbs at the time, on account of interior troubles in Mexico and lack of transportation facilities, cause[d] this demand."[53]

As World War I turned flesh into soil, the US's British allies ceased exporting the hash they received from India. In response, American pharmaceutical giants began cultivating their own and shipping it to, among other places, *border* towns.[54]

Locoweed wasn't local weed.

Locoweed was medically-manufactured, hardcore hash coming from Big Pharma institutions.[55] Local (but still sizable) Texas companies like the Huston Drug Co., J. Armengol, and San Antonio Drug Co. also distributed Indian Hemp to smaller pharmacies along the border. The locals, presumably used to the milder effects of wild cannabis, were perhaps not ready for the awesome strength unleashed by hash—especially if they were using it in just as high of doses as their usual fare (or were first-time users). Even Harry Anslinger (1892–1975), the notorious anti-cannabis crusader who we will meet in great detail in the following chapter, differentiated between the two strains while testifying before the House Ways and Means Committee of 1937. When asked, "Is [hash] the same weed that grows wild in some of our Western states which is sometimes called the locoweed," Anslinger replied "No, sir, that is another family."[56]

This wasn't a one-way street, though. Cannabis was also coming into the United States via companies like the Mexican Product Company.[57] Pharmacies aside, evidence of personal curiosity about cannabis turns

52. Quoted in Smith, "Report . . ." (1917), p. 41.
53. Quoted in Smith, "Report . . ." (1917), p. 40.
54. Smith (1917), p. 14.
55. E.g., Allaire, Woodward, and Co. based in Peoria, Illinois; Parke Davis and Co. from Detroit, Michigan; Murray and Mickell from Chicago, Illinois; Moyer Brothers Drug Co. based in St. Louis, Missouri; and Lehn and Fink, with offices in both St. Louis and New York, among others; see Smith (1917), p. 14.
56. "Statement of H. J. Anslinger," Hearings on H.R.6385, *The Washington Post* (November 23, 1936).
57. Smith, "Report . . ." (1912), p. 10, 12.

up James Love who "introduced [cannabis] into Texas from Mexico by special permission of the state agricultural department." Love brought "ten pounds of the seed of the plant" over the border to cultivate.[58]

One can get a feel for how this locoweed, this Big Pharma hashish, affected the locals. So-called *marihuanos* (or "cannabis-smokers") appeared in one Mexican newspaper after the next, giving us some of our best evidence. A *Mexican Herald* article from 1899 mentions a "curious scene" at the civil registry office. A "marihuana fiend" stormed into the office while a crowd of new mothers waited to have their babies added to the census. He attacked the bystanders with a knife screaming that he was King Herod "and that his mission was the extermination of new-born infants."[59] Chaos ensued as mothers ran for their and their children's lives. The assailant was eventually subdued by the police.

Another report from the *Mexican Herald* a few years later speaks of Manuel Guerrero and Florencio Pino, who smoked cannabis and "ran amuck. Then they went into the street . . . attacking everybody." The two men proceeded to break into a fistfight between themselves. Eventually detained, they were sent to the hospital in "straitjackets. It [was] feared that the two men . . . w[ould] lose their minds permanently."[60] Still another man, fueled by "much talk against the Americans and a dose of marihuana," decided to cross the International Bridge in El Paso "[f]iring a rifle at all and sundry . . . he had decided to invade the United States by himself." He was quickly taken out by a bullet courtesy of the bridge guard.[61]

Other stories are equally bizarre. Take one about a priest from Zacatecas, Jesus Molinez, a holy cannabis-smoker that "exorcised the body of a dead man, who in life had been accused of being a wizard, and was said to hold conversation with the devil." Molinez mercilessly beat the sin out of the corpse and then later committed suicide by "smoking several enormous cigarettes of marihuana, while lying in a pool abound-

58. "Use for Deadly Weed," *The Florida Star* (October 16, 1908), p. 3.
59. "Across the Border," *The Oasis* (July 15, 1899), unpaged.
60. "Dangerous Mexican Weed to Smoke," reprinted in *Phillipsburg Herald* (August 18, 1904), unpaged.
61. "Character of the Mexican: Proper and Improper," *The Sun* (May 17, 1914), p. 7.

ing with venomous insects."[62] The author was incredulous: "And this is the nineteenth century!" she exclaimed. According to one scholar, of the 424 mentions of cannabis use reported in Mexican newspapers between 1854 and 1920, *200* mention violent crimes associated with smoking it and *140* note that it causes madness.[63]

Additional supercilious misogyny courtesy of Mexican doctors towards the local *herbolarias* (roughly: "wise-women skilled with herbs") as superstitious "rebels against civilization" only made matters more oppressive.[64] *El Imparcial* reported in 1903 that "the witch . . . during certain hours of the day sells in the markets herbs to cure 'the air,' others against indigestion, others in order to bewitch or unbewitch . . . in reality if they produce one effect it is madness, like marijuana." Some *herbolarias* were even said to conduct "black masses" that included smoking cannabis.[65] José del Moral, who found himself arrested for possessing a boatload of the good stuff, noted how "witches [*las hechiceras*] of many mountains go into ecstasies by smoking cannabis between prayers and dances, events which only the initiated attend."[66] The parallels between European witches and these Mexican *hechiceras* are quite noticeable: psychedelic sacraments, a mountainous setting, and ecstatic rites.

Regular, law-abiding Mexicans reviled cannabis smokers: "In Mexico a 'Marihuana fiend' is ostracized from all society. No one will have anything to do with him or trust him. He is absolutely unreliable and irresponsible," claimed F. A. Chapa, a Mexican-born pharmacist living in San Antonio; he adds, "I believe that the Government should pass a law of some sort to prohibit its [meaning "Parke-Davis Indian hemp"] sale."[67] Imported into the southern United States from Mexico was a view of cannabis as a drug that caused insanity and violence. Chapa was echoed by another Mexican-born pharmacist living in Texas. Dr. Fernando Lopez (also of San Antonio), wished to see anti-cannabis laws al-

62. "Senseless Brutality: A Mexican Priest Flogs the Corpse of a Dead Wizard," *The Memphis Appeal*, Vol. XLVII, No. 1 (April 25, 1887), unpaged.
63. Campos (2012), p. 89.
64. Quoted in Labate, Cavnar, and Rodrigues (2016), p. 36.
65. Quoted in Campos (2012), p. 150.
66. Quoted in Campos (2012), p. 165.
67. Quoted in Smith, "Report . . ." (1917), pp. 16–17.

ready on the books in Mexico applied to the United States.[68] Del Moral, who wrote of the cannabis witches of the mountains, claimed that "when common people ... see even just a single [cannabis] plant, they feel as if in the presence of a demonic spirit.... [T]he ignorant masses curse and scorn it."[69] (We are reminded of the Tarahumara that we met earlier who were so scared of peyote that they refused to so much as touch it.)[70] Broadside cartoon characters, like the foreigner "Don Chepito Mariguano," popular with the illiterate people of Mexico City, contrasted the maniacal, cannabis-smoking foreigner with the good citizens of the city who abstained from such vices.[71]

Three high-profile cases also helped cement this image of the villainous cannabis-smoker in Mexico: Enrique Cepeda, Governor of Mexico City; Presidente Victoriano Huerta (1854–1916),[72] and Charlotte Carlota, Queen of Mexico (1840–1927).[73] Governor Cepeda had been accused of committing homicide after smoking cannabis. During his trial, legal experts commented that cannabis was "capable of producing mental derangement."[74] Huerta, not-so-affectionately called "Presidente Mota" (i.e., "President Cannabis"), achieved his most lasting defamation as the subject of the well-known verse "*La Cucaracha*" or "The Cockroach." The famous verse goes in this wise:

> *La Cucaracha, la cucaracha* (The Cockroach, the Cockroach)
> *Ya no puede Caminar* (Cannot walk)
> *Porque no tiene, porque no tiene* (Because he lacks, because he lacks)
> *Marihuana que fumar* (Marijuana to smoke)

It was Huerta who, according to the soldiers in Pancho Villa's army, "Cannot walk because ... he lacks Marijuana to smoke."[75] Pancho Villa was seen as a hero of the common people; anything that he did not ap-

68. Smith, "Report ..." (1917), p. 17b.
69. Quoted in Campos (2012), p. 165.
70. La Barre (1989), p. 24, n. 8.
71. Campos (2012), pp. 156 *ff.*
72. President of Mexico, 1913–1914.
73. Queen of Mexico, 1864–1867.
74. Quoted in Campos (2012), p. 167.
75. Campos (2012), pp. 162–63.

prove was also shunned by the lower classes.

At the top of that list was cannabis.

As for Queen Carlota, rumor had it that she had been driven insane after some unknown enemy of her husband (King Maximilian I) spiked her morning tea with "deadly marihuana." Dubbed "the mad queen," she spent the rest of her days "alone in a castle in France, still hopelessly insane, 50 years after the potion was administered," as one newspaper reported.[76]

By 1907 the Mexican government had already moved to "exterminate the plant throughout [the country]."[77] It would not succeed until 1920, almost two decades before cannabis became federally illegal in the United States.

Scholars of drug history agree that the majority of Mexican cannabis use was relegated to prison inmates and soldiers fighting in the Mexican War for Independence. As one example of the latter, we read of soldier José Solas, whose "uncontrollable desire for the weed," caused him to desert the Fifteenth Battalion in hopes of scoring. Finally getting his hands on some, "while under the influence of Marihuana [he] killed Maximo Salazar. . . . Solas was violently insane when he committed the murder."[78] *El Imparcial de Texas* noted how cannabis use was "growing even in the army among members of distinguished families. . . . This, of course, is doubly lamentable." *El Imparcial* was resolute: the cannabis user was "always aggressive" and the plant itself was "terribly noxious when used as a narcotic, from which a dangerous vice is acquired."[79] Another paper detailing cannabis's effects on the Mexican Army stated, "More than one riot among the soldiers has been caused from smoking weed."[80]

The Mexican army decided to crackdown on cannabis. And these crackdowns were, at times, brutal. Under General Porfirio Diaz (1830–

76. "Is the Mexican Nation 'Locoed' by a Peculiar Weed?" in *Ogden Standard* (September 25, 1915), unpaged.
77. "War on Marihuana Smoking," *The Sun*, Second Section (May 26, 1907), unpaged.
78. "War on Marihuana Smoking" (1907).
79. Quoted in Smith, "Report . . ." (1917), p. 18.
80. "Use for Deadly Weed" (1908), p. 3.

1915), who would go on to become the president of Mexico,[81] soldiers who used cannabis found themselves blindfolded, hands tied behind their back, standing before a firing-squad. According to a former soldier turned pharmacist who carried out these orders for General Diaz, "Sometimes as many as 8 or 10 soldiers in our regiment a week [were executed] when they went crazy from Marihuana."[82]As a result, Mexican soldiers (who were barred from purchasing cannabis), would have their wives buy it and smuggle it into the barracks.[83]

Sometimes these *soldaderas* (soldier's wives) also partook of the herb. We know of a certain Laura Veraza who entered a Mexico City barracks in May 1898. Under the influence of cannabis, she attacked some of the soldiers with a knife. She managed to kill one; two more were severely injured. *El Imparcial* noted that Veraza seemed less a human and more a "wild beast." They even gave her a nickname: *La Fierita* "The Little Wild Animal," commenting that such behavior was common among the lower classes.[84] Though, one also wonders what kind of harassment, if any, *La Fierita* endured as she strolled through the barracks.

One might also wonder if we are getting a glimpse into the effects of hash on those suffering from mental illnesses that were poorly understood at the time. Consider that the two groups most known for consuming cannabis in those days, prisoners and soldiers, had no doubt experienced serious trauma in life that led them to either commit violent acts (in the case of prisoners) or had seen such horrors on the battlefield that it fundamentally changed their worldview (soldiers suffering from PTSD).

Getting back to Reginald Smith's Treasury Department investigation at the Southern border; the majority of his report mentions that sales of both "Marihuana and Indian Hemp" went to Mexicans, who had already been familiar with the herb. But he also reports transactions to both black and white Americans and "East Indians."[85] In Houston, for

81. President of Mexico, 1884–1911.
82. Quoted in Smith, "Report . . ." (1917), p. 45.
83. Smith, "Report . . ." (1917), p. 71.
84. Quoted in Campos (2012), p. 100.
85. Smith, "Report . . ." (1917), p. 80.

instance, the bulk of patrons visiting Smith Drug Stores Incorporated to purchase Indian Hemp (supplied by Big Pharma), were "well-dressed American men . . . known as gamblers, 'hop heads,' and pimps." These men were joined by "American and Spanish sporting women" (i.e., sex workers). A certain Mr. Cummingham, proprietor at Smith Drug Stores, stated frankly: "We used to sell [hash] to quite a few Mexicans[,] but I have noticed lately in the last year that the trade in this article has changed and that we [are] selling fewer Mexicans and more whites."[86] Story after story of continued cannabis consumption made Smith realize that "Treasury Decision No. 35719 [was] proving ineffective."[87]

One thing that strikes the careful reader of Smith's report is the total lack of racism on his part or the variety of people he interviewed. All his informants spoke openly and honestly about their experiences dealing in the cannabis trade along the Mexican-US border at the turn of the 20th century. These include Mexican druggists and doctors who carried the stereotype of the locoweed over the border and into the US in the first place. Smith was not a racist man trying to convince Mexicans that cannabis caused violence and insanity; quite the contrary—it was the Mexican people along the border convincing him of the same. Smith's report, when read in full, cares nothing about race. He was far more interested in upholding Treasury Decision No. 35719 than he was in racializing the issue. The stereotypes about the locoweed started in Mexico; the idea that cannabis made someone insane began in Mexico; and cannabis's reputation for violence also started in Mexico. North Americans merely adopted the preexisting Central American vanguard.

As we close out this chapter, let's recall the claims addressed at the beginning. We heard from the NYCLU, "As early as the turn of the 20th century, marijuana was framed by the dominant culture as dangerous and associated with Black and Brown people."[88] This is palpably false. Black and Mexican Americans played no role whatsoever in the creation of cannabis laws or seller/addict stereotypes, of which the earliest concerns

86. Quoted in Smith, "Report . . ." (1917), p. 76.
87. Smith, "Report . . ." (1917), p. 12.
88. Smith-Thompson and Abdul-Qadir (2021).

dealt with curtailing youthful vices; the first widescale arrests for such infractions were of white Americans (particularly doctors).

Journalist Olivia B. Waxman quotes Smith's report this way: "... a 1917 Treasury Department report ... noted that its chief concern was the fact that 'Mexicans and sometimes Negroes and lower class whites' smoked marijuana for pleasure, and that they could harm or assault upper-class white women while under its influence."[89] Waxman's assessment misses the larger context. The "chief concern" of the report had nothing to do with black or Mexican American people, and everything to do with uncovering whether or not the new T.D. 35719, enacted two years earlier in 1915, had been effective. Waxman's conclusion was born in a vacuum.

To be sure, *some* of Smith's informants did reference black and Mexican Americans as the major purchasers of cannabis products. However, of the three pharmacists who made direct mention of black and Mexican Americans, two of them (Ruis and Ramirez) were themselves Mexican American; the third, Schaffer, was German American. F. A. Chapa, the Mexican-born pharmacist we met earlier, also references "several American negroes and whites of the lower class." Incidentally, Chapa received his cannabis from an Italian druggist named Francisco Pizzini, "the largest dealer of marijuana in San Antonio."[90]

Our story is far more nuanced than the usual Racist Narrative.

More truly creative narrative-weaving comes from the Reefer Madness Museum, the curators of which pulled the ultimate race-bait and switch when they erroneously claimed that the majority of people arrested for cannabis use "all seem to have Mexican sounding last names." Putting aside the questionable veracity of such a statement, somehow the museum curators used this information to conclude that the "War on Drugs" most probably is a "War on Blacks."[91] How exactly Mexican surnames implicate black Americans is anyone's guess.

I have no doubt that some of the US government pencil-pushers drafting anti-cannabis laws were racists themselves. However, I have yet to see any evidence that their private racism played into forming any ear-

89. Olivia B. Waxman, "The Surprising Link Between U.S. Marijuana Law and the History of Immigration," *Time* (April 19, 2019).
90. Quoted in Smith (1917), p. 16.
91. Reefer Madness Museum, "Is it the 'War on Drugs' or the 'War on Blacks?'"

ly cannabis laws in the United States. These initial laws had nothing to do with a stereotype that linked cannabis with criminal activity among Mexicans or black Americans and everything to do with the idea that drugs were a "vice" from which children should be protected. Since the Racist Narrative is so all-encompassing, we have to tease out the fact from the fiction. While we cannot deny the fact of America's racist past, we need not accept the fiction that this included passing anti-cannabis laws in an effort to oppress black and Mexican Americans.

9

Like Dandelions: Racism and the Marihuana Tax Act of 1937

Yes, marijuana prohibition began with clear racial undertones, reflecting the views of 1930s US society.

—Chris S. Duvall, "Decriminalization Doesn't Address Marijuana's Standing as a Drug of the Poor"

Harry Anslinger conflated drug use, race, and music to criminalize non-whiteness and create a prison-industrial complex.

—Laura Smith, "How a Racist Hate-Monger Masterminded America's War on Drugs"

The Commish

He didn't care much about cannabis. If anything, cannabis policing would mean that some of the nearly two-million-dollar annual budget[1]

1. The exact amount comes in at $1,712,998; see John C. McWilliams, *The Protectors: Harry J. Anslinger and the Federal Bureau of Narcotics 1930–1962* (Newark: University of Delaware Press, 1990), p. 47.

granted the Federal Bureau of Narcotics (FBN) would now be diverted from harder substances like cocaine, opium, and heroin and towards a common, harmless weed, he reasoned. Due to the Great Depression, his budget would not be increased to fight this new menace *and* he would have Congress breathing down his neck. The logistics made no sense either. He had only 250 agents that were somehow supposed to police 4,000 miles of terrain and—even more daunting—20,000 miles of seaboard. "To achieve full enforcement," a historian writes of the scenario, "one agent would have to maintain the security of 100 miles of the United States border."[2] A truly insurmountable task.

He was no stranger to substance issues in the United States as he had already made a name for himself as assistant commissioner during Prohibition. He knew how little arbiters of justice cared about private drinking. "Why are you in here with the minor case of someone dealing with alcohol?" a judge might ask.[3] He found such questions embarrassing—a jab at his professionalism.

He wasn't pro-cannabis by any means, but he also didn't feel a federal ban was necessary. Let each state decide its own laws, he preferred. He didn't want a bloated bureau, but rather a "very lean, simple, administration."[4] Driving along a lone road one day he stopped and got out of his car, his eyes bewildered by the amount of wild cannabis growing along the upper Potomac. *This, they want me to stamp out*? he might have asked himself . . . *these ample waves of green, from sea to shining sea*? This stuff grows "like dandelions," he lamented.[5] Eschewing moral bullhorns and propaganda hit pieces, he initially opted for a protocol of "silence" as "a very important element of the drug strategy." He did not "want to wake sleeping dogs" as one of his biographers recalls.[6] Don't promote it, don't talk about it, don't make a big deal about it and cannabis will just go away, he hoped.

2. McWilliams (1990), p. 47.
3. Quoted in "Dr. David F. Musto Interview," *Frontline* (Winter, 1997–98).
4. "Dr. David F. Musto Interview."
5. Quoted in Mike Gray, *Drug Crazy: How We Got into this Mess and How We Can Get Out* (NY: Random House, 1998), p. 75.
6. "Dr. David F. Musto Interview."

Despite his early indifference to the Lord's plant, Harry J. Anslinger, Commissioner of the FBN during the 1930s, would one day wage a war against cannabis that would change the course of American drug policy. And due to lacking the funds to fight cannabis through law enforcement, Anslinger would eventually go against his own strategy of silence and wage this war with the only free resource he had available: the American media.

As we saw in the last chapter, contemporary popular opinion takes it as a given that anti-cannabis legislation began as a racist endeavor and continues as such to this day. First, writers with a critical social justice bent link the origin of cannabis laws to the racist motives of Harry Anslinger and place the beginning of stringent codification with the Marihuana Tax Act of 1937. Second, they claim that this unfounded racist-inertia accounts for the majority of black Americans in prison today. Third, they argue that despite equal usage of cannabis by white Americans, more black Americans are in prison for consuming it.[7] And of course, Anslinger must be compared to Donald Trump at least once for good measure.[8]

The thrust of their articles seeks to link the very real moral crimes of the past like slavery, Jim Crow, and anti-Mexican racism to the anti-cannabis laws of yesterday and today. The span of this narrative can be seen in a single title of one such article, Nick Wing's "Marijuana Prohibition Was Racist from the Start. Not Much Has Changed."[9] Wing's article is the usual fare: Anslinger was racist + black Americans = anti-cannabis laws.

These views have seeped into contemporary psychedelic spaces. Columbia professor and bestselling author of *Drug Use for Grown-Ups* (2021), Dr. Carl Hart, claims, "Back in the 1930s, numerous media reports exaggerated the connection between marijuana use by blacks and violent crimes. . . . These fabrications were used to justify racial discrimination and to facilitate passage of the Marijuana Tax Act of 1937." The

7. Kyle Schmidlin, "Column: 'War on Drugs' Merely Fights the Symptoms of a Faulty System," *CBS News* (September 13, 2008); see also, Wing (2014); Duvall (2015); Smith (2018); *News Beat* (2017).
8. Vitiello, "The War on Drugs . . ." (2021) p. 6.
9. Wing (2014).

culprit? Harry Anslinger.[10] Soap entrepreneur David Bronner, who has made no secret about his support for psychedelics, posted a message on his Instagram page that read in part: "Cannabis prohibition has always been rooted in racism—dating back to 1937, when Harry J. Anslinger used bigoted rhetoric to convince Congress to pass the Marijuana Tax Act, which effectively criminalized possession of cannabis."[11]

This chapter will explore the history of cannabis legislation in the United States on a federal level, as outlined in the Marihuana Tax Act of 1937, and untangle where race did and did not play a role.

But first, we have to clear some things up about Harry Anslinger.

Assassin of Truth

A giant, demonizing spotlight has been projected upon Anslinger, the now infamous anti-cannabis crusader of the 1930s, who famously called the Lord's plant the "Assassin of Youth."[12] And let me be clear—Anslinger knew absolutely nothing about cannabis and unapologetically exaggerated its dangers. But a more nuanced (and I feel, more interesting) investigation would seek to uncover whether Anslinger was racist and if his racism had a direct correlation with unconscionable cannabis laws.

First we must deal with two widely circulated quotes that supposedly originate with Anslinger, which appear on, among other places, the Twitter feed of the National Organization for the Reform of Marijuana Laws (popularly called NORML).[13] And while it is true that Anslinger had many flaws and lied about the harms of cannabis for political status, some of his most notoriously racist "quotes," pushed by unscrupulous media outlets and Ivy League professors, deserve special attention if for nothing more than to show how pervasive this problem of falsely attributed quotation (*à la* María Sabina) is today.

They read as follows:

1. *Reefer makes darkies think they're as good as white men.*

---

10. Hart (2021), p. 141.
11. David Bronner, "End the Racist War on Drugs."
12. Harry J. Anslinger and Courtney Ryley Cooper, "Assassin of Youth," *Schaffer Drug Library*.
13. @NORML.

2. *There are 100,000 total marijuana smokers in the U.S., and most are Negroes, Hispanics, Filipinos and entertainers. Their Satanic music, jazz and swing result from marijuana use. This marijuana causes white women to seek sexual relations with Negroes, entertainers and any others.*[14]

As it turns out, there is no evidence Anslinger wrote or said these words. For starters, the language is wholly anachronistic. "Darkies," although certainly used during Anslinger's lifetime, was not a common term during the 30s but rather a reprehensible slur that only caught on to the tongues of racists later in the century. Additionally, Anslinger rarely (if ever) used the word "Hispanics" and opted for "Mexicans." Finally—and this one is subtle—"marihuana" (with an *H* instead of a *J*) was the common spelling of the time. Further, when these quotes are attributed to Anslinger, they are often shared without any kind of citation, and in those cases when a secondary source gives a primary source, the provided primary source does not contain the actual quotes. For example, some writers and CSJ activists say that Anslinger uttered these words during congressional testimony in 1937, but Anslinger said nothing of the sort in his three testimonies that year.[15] (In fact, he made little to no mention of race at all in his testimonies—more on that later in the chapter.) And in those cases when a secondary source is cited, the secondary source either does not provide a legitmate primary source or does not even include those quotes. For example, a public service advertisement published by the organization Common Sense for Drug Policy (CSDP) cites Mike Gray's book *Drug Crazy* (1998) as a source for these quotes. I'm not sure how the ad creators at CSDP decided upon them,

14. Quoted in Smith (2018); Vitiello (2021), p. 6.

15. Although I have yet to discover the origin of these quotes, the earliest publication I uncovered that approximates them and cites Anslinger's testimony is Jack Herer's *The Emperor Wears No Clothes* (HEMP/Queen of Clubs Publishing, 1995). Herer writes, "In 1937, Harry Anslinger told Congress that there were between 50,000 to 100,000 marijuana smokers in the U.S., mostly 'Negroes and Mexicans, and entertainers,' and their music, jazz and swing, was an outgrowth of their marijuana use. He insisted this 'satanic' music and the use of marijuana caused white women to 'seek sexual relations with Negroes'" (p. 69). As noted, Anslinger didn't say anything like this in his three testimonies in 1937. Elsewhere, Herer writes that, to officials and newspapers in New Orleans between 1910 and the 1930s, "marijuana's insidious evil influence apparently manifested itself in making the 'darkies' think they were as good as 'white men' (p. 67). Here, he makes no reference to Anslinger.

but it wasn't from reading *Drug Crazy*, because those alleged quotes from Anslinger appear nowhere within its pages. And yet, the CSDP ad has likely been seen by millions over the years, having appeared in several media outlets, including *New Review*, *New Republic*, *American Prospect*, *The Nation*, *Reason Magazine*, and *The Progressive*.[16]

This phenomenon—whereby ideas are spread without checking their authenticity first—has a name: the "citation circle-jerk." This phenomenon occurs when lazy journalists and pampered professors merely lift article formatting and unverified quotes from each other, all while never pointing to an accurate primary source. Such an approach only serves to create a deeper racial divide in the psychedelic Renaissance and beyond.

I tracked down two actual quotes from Anslinger that show a more complex, and much fuller, picture of the man.

When Anslinger caught word of interracial cannabis parties occurring at a certain Midwestern university, he doesn't seem to have been bothered that such soirées were used to "improve race relations." He writes, "[t]here seemed to be, at the time, a brief commitment on the part of many people to explore and better [racial] conditions; Hollywood produced a rash of movies dealing with this theme. News organizations made it their business to call attention to the inequities existing between black and white Americans. Moves like this should be applauded."[17]

While Anslinger didn't like that those college students were using cannabis to heal race relations, his overall tenor doesn't sound very racist to me. In fact, the source of Anslinger's concern dealt with the "unthinking selfish few" [i.e., cannabis-smokers] who had "clouded the genuine efforts of others to find a solution so that all races could live in harmony."[18] Anslinger's concern that cannabis would ruin race relations, while wholly misplaced, in the very least shows a man who cared about healing race relations.

As for claims that Anslinger used "jazz music" and interracial mingling to stir cannabis controversy, his tactics show a very different approach. When a young woman offered her services to act as an informant for the FBN, Anslinger turned her away. His reason: "[W]e did not want

16. Common Sense for Drug Policy, "The Devil Weed and Harry Anslinger" (2003).
17. Harry J. Anslinger, *The Protectors: Our Battle Against the Crime Gangs* (NY: Farrar, Strauss, and Company, 1964), p. 100.
18. Anslinger (1964), p. 102.

to create the specter of wild sex and drugs with the girl and her Negro contacts."[19] In other words, Anslinger consciously *avoided* doing what unscrupulous journalists claim.

Does this mean that Anslinger harbored no racial prejudices? Of course not. We will see in a moment that he did. However, for the while, it's fairly safe to say that Anslinger's irredeemable racism has been grossly exaggerated.

The surprising fact is that racial epithets are almost entirely absent from his public testimonies and speeches. In fact, one of Anslinger's *only* racist remarks was met with such a serious backlash that it almost ended his career. The slur began with an internal memo written by Anslinger to the FBN's district supervisors about a certain unreliable informant named Edward Jones. Therein, Anslinger labeled him a distrustful "ginger colored n[****]r."[20] Through avenues unknown, the memo leaked out of the bureau's circulation and ended up causing quite a stir amongst the American public. Anslinger's state Senator called for his immediate termination. "[A]n avalanche of protest" flooded the office calling for Anslinger's removal.[21]

Reasonable people might consider that just because Anslinger used a racial slur does not mean that everyone at the FBN approved of his language. Some of his colleagues found his comment as racist as we do. Unfortunately, one biographer notes that Anslinger "cultivated and sustained ties with key members of both parties . . . interest groups and lobbies . . . making him virtually immune to opposition."[22] As such, he managed to hold onto his job.

The Marihuana Tax Act of 1937

There are a number of conspiracies regarding how cannabis became federally illegal via the Marihuana Tax Act of 1937—some of which I once believed myself. For instance, it has been argued that the true thrust of

19. Anslinger (1964), pp. 101–02.
20. Quoted in Gray (1998), p. 74.
21. Fisher, "Racial Myths . . ." (2021), p. 944.
22. McWilliams (1990), p. 47.

federal anti-cannabis laws came from the fresh-out-of-Prohibition alcohol industry. This conspiracy holds that alcohol manufacturers feared that "if you could grow marijuana in your backyard, [it] would cost you simply nothing to get high, you wouldn't buy alcohol." Others hold tycoon Lammot Du Pont responsible. Du Pont had invested in nylon and was "very fearful of competition from hemp."[23] Still others believe that publisher William Randolph Hearst was behind the laws. Hearst had much the same concerns as those coming from Du Pont; only his interests were in paper production, not garments. Since paper products are just some of the various industrial uses for the hemp plant, some authors have advanced the idea that, as Jack Herer writes in *The Emperor Wears No Clothes*, Hearst "stood to lose billions of dollars and perhaps go bankrupt" if the hemp plant were protected from the law.[24] Seeing how much more sturdy was cannabis to other natural fibers, Du Pont urged Congress to ban the plant and ensure his hemp-growing rivals would end up on breadlines.[25]

Attractive as these conspiracies prove, there is no evidence for any of them. And while some conspiracies *do* happen at times[26] and corporatism remains a vile and sinister enterprise, the story of federal anti-cannabis laws is far too vast and nuanced to leave much room for such conjecture.

Still, there is a fourth conspiracy, one awash with racism. This conspiracy states that cannabis laws were a white supremacist measure to keep black and Mexican Americans oppressed in the age of Jim Crow. Dr. Carl Hart believes this one, alleging, "media reports exaggerated the connection between marijuana use by blacks and violent crimes. . . . These fabrications were used to justify racial discrimination and to facilitate passage of the Marijuana Tax Act of 1937."[27]

But when I examined those media reports I found something very different.

News stories from the early twentieth century show a medley of canna-

23. "Dr. David F. Musto Interview."
24. Herer, *The Emperor Wears No Clothes* (1995), p. 24.
25. "Dr. David F. Musto Interview."
26. The Gulf of Tonkin incident serving as an obvious example from living memory.
27. Hart (2021), p. 161.

bis-using and peddling ethnicities. *The New York Times*, for example, did specifically mention cannabis use among "Latin Americans" (not black Americans), noting that it was "the same weed from which Egyptian hashish is made."[28] But other stories mention white Americans.[29] In still other stories, the arrested youth was Italian American, an ethnicity considered to exist somewhere between black American and white American during the 1930s.[30]

In one such case, an Italian American, Benito Sarego, bought "narcotic cigarettes" from a man (not otherwise identified). Sarego supplied the smokes for his peers. Not too business-savvy, he sold the reefers for the same price he bought them: 10 cents apiece. The largest "narcotic garden" discovered in Brooklyn was operated by two white American men, Robert Arnold and Louis Kelly, who sold the cigarettes to soldiers stationed at Governors Island. Police raided Arnold and Kelly's grow-op, seizing $50,000 worth of cannabis—their biggest bust in the city at that time.[31] The demand at Governors Island did not cease with the arrest of Arnold and Kelly. Two other young men, Joseph Lopez and Patrick Keenan (a Mexican and Irishman respectively) worked side by side to ensure the soldiers wouldn't be left un-high and dry. Sadly, they too were arrested for doing the good work.[32] One black American man was wrongfully arrested in White Plains, NY, for selling "reefers"; however, he was booked alongside an Italian American man and several others of unknown ethnicities. And as it turns out, the supposed "reefer" cigarettes contained nothing more than "tea leaves and tobacco."[33] They were released.

We might also point to actors like Robert Mitchum who spent thirty days in lockup due to a cannabis arrest. All his fame and fortune and privilege counted for nothing when the feds came calling. By the

28. "Use of Marijuana Spreading in West," *The New York Times* (September 16, 1934), p. 6E.
29. "Narcotic Garden Found in Brooklyn," *The New York Times* (October 18, 1934), p. 4.
30. "Boy, 16, Says Man Sold Narcotic Cigarettes," *The New York Times*, Section N, p. 4 (Oct. 7, 1928).
31. "Narcotic Garden Found in Brooklyn" (1934), p. 4.
32. "Two Seized for Selling Opiate to Troops: Two Accused of Peddling Loco Weed Cigarettes Daily on Governors Island," *The New York Times*, Financial Section (January 23, 1935), p. 38.
33. "Westchester Hunts Marijuana Sources," *The New York Times* (May 24, 1938), p, 21.

1930s, the crucial decade of cannabis legislation, reports of muggleheads came from all corners of society. Anslinger biographer John McWilliams paints the scene: "By 1936 [cannabis] was said to have replaced liquor [from] "Harlem . . .. [to] affluent Westchester County, New York." McWilliams continues, "What caused perhaps the greatest concern was the ease and speed which marijuana seemed to gain popularity among a totally new and different group of users—young people."[34] The fears from the early 1900s over youthful vices had not changed by the 1930s. Tying cannabis use specifically to black and Mexican Americans did not exist in the 1930s in any profound and widespread way; it is a product of *our* time—a product of our overcorrection for the real racist sins of the American past.

Curious readers can check the newspapers for themselves—most have been digitized on various website collections cited in this book. There does not seem to be any racial agenda on the part of police enforcing anti-cannabis laws. News stories portray a diversity of cannabis users and sellers—Irish, black, Italian, Indian, and Mexican American. Now where we *can* spot a form of racism is in the following way: journalists of the era took the time to mention if a suspect was black American or not. This rule sometimes applied to Latin and Italian Americans too; though, sometimes reports would simply let the name speak for itself (Lopez, Rodríguez/Grassi, La Rosa). Cringe as that was, the practice helps us today distinguish one ethnicity from another in the stories.[35] Notwithstanding that racism from a bygone era, there is simply no sign of a marijuana-crazed, homicidal, specifically black American man anywhere in the historical record. In fact, one paper of the time spoke of the "Marihuana-Crazed *Madman*," wholly untethered from any ethnicity.[36]

If anything, Anslinger had a bug up his ass about—more so than any other ethnic group—*Italian Americans.* Anslinger hated Italian Americans, viewing them as prone to criminal activity (a common trope in the 1920s and 30s) due to the rise of the Mafia in the late 1800s. Anslinger had already tangled with the Mafia during its days bootlegging illegal liquor during Prohibition. The Mafia returned the sentiment in kind,

34. McWilliams (1990), pp. 49–50.
35. As we will see in a later chapter, this same practice is still used by journalists today; only now the tactic is meant to skew crime and police shooting statistics.
36. Quoted in Gray (1998), p. 76; *italics* mine.

dubbing him "that bastard Anslinger."[37] When Prohibition ended, Anslinger knew exactly how the Mafia would change up tactics: "the gangs would convert to the procurement and sale of illegal drugs; they had the organizations, the contacts, the personnel."

His target? Neither black nor Mexican Americans; instead, Anslinger focused on the Parmagini and Balestreri crime families.[38] During a speech delivered at Dickinson College in 1932, Anslinger stated that the FBN would not "concentrate on individual peddlers and addicts." Instead, he felt that the FBN "should break up international rings of narcotic runners, and stop interstate commerce traffic."[39] Impoverished black and Mexican Americans hardly made up the personnel of international drug rings; it was specifically Italian Americans. In fact, the "cannabis-crazed" story Anslinger pushed the most in public consciousness dealt with an Italian American who we will meet in a moment.[40]

Italian Americans aside, even if Harry Anslinger also had visions of evil Mexican Americans smoking cannabis and poisoning the precious white American youth with muggles (and there is no evidence that he did), the average United States civilian would have disagreed. This is not to suggest that racism did not exist in those days. Of course it did. It is rather to say that racists simply weren't concerned about black or Mexican American drug dealers. They were worried about *white American* drug dealers. The United States was still a segregated country in those days. Anslinger *knew* he couldn't manipulate race to sell fear. Anyone caught selling cannabis to white American schoolkids would likely have been white American as well.

Racism serves as an unfounded impetus behind the creation of the Marihuana Tax Act. The true purpose of the Act, as outlined in the very testimonies of those who sought to pass it, was "to employ Federal taxing power to raise revenue by imposing occupational and transfer taxes upon

---

37. Quoted in Frederic Sondern, *Brotherhood of Evil: The Mafia* (NY: Farrar, Straus and Cudahy, 1959), p. 90.
38. McWilliams (1990), pp. 20–21.
39. McWilliams (1990), p. 47.
40. Larry Sloman, *Reefer Madness: A History of Marijuana* (NY: St. Martin's Griffin, 1998), p. 60; Fisher, "Racial Myths . . ." (2021), p. 937.

dealings in marihuana and to discourage the widespread use of the drug by smokers and drug addicts."[41] According to Dr. Carl Hart and a gaggle of journalists, this is the moment that racism became enshrined in all future American drug laws.

But there is a problem with that narrative.

Federal cannabis prohibition, as it turns out, began as an extension of earlier gun laws—specifically the National Firearms Act of 1934. The Act stated that a gun owner could not gift, sell, or lend an automatic weapon until she had purchased a "machine gun transfer stamp." But no such stamps were ever produced, so the problem, so to say, fixed itself. This strategy was then applied to cannabis. At one of the first Treasury Department meetings about cannabis legislation, which we will examine in a moment, a certain Mr. Peirce said, "We are attempting to thrust the marihuana traffic into legal channels where it will be taxed some."[42] A farmer could not grow cannabis without the stamp and the FBN ensured that such vouchers would be minimally produced.[43] Purchase of the stamp was so expensive ($100 per ounce of cannabis), that the original intention of raising federal funds through evermore taxation became moot.

Three hearings in 1937 would push the Marihuana Tax Act from Anslinger's personal fantasy into a nightmarish federal reality: The Conference on Cannabis Sativa Linne in January; the House Ways and Means Committee in April; and the Hearing Before a Subcommittee of the Committee of Finance (where the infamous Tax Act was finally approved) in July.

Anslinger attended all three.

Let's see what he had to say.

41. "Taxation of Marijuana," Hearing Before a Subcommittee of the Committee on Finance, United States Senate, Seventy-Fifth Congress, First Session, *United States Government Printing Office* (July 12, 1937), p. 5.

42. "Conference on Cannabis Sativa L.," *Schaffer Library of Drug Policy* (January 14, 1937).

43. "Dr. David F. Musto Interview."

The Conference on Cannabis Sativa Linne

The legislators found themselves in a bind. Mr. H. J. Wollner, consulting chemist of the treasury secretary, articulated the problem right from the start: the fourteen delegates at the Conference of Cannabis Sativa Linne were "[t]o see the marijuana problem ... from an enforcement point of view" all the while remaining "mindful of the legitimate uses of the product.... For every negative statement made [about cannabis] there is a positive one made to counteract it."[44] The entire meeting revolved around how to define the parts of the cannabis plant that were known "to produce deleterious physiological effects upon the human body."

Anslinger wasn't having it. He wanted a law that would be "all-inclusive." He was echoed by Mr. A. L. Tennyson, also from the FBN, who had found a field of cannabis growing in Massachusetts, where the plant had been illegal since 1911. However, the laws of the time only spoke of *cannabis indica*. This Bay State farmer was growing *cannabis sativa*, or as the delegates called it on that cold January day, "Cannabis Americana." Tennyson worried that the difference between *sativa* and *indica* "might have availed him something in court if there is any distinction between Indian hemp and American." But Tennyson was also more pragmatic than Anslinger, which might have caused some friction between the two gents; for Tennyson was resolute: "There is a use for fiber, for bird-seed, and for oil in the varnish industry. Those people will probably come in and complain about what they consider a foolish attempted control if we try to make this all-inclusive," he stated. Dr. Peter Valaer, of the Alcohol Tax Unit Washington Laboratory—who was a cannabis cultivator himself—agreed, cautioning: "If we go too far[,] I am afraid we are going to get into trouble."

Far from notions of Anslinger slinging racist comments throughout the hall, the majority of the hearing is filled with talks of chemistry, studies conducted on both female and male plants, whether seeds and leaves contain active alkaloids, legal names for the intoxicating parts of the plant, bioassays, and definitions, definitions, *definitions!* The delegates knew the upcoming Committee Hearing in July would require their

44. Quotes in this section taken from *Schaffer Library of Drug Policy* unless otherwise specified.

lawful definitions of what constituted *illegal* cannabis to have already been settled. Anslinger, a former Prohibition officer whose knowledge of cannabis amounted to *nil*, sat in silence for the majority of the hearing.

That was, until his feelings of inadequacy got the best of him. He finally took some initiative towards the end of the meeting and asked, "What are the proofs . . . that such addiction develops socially undesirable characteristics in the user?" But this was just the bait. The hook came when Anslinger decided to answer his own question, telling the story of a fifteen-year-old lad from Finley, Ohio, who received cannabis from some playground supervisors. Unfortunately, the stenographer simply records "reads from report of case." However, in Anslinger's recorded words about the incident, he says nothing of the boy's ethnicity or that of the playground supervisors.

Larry "Ratso" Sloman's book, *Reefer Madness* (1998), is interesting in this regard. Sloman claims that after Anslinger spoke about the Ohio teenager, he received a "green light from his superiors, [and] gave full rein to the seamiest . . . most heinous cases. . . . And, not surprisingly, many of these stories involved interracial contact."[45] Sloman then lists off a battery of cases that he believes Anslinger addressed before the attendees.

Sloman is wrong. Anslinger did not mention other cases at the conference; they simply do not appear in the meeting minutes. There is also a fairly obvious hiccup here. While it's true that many gruesome stories appear in Anslinger's "Gore File"—his collection of news clippings that linked cannabis with criminal activity—the reports feature various ethnicities. Of the nine cases that Sloman reproduces from the Gore File, only *three* deal with black American perpetrators. All the rest dealt with white Americans. Anslinger says zilch about Mexican Americans. In light of this fact, we might conclude that Anslinger's point wasn't about race; it was about this new scourge that he imagined was corrupting America's youth called, now legally, Cannabis Sativa Linne.

But he wasn't done yet.

45. Larry Sloman, *Reefer Madness: A History of Marijuana* (NY: St. Martin's Griffin, 1998), pp. 58–60.

The House Ways and Means Committee

Anslinger would have another chance to weaponize race through his Gore File at the House Ways and Means Committee three months later (in April 1937). Since local newspapers at the time often mentioned if the perp was black American, Anslinger could marshal all the lewdest and most abhorrent stories to read before his colleagues. Only Stanford law professor George Fisher compared the local reports to Anslinger's statements and found a curious disconnection between the races mentioned in the news and how Anslinger relayed them in his public testimonies.

For example, one report from his Gore File addressed a twenty-five-year-old Puerto Rican cannabis smoker from Baltimore, Maryland, who was sentenced to death after assaulting a ten-year-old girl. When Anslinger referenced this terrible incident while speaking before the House Ways and Means Committee, he only mentioned "a young man." He says nothing of the man's ethnicity—not once. In his entire testimony, Anslinger referred to Mexico exactly twice (and only in his opening remarks), simply to clear up some linguistics, saying, "Marihuana is the Mexican term for cannabis indica. We seem to have adopted the Mexican terminology, and we call it marihuana, which means good feeling." He says nothing about Mexican people. Notwithstanding a reference to "a great deal of use [of cannabis] in Egypt," and another to the Hottentots of South Africa, he makes *zero* mention of black Americans, jazz clubs, Devil's music, or interracial mingling.[46]

Hearing Before the Committee on Finance

During the course of Anslinger's testimony at the third and final conference devoted to cannabis, several moments presented themselves for him to share some truly racist ideas. And yet, the only time race got mentioned was when Anslinger read a letter sent to him from a member of the Interstate Commission on Crime, Richard Hartshorne, which references "one colored young man [who] killed another." I should note that Hartshorne does not tie cannabis use with black American crimi-

46. "Statement of H.J. Anslinger," House Ways and Means Committee (1937).

nality, but rather to a kind of temporary madness, to which *anyone* could be susceptible. Hartshorne further states in his letter that he believes cannabis so corrupted the young man's brain "that he did not know what he was doing."[47] We might also consider that what we are really talking about here is a *murder* case. Is it really so odd, considering the Mexican-born locoweed stereotype, that an investigator might believe such a connection between cannabis and homicide if cannabis was involved in a homicide? When Dr. Carl Hart says that media reports exaggerated the connection between cannabis use and black American crime, I'd like to believe that he is not suggesting that the homicides and sexual assaults were figments of the imagination.

In any event, so far as concerns Anslinger, this is a lone mention of race in an otherwise race-less testimony. Just as he had done when he previously testified before the House Ways and Means Committee and the Conference on Cannabis Sativa Linne, when Anslinger spoke before the Committee on Finance—the final assembly to discuss the Marijuana Tax Act of 1937—he never once racialized cannabis use. He never once links black or Mexican Americans to criminality. For example, he mentions seven boys who smoked cannabis and "conceived a series of crimes in a state of marihuana intoxication."[48] These boys could have been Irish, African, Italian, Mexican, or Asian (including Southeast) American, or a mix of two or more.

Anslinger had other things on his mind besides race at the conference—like bird feed.

Here's what happened:

During the 1930s, bird feed, then as today, was composed of various seeds. One of those kernels was "Hempseed." Recall our Arab and Turkish brothers from the previous chapter who sold their cannabis seeds for just that purpose. Tens of thousands of bird-feeding Americans, in tens of thousands of parks, yards, and other outdoor areas, had inadvertently planted millions of cannabis plants all over the United States! These plants then grew and seeded thousands more. In Philadelphia alone, po-

47. Quoted in "Taxation of Marihuana" (July 12, 1937), p. 11.
48. "Taxation of Marihuana" (July 12, 1937), p. 14.

lice forces seized 200,000 pounds of the plant "as the result of dissemination of birdseeds." Criminals grew wise to where cannabis crops were planted and starting harvesting and selling it, keeping all of the profits. No overhead. They just had to wait until spring when Americans started feeding their birds again.

"The plant reseeded itself," Anslinger groaned.[49]

When committee members asked what distinguished an opium user from a cannabis user, Anslinger rested his argument on age, not ethnicity, saying, "The opium user is around 35 to 40 years old. [Cannabis] users are 20 years old, and know nothing of heroin or morphine."[50] A most telling exchange occurred when a Senator Brown gave Anslinger a wide-open shot to spout some truly racist claptrap before the committee. "What has caused this new dissemination of [cannabis]?" he asked.

All of Anslinger's professional life had been building towards this moment—building towards this question. He could finally sound off about the dangers Mexicans and jazz musicians brought to society when they smoked cannabis and explain why the Marihuana Tax Act would be a boon to ensuring white supremacy remains forever enshrined in American drug laws. And yet, his answer is most surprising: "I do not know just why the abuse of marihuana has spread like wildfire in the last 4 or 5 years," Anslinger replied.[51] So where is all the racism supposedly preserved in the Marihuana Tax Act of 1937?

The historical record turns up nothing.

Assassins

After the Marihuana Tax Act passed, Anslinger (along with coauthor Courtney Ryley Cooper) published the infamous essay "Assassin of Youth" (1937) in *American Magazine*. The title reinforces the fact that Anslinger was less concerned with race and more concerned with youthful vices. Therein, he once again mentions the Baltimore Puerto Rican but only as "a young marihuana addict"—no mention of ethnicity. Anslinger also notes "two boys" from Chicago who killed a police officer

49. "Taxation of Marihuana" (July 12, 1937), p. 13.
50. "Taxation of Marihuana" (July 12, 1937), p. 15.
51. "Taxation of Marihuana" (July 12, 1937), p. 15.

"while under the influence of marihuana." What Anslinger doesn't say is that the two Chicagoans were black Americans. He also tells of a Colorado man who attacked a young girl.[52] The man who sent Anslinger that last report, Floyd Baskette of the *Daily Courier*, opted for a racist angle, writing, "I wish I could show you what a small marihuana cigarette does to one of our degenerate Spanish speaking residents. That's why our problem is so great; the greatest percentage of our population is composed of Spanish speaking persons, most of whom are low mentally, because of social and racial conditions."[53] Baskette offered Anslinger plenty of unapologetically racist ammunition right there to fire into the Mexican American population publicly, exposing them for the evil dope peddlers they were. And yet, Anslinger never did, referring to the Colorado predator only as a "sex-mad degenerate."[54]

There was also a "young man" from Florida who had "become crazed from smoking marihuana," and slaughtered his family with an axe.[55] This last kid, Victor Licata, was the Italian American of whom Anslinger spoke more so than any other case from his Gore File.

What Anslinger didn't reveal was that Victor Licata had been suffering from mental health issues, specifically "Dementia Praecox with homicidal tendencies," which left him "subject to hallucinations accompanied by homicidal impulses and occasional periods of excitement."[56] His condition was most probably hereditary, coming as he did from a long line of institutionalized family members; it probably didn't help that his mother and father were first cousins either. He became convinced that his parents intended to chop off his arms and replace them with wooden ones. On the night of 17 October 1933, he took an axe to his parents, two brothers, and sister; authorities found him in the bathroom muttering gibberish to himself. He was committed to the Florida State Mental Hospital a few weeks later.

Perhaps most devious was that Anslinger *knew* full well about Licata's mental health history. But instead of addressing the dementia

52. Fisher, "Racial Myths . . ." (2021), p. 942.
53. Quoted in McWilliams (1990), p. 53.
54. Quoted in Fisher, "Racial Wars . . ." (2021), p. 942.
55. Anslinger and Cooper, "Marijuana: Assassin of Youth," *The Reader's Digest* (February 1938).
56. Quoted in Sloman (1998), p. 62.

praecox in "Assassin of Youth," (which would take the focus away from cannabis), he decided to cast him as a once "sane, rather quiet young man" who was now "crazed." And the catalyst that flipped him from a quiet kid into a psychotic murderer was cannabis.[57] Victor Licata, not any black or Mexican American, became the face of American cannabis "addiction" and the violence that Anslinger believed followed.

Notwithstanding a passing reference to "musicians" who brought the plant from the southern border up North,[58] the only time Anslinger references any kind of specific ethnicity in conjunction with cannabis use in "Assassin of Youth" occurs when he points not to Mexicans but to ancient Greeks and Persians. According to Anslinger, but not confirmed by any historical source, ancient Grecians believed that cannabis transformed people into pigs, which made them forget their responsibilities.[59] He mentions Persians to link "hashish" to the Assassins, who "engage[d] in violent and bloody deeds."[60] For Anslinger, the myth that cannabis made people degenerates or homicidal maniacs had nothing to do with black or Mexican Americans and everything to do with Greeks and Persians! "In Persia, for thousands of years before Christ," Anslinger tells us, "there was a religion and military order founded which was called the Assassins, and they derived their name from the drug called hashish."[61] There is a reason he settled on the word *assassin* for the title of his article—to inspire images of marauding bandits high on cannabis attacking and robbing youthful innocence. Indeed, earlier news reports from the turn of the 20th century offered Anslinger historical precedent for this conclusion. One article from 1895 titled "Local Hash-Eaters," had this to say about Middle Eastern muggleheads:

---

57. Anslinger and Cooper, "Marijuana . . ." (1938).

58. Presumably, he means specifically black American jazz musicians here. But again, he doesn't associate any antisocial or criminal activity with the use, noting only that cannabis helps musicians because "it had long been known that the drug has a strangely exhilarating effect upon the musical sensibilities"; see Anslinger and Cooper, "Assassin . . ." (1938).

59. Here, Anslinger seems to have conflated the story of Circe from Homer's *Odyssey* with some other Greek lore unknown to this author.

60. Anslinger and Cooper, "Marijuana . . ." (1938).

61. Anslinger and Cooper, "Marijuana . . ." (1938). Note: The Order of the Assassins operated between 1090–1275, a thousand years after Christ.

> The desert Arabs grinds [*sic*] the leaves to a powder, which they swallow with a mouthful of water. . . . the fellows run amuck. It is dangerous . . . to meet one of these desert Arabs while the drug is acting on him. The Dervishes grow so wild that many instances are told of where they literally tore their horses and camels to pieces and devoured the flesh while the animals were yet alive.[62]

Such headlines like an article titled "Greek Hashish Drug" from the 1908 *Springfield Daily Republican* speaks of a "strange drug which has given our language its word assassin." Another article, "Do You Smoke Hemp?" from the *Boston Daily Globe* (1893) mentions "a secret society established at Cairo for the purpose of exterminating all enemies."[63]

For those reasons, Anslinger speaks of high volumes of use in Egypt, Greece, and India and calls it "Indian hemp."[64] Cannabis may have entered the US via Mexico *en masse*, but it was not exclusively a Mexican plant—especially not to early anti-cannabis crusaders like Anslinger. In fact, back at the meeting before the Department of Finance, Anslinger told those assembled that cannabis came mostly from Europe and Persia.[65]

In all, Anslinger retold over a dozen stories of cannabis-crazed crimes in "Assassin of Youth" and never once revealed an ethnic identity for any of them. However, so far as the cannabis vendors were concerned, Anslinger refers only once to ethnicity when he mentions "an Italian." Also mentioned were "a hot tamale salesman" and a "hot tamale vendor."[66] Let's focus on the latter two. The original newspaper that reported on the tamale/cannabis slinger, who had established a "dope den" for high school kids, made explicit reference to a "*Mexican* hot-tamale salesman."[67] It's hard to know what to make of this. Did Anslinger believe that the "tamale" part would be enough to instill fears of Mexican Americans into the minds of white Americans *or* was it just *du rigueur* for him to avoid ethnicity when speaking publicly about the canna-men-

62. "Local Hashish-Eaters," *San Francisco Call* (June 24, 1895).
63. Fisher, "Racial Myths . . ." (2021), p. 936.
64. Anslinger and Cooper, "Assassin . . ." (1938).
65. "Statement of H.J. Anslinger" (1937).
66. Quoted in Fisher, "Racial Myths . . ." (2021), p. 940.
67. "Mexican Arrested here for Selling Marihuana Plants," *Tulsa Tribune* (September 1929), p. 3; *italics* mine.

ace? We may never know for certain. What we do know, however, is that these few examples aside, the overwhelming majority of Anslinger's public pronouncements left ethnicity unaddressed (except, in this instance, when it came to those hated Italians).

According to one Anslinger historian, Alexandra Chasin, the whole of the Gore File includes "only examples of people of color."[68] This is provably false. William Gardner, a Chicago janitor, a New Jersey murderer, among many others arrested for cannabis use and/or distribution, were all white American.[69] And while the first person arrested under the new federal Marihuana Tax Act of 1937 was Moses Baca (born c. 1914), a Mexican American of twenty-three years, the second person arrested was a white American man, fifty-seven-year-old Samuel R. Caldwell (1880–1941). But this was just a timing-issue. Had Caldwell's arrest taken place a mere forty-eight hours earlier, he would hold the title of—as a popular tee-shirt erroneously calls him—"the first pot POW" of federal anit-cannabis regulation.[70] Incidentally, Caldwell received the harsher prison sentence because he was a *grower* while Baca was a *buyer*. It's almost as if the authorities cared more about the nature of the crime than they did about the ethnicity of the perpetrator. And anyway, Baca was first confronted by the police because he "was drunk and beat his wife."[71] Ethnicity had nothing to do with his cannabis arrest.

Journalists have the story backwards. A writer at *News Beat* tells us, "It's near-impossible to exaggerate Anslinger's contributions to the now-global drug war. . . . Anslinger successfully strong-armed entire countries to wage this war, his way. To best illustrate Anslinger's intimidation tactics, Mexico, for example, initially refused to comply with his demands until

68. "Alexandra Chasin Discusses Assassin of Youth: A Kaleidoscopic History of Harry J. Anslinger's War on Drugs," Cambridge Community Television (January 6, 2017).
69. See "Electrocution Death of Murderer," and "Janitor Selling Marijuana to High School Students," *Reefer Madness Museum*.
70. Daniel Glick, "Marijuana Prohibition Began with these Arrests in 1937," *Leafy* (July 28, 2020).
71. Quoted in Glick, "Marijuana Prohibition . . ." (2020).

the United States threatened to withhold painkillers from Mexicans."[72] This is total nonsense. Historian Isaac Campos tells us, "One of the really important things people often presume is that Mexicans have had a more tolerant attitude towards cannabis than Americans, and that's just not the case.... Cannabis was demonized in ... Mexico. The history of these kinds of regulations is way more similar between Mexico and the U.S. than different."[73] The journalists at *News Beat* effectively prove that it is totally possible to exaggerate Anslinger's role in the drug war.

Anslinger also never believed that cannabis served as a gateway to harder drugs. Despite Eric Schlosser writing in *Reefer Madness* (2003) that Anslinger viewed cannabis as a "stepping stone" to harder substances, he never offers a citation for this claim in his endnotes.[74] And there is a good reason for that. When asked "whether the marihuana addict graduates into a heroin, an opium or cocaine user," Anslinger replied, "No sir; I have not heard of a case of that kind. I think it is an entirely different class. The marihuana addict does not go in that direction."[75]

What really motivated Anslinger was not racism, but instead keeping his job. With the Great Depression, government spending slowed to a crawl, including funds usually directed towards the FBN. Additionally, the repeal of Prohibition in 1933, from which Anslinger made his reputation, meant a new intoxicating menace needed attention.

Anslinger's testimonies further demonstrate that he knew cannabis was not necessarily destined to drive a person insane, "It affects different individuals in different ways.... Some people will fly into a delirious rage ... and may commit violent crimes. Other people will laugh uncontrollably. It is impossible to say what the effect will be on any individual."[76] This is hardly a man inflating a connection between black American crime and cannabis, as psychedelic Theorists would have us believe. In any event, Anslinger was successful in getting anti-cannabis

72. *News Beat*, "Racism, Weed & Jazz ..." (2017).
73. Quoted in Waxman (2019).
74. Eric Schlosser, *Reefer Madness: Sex, Drugs, and Cheap Labor in the Black Market* (NY: Houghton Mifflin Company, 2003), p. 21.
75. Quoted in Richard J. Bonnie and Charles H. Whitebread, "The Forbidden Fruit and the Tree of Knowledge: An Inquiry into the Legal History of Marijuana Prohibition," *Schaffer Drug Library*.
76. "Statement of H.J. Anslinger," House Ways and Means Committee (1937).

legislation passed; his crowning achievement, the Marihuana Tax Act of 1937.

Looking carefully at Anslinger's source material, a certain thread emerges that tells a story beyond race—one not of a growing fear of black or Mexican Americans, but fear of the *addict.* The addict was bound by no race, class, or sex. The addict was stereotyped as either a deranged man of any ethnicity carrying out violent acts or as a promiscuous woman of any ethnicity who would sell her body to the devil for just one puff of the infernal grass.

Don't get me wrong. Anslinger absolutely and knowingly lied about the "dangers" of cannabis, which still affects people to this day. And if that were my question it would have been settled pages ago. But that is not my question. My question is whether or not federal cannabis legislation was born of a racist desire to keep black and Mexican Americans under boot.

So far, a careful look at the evidence turns up nothing of the sort.

Anti-Cannabis Propaganda in Popular Culture

If we can't find racism in any public statements from Anslinger or related legalese, or any news reports exaggerating criminality with black or Mexican Americans, perhaps we will find some in the popular anti-cannabis propaganda of mid-century America. Again, we hit a brick wall rather quickly. The American public—by and large—did not seem to care about race when it came to protecting their children against any kind of drug "menace"—real or imagined. Many parents of the 1930s had grown up during the first wave of popular substance use around World War I and already had a visceral reaction to over-indulgence. They watched their parents struggle and did not want their children to experience the same.

The United States also saw a surge of new health trends at the time; substance use was seen as an extension of the growing fitness and wellbeing industry. President Calvin Coolidge knew the problem: the expansion of office jobs and creation of the stale, inhumane corporate environment. Addressing the National Conference on Outdoor Recreation, the president stated, "With the development of our industrial and commercial life there are more and more of those who are engaged in purely clerical activities. All of this makes it more necessary than ever that we should stimulate every possible interest in out of door health giving recreation." And, of course, the main concern revolved around the youth: "Too much emphasis can not be placed on the effort to get the children out of the alleys and off the streets into spacious open places where there is good sunlight and plenty of fresh air."[77]

This fitness and health trend directly tied to the public's concern over drug use. As one Anslinger historian reflects: "We have in this country a pattern of looking at drugs and other substances, such as food, almost as an instrument to improve ourselves . . . what we call an anti-drug movement, you could, at the same time, call it a pro-health movement." In other words, it was the public, not bureaucrats, that "demanded laws against drugs."[78]

One need only look at popular movies of mid-century America like *Devil's Harvest*, *Tell Your Children* (later rechristened as *Reefer Madness*), *Marihuana*, *The Devil's Weed*, *The Burning Question*, and scores of other over-the-top films, which show white Americans as both the dealers and the users. Take the most popular (then and today) of these ridiculous films, *Reefer Madness*. In the movie, the closest we get to any non-white American character is a piano player in a soda shop, Hot-Fingers Pirelli, who would excuse himself between songs to get high. His surname, coupled with an olive complexion, suggests an Italian background. And while he plays no major role in the film, one scholar believes Pirelli's character "represent[s] the dread drug itself."[79] And perhaps there is something to this hypothesis. After all, Pirelli smokes his cannabis and then plays both the *black* and *white* keys. He has the town's children under his fingertips (despite the absence of a single black American kid in the movie). In fact, the only thing racist about these propaganda films is the complete lack of ethnic diversity!

The same rule holds when we look at anti-cannabis propaganda in the form of comic books. An anthology of these cartoons collected by Craig Yoe, much like the abovementioned films, shows a more realistic

77. Calvin Coolidge, "Address to the National Conference on Outdoor Recreation in Washington, DC: 'The Democracy of Sports,'" *The American Presidency Project*.
78. "Dr, David F. Musto Interview."
79. Fisher, "Racial Myths . . ." (2021), p. 977.

picture. Only a *single* comic (out of twenty-one) uses racist language. Titled "The Border Patrols' Never Ending Fight Against Narcotics!," the author uses the term "wetbacks" a total of five times to describe our Mexican sisters and brothers.[80] However, the real crime lord who hired Mexicans to smuggle cannabis across the border in this particular comic was a fictional white American mobster named Mike Joyce.[81]

Another comic titled "I was a Musician's Girl," shows the influence of cannabis on jazz musicians. Only the featured jazz band of the story is comprised solely of white American players.[82] Notwithstanding one black American kid appearing in a Public Health Service Proclamation comic in 1969 (and "The Border Patrols Never Ending Fight Against Narcotics!"), all the other vendors and "addicts" in all the other comics are portrayed as white Americans.[83] This lone, young black American man is never called a racial slur, never associated with cannabis due to his race, and is surrounded by friends who are all white American "addicts." Like popular propaganda films of the time, the only real racism here is a near total lack of ethnic diversity.

While the United States was undeniably a white supremacist country during the 1930s, this doesn't seem to have affected cannabis legislation on a federal level any more than it did on the state level. The Supreme Court ruled the Marihuana Tax Act unconstitutional in 1969 after LSD guru Timothy Leary (1920–1996) cleverly pointed out that a person could not obtain a stamp without criminalizing herself.

Not a single document pertaining to the passing of the Marihuana Tax Act of 1937 says anything much about race, which is reflected in the historical reality that saw many white Americans arrested for cannabis use and distro. The historical linking of black and Mexican Americans to cannabis use under the law appears to be, at best, a modern exaggeration of the Racist Narrative.

---

80. Craig Yoe (ed.), *Reefer Madness Comics* (OR: Dark Horse Books, 2018), pp. 95–6, 98.
81. Yoe (2018), p. 100.
82. Yoe (2018), pp. 180–87.
83. Yoe (2018), p. 95.

10

Genie in the Glass Bottle: The Legacy of White Supremacy

There is a leaf of a small tree . . . the Indians always have in their mouths when walking, and they say it sustains and refreshes them in such a way that when they walk in the sun they feel no heat; and in this country it is worth gold and is the principal tax for tithes.[1]

—Cristóbal de Molina, Bishop of Cuzco

There aren't any fistfights in the city anymore. People just kill each other.[2]

—homicide detective, Washington, DC

Broken Windows Policing

In the summer of 1999, I found myself in the East Village attending a Crisis[3] show at CBGB, hanging outside the venue drinking a 40 oz of

1. Quoted in Gerald T. McLaughlin, "Cocaine: The History and Regulation of a Dangerous Drug," *Cornell Law Review*, Vol. 58, Issue 3 (March 1973), p. 540.
2. Quoted in Nancy Lewis and Sari Horowitz, "Hundreds Flee Fatal Shootout Near SE Club," *Washington Post* (October 28, 1988).
3. 90s Hardcore band from New York.

Olde English[4] making friends, when a person about my age, Dave, approached and asked if I wanted to smoke cannabis. "Sure!" I exclaimed. This would be the last Crisis show before the band headed to California, so getting high before they hit the stage (and the road) seemed like the only option for a proper send-off. Dave asked if I had any cannabis to which I replied in the negative. "Let's try to find some," he suggested. I took my last swig of Olde English and told him that I had already spent my money on admission to the show and the 40 oz. I had a dollar to my name. He didn't care. He just wanted company . . . and someone who could find the Lord's plant. I knew exactly where to go: Astor Place.

I'd always been able to find cannabis at Astor Place; skateboarders hung around the giant cube and were happy to oblige a sale. Dave bought a dime from one of the skaters and as we were walking away a homeless man asked if we had any change. Dave had just spent the last of his money on the dime bag, so I handed the man my last dollar. Before I knew it—wham!—two undercover officers had me pegged against a wall outside the McDonald's on the corner of Astor and 8th Street, one of their forearms digging into the back of my neck forcefully; two others had Dave; and another had the homeless man. They searched the three of us, finding the cannabis on Dave. Handcuffed and thrown in a police van I couldn't believe what was happening—what law had I broken?

I later found out exactly what transpired. The cops hadn't actually seen Dave's purchase of cannabis from the skater. They saw me giving the homeless man a dollar and thought it was a drug deal. Dave and I were searched because the police believed I had just bought cannabis; then we were both arrested because Dave had a negligible amount of cannabis on him.

That night I was arrested for giving a homeless man a dollar and spent the night in lockup. Dave, every inch as white American as me, was arrested for an insignificant amount of cannabis. Such were the realities of the Broken Windows policing experiment of the mid- to late 90s.

4. Before the terrorist attacks on my home city on September 11, 2001, most Manhattan bodegas did not check IDs. You needed only "look" 21 (whatever that means to you) and you could buy alcohol.

Broken Windows policing ignited a revolution in NYC's law enforcement strategies. The idea was to focus police resources on small crimes like graffiti, public intoxication, and panhandling. The NYPD wagered that this strategy would send a message to more violent criminals that armed robbery, rape, and murder were no longer welcome in the city. Stopping misdemeanors, it was reasoned, would preemptively stop felonies. If some nineteen-year-old punk could get arrested for, say, giving a homeless man a dollar—this would incentivize more hardcore criminals to think twice before committing violent offenses. This model was coupled with a radical new protocol that was data-driven. No longer content to simply wait for crime to happen and then respond, the NYPD deployed officers based solely on local crime statistics, focusing the bulk of their resources on high-risk neighborhoods. They knew the crime hot spots; they knew the repeat offenders; they knew the perpetual victims. The NYPD also saw a dramatic increase in police officers—upwards of 45%—between 1991 and 2001.[5] This coupling of Broken Windows and data-driven enforcement, along with a robust police department, led to an astonishing drop in New York City's crime rate during the 1990s. One by one, other police departments around the country started to employ those former two tactics and saw similar results.[6]

As I sat in a holding cell listening to a murderer tell me what he was in for I seethed with anger for the NYPD. However, with the perspective that only twenty years of hindsight can sort, I understand it today. Broken Windows and data-driven policing saved a lot of lives and improved the quality of life for many residents living in high crime areas, despite me getting caught up in the crossfire that hot summer night way back in 1999. There were far greater forces at play, of which I have only recently become aware.

---

5. Steven D. Levitt, "Understanding Why Crime Fell in the 1990s: Four Factors that Explain the Decline and Six that Do Not," *Journal of Economic Perspectives* Vol. 18, No. 1 (Winter, 2004), p. 173. Note to reader: Levitt disagrees that Broken Windows policing was effective.

6. See Mac Donald (2017); *cf* Levitt (2004).

Racism

As shown in the previous section, the various kinds of prejudice that existed in diverse communities all over the globe were mostly based on climate and culture. However, none of those discriminatory views amounted to racism, a purely Western invention. We are all familiar with the abhorrent history of scientific racism in the United States, but we might not be aware of how it originated.

In 1859 Charles Darwin (1809–1882) published his groundbreaking work *On the Origin of Species*. The book sparked a revolution in how scientists thought about biology and its medley of mutations over time. For centuries, atheists had denied the existence of the supernatural, but not until Darwin could a solid case for a godless natural world be made. *On the Origin* has proven to be perhaps the most influential book since, well, the Bible.

Though, one aspect of *On the Origin* that isn't talked about so much is that it invigorated a new kind of prejudice, one that couldn't be escaped, no matter the climate or culture. Darwin believed that internal biology could account for external cultural achievements. A century earlier, Auguste Comte (1798–1857) considered that human civilization progressed through three stages of development: first theological, then metaphysical, then scientific. Others of the time, like anthropologist Lewis Henry Morgan (1818–1881) preferred to label the three stages savage, barbaric, and civilized. This assumed cultural progression would one day be called "social Darwinism."

To the social Darwinist, so-called "primitive peoples" had never left the first theological (or savage) stage. For many enlightened Europeans, tribal societies represented "the way we [meaning Europeans] were" in the past.[7] But the question thus arose: why didn't these cultures evolve into great seafaring, technological, architectural, and scientific empires? Anthropologists and historians today are well aware that contact with other groups and sharing knowledge—what might be called "cultural appropriation" through a critical social justice perspective—are what lead

7. Quoted in D'Souza (1995), p. 131.

civilizations to evolve.[8] Only this wasn't known to social Darwinists in the 19th century. The greatest champion of this flawed perspective was Herbert Spencer (1820–1903), who coined the phrase "survival of the fittest" (which has been falsely attributed to Darwin). Spencer believed that the differences among various cultures were the results of hereditary factors. Poverty, crime, ignorance, and other "social ills" were not the result of external societal forces, but instead defects of which some people were born.[9] Biological inferiority, not cultural or climate circumstances, allowed advanced cultures to lord over those they saw as primitive. As Darwin wrote in *The Descent of Man* (1871), "Viewing such [primal] men, one can hardly believe that they are fellow-creatures, and inhabitants of the same world. . . . The difference between savage and civilized man is the difference between a wild and tame animal."[10]

Scientific racism was born. From there, it was only a short step for scientific racism to morph into white supremacy. But therein we find an issue with the Racist Narrative, which holds that racism is everywhere and everlasting. Considering that we have a good idea about how racism started means there is nothing intrinsically racist about Europeans or white Americans (no matter what your DEI or JEDI master tells you). Racism can't be both everywhere and everlasting if it's confined to only a specific time and place.

And very much, thankfully, seems to be choking on its last breaths.

In order to navigate our way towards understanding the fullest picture of our current social troubles, including whether or not critical social justice has a place in the psychedelic Renaissance, it is imperative that we explore the role white supremacy played in creating the issues around race that media outlets like Chacruna Institute and Psymposia promote. Like the Decolonize Narrative, the Racist Narrative has a solid foundation in unassailable historical truths. For just shy of 400 years, governmental authorities, slave-holding entrepreneurs, and ordinary bigots have worked themselves tirelessly to abuse the black American man, dehumanize the

8. See Harari (2011).
9. D'Souza (1995), p. 132.
10. Quoted in D'Souza (1995), p. 130.

black American woman, and marginalize the black American child.

Freed slaves in the United States had only been emancipated from physical bondage. Cultural bondage remained fully intact. The Thirteenth and Fourteenth Amendments (ratified 1865 and 1868, respectively)—two of the Reconstruction Amendments of the US Constitution—were hampered by some white Americans' pathological need to keep black Americans submissive and shackled without chains. Political disenfranchisement grew rapidly, with Mississippi adopting poll taxes, grandfather clauses, and "good character" assessments meant to keep black Americans away from voting booths.[11] Mississippi's black American population reached over 900,000 in 1900, the second highest behind Georgia.[12] And yet, the black American vote in Mississippi around that time didn't breach 1,000 ballots. Other Southern states followed Mississippi's oppressive lead, implementing similar racist tactics. Alabama, the US state with the third highest black American population, churned out only 3,500 votes. Between 1896 and 1900, the black American vote in Louisiana dropped 96 percent.[13]

Black American children felt this crushing of the spirit too. Southern states allocated a paltry $2.89 for each black American student, while giving the lion's share of the spoils to white American children, who enjoyed $10.32 per student.[14] The Reconstruction Amendments had done little more than fuel white supremacist sentiments. The troops sent south to protect black American civil rights were helpless in the face of this ugly white supremacy, some of them no doubt siding with the racists. Lower-class white Americans, almost as destitute and powerless as black Americans, hated these newly freed people.[15] A shaky masculinity seems to emerge in any men that society has forgotten. Even a hint of black

11. Harvard Sitkoff, *The Struggle for Black Equality: 1954–1992* (NY: Hill and Wang, 1993), pp. 4–5.
12. Walter F. Wilcox, "The Negro Population," p. 19.
13. Sitkoff (1993), p. 5.
14. Sitfoff (1993), p. 6. In today's dollars that amounts to roughly $108 dollars for every black American kid verses roughly $386 for every white American kid (based on numbers from 1900).
15. Booker T. Washington, *Up From Slavery* (NY: Airmont Publishing Company, Inc., 1967), pp. 28–9.

American success would be met with violence and murder at the hands of impoverished, bed sheet-wearing, goofy Klansmen. With the promise of emancipation nothing more than a hose job, racism intensified throughout the South.

Between roughly 1910 and 1970, many black Americans fled North hoping for a better life away from the plantations—a move historians recognize as the "Great Migration." But white supremacy was not limited to the South. It reared its ugly head in the North through segregation, unfair housing practices, and police indifference to crime.

In *Up from Slavery* (1901), Booker T. Washington (1856–1915) notes how black Americans, upon achieving their "freedom," fled not to the ale houses but to the universities.[16] Only the doors of higher learning remained closed to them. Without access to books, many turned to the bottle. Alcoholism and drug use ran rampant. The frustration, the struggle, the crippling injustices were all too real and any relief, whether through syringe, pill, or gin seemed the only way to cope.[17] With hard substance abuse came increased crime. Thought-leaders like Marcus Garvey spoke truth to power—black Americans were not failing due to any inherent problem in their genetic code; they were failing due to white supremacy.[18] He was right. Despite the election of the first black American to Congress in 1928, Oscar Stanton De Priest (1871–1951), the problem of white supremacy would outlast Garvey's lifetime.

Culture of Revenge

As more and more black Americans fled the South seeking a better life, they found that they would not receive the same police protections as their white American counterparts. In this sense, the notion "black lives matter" rings an air of truth to it. Only the BLM movement of today has the story backwards. It wasn't that police were ever killing black Americans willy-nilly in the streets (more on that later); it was the police's *indifference* to black-on-black American crime that was racist. Swedish economist Gunnar Myrdal noted in *An American Dilemma* (1944) that

16. Washington (1967).
17. Jill Leovy, *Ghettoside: Investigating a Homicide Epidemic* (London: Penguin Random House, 2014), p. 50.
18. Sitkoff (1993), p. 10.

black Americans found themselves in an odd position somewhere between the devil and the deep blue sea. They both distrusted the police (due to the understandable fears that came when white supremacy was wed with gun and shield) and wanted more police (to protect them from their neighbors).[19] Out of this precarious middle ground between Hell and high water, a culture of revenge evolved within minority communities.

Cultures of revenge historically flourish in places without much or any police protection.[20] Needing a sense of justice is a fine human trait, one the majority of us harbor. We don't like it when the bad guy gets away with it. We like to see the bad guy face justice. But what to do when there is little to no possibility of justice? That stinging feeling that forms in our guts knowing that the bad guy got away with it never sits right. Victims of street crime can only be pushed so far—especially if the courts and police ignore them. This was the situation for minority neighborhoods in the early 20th century. As such, many turned to seeking justice on their own.

One of countless examples of this phenomenon took place in June 1925 when a black American mugger, Jay Eva Harris, was murdered by two of his Japanese American victims, H. Nishikawa and I. Hatawaka. Harris had robbed Nishikawa over $1.50. This wasn't his first offense. Harris had been mugging Japanese Americans in Los Angeles since December 1924. He had also been brought in for questioning about a murder a week before robbing Nishikawa. Harris simply showed the investigators the large-sum paystubs he had earned as a screenwriter, claiming he didn't need to murder anyone for money. This sufficed for the investigators of the time (likely because the victim was not white American).

Back on the streets, Harris continued to prey on Japanese American residents until he picked the wrong fight with Nishikawa, who, along with Hatakawa, grabbed a couple of shotguns and returned to the place of the mugging. Harris jumped out at them with a steel bar, yelling for them to "throw their hands up." Nishikawa and Hatakawa calmly raised their shotguns, aimed, and fired.

19. Leovy (2014), p. 50.
20. Leovy (2014), pp. 334–35, n. 41.

The police were apathetic about the killing. In fact, when called in for questioning, Nishikawa and Hatakawa were "surprised that the matter had even evoked the attention of the peace officers." Harris had "robbed many of their friends," the Japanese men explained. And, since the police ignored it, "[t]hey had merely taken the law into their own hands." Investigating officers Modie and Hanby were satisfied and pressed the matter no further. Nishikawa and Hatakawa were released.[21] Thoughtful readers might consider that if Harris had been white American perhaps the story would have gone another way; Nishikawa and Hatakawa no doubt would have faced severe penalties. But police in the early 20th century simply did not much care if a black American man was murdered. A sheriff in Alabama shrugged off black-on-black American homicide in this grotesque way, "If a n[***]er kills another n[***]er, that's one less n[***]er."[22] This, more or less, was the general sentiment of American police forces up until only recently. Drug researcher Claire E. Sterk, who interviewed several women for her exposé on crack addiction in inner cities, found "a frequent complaint concerned the lack of police in their neighborhoods.[23]

This police indifference to black American lives fed the culture of revenge. As the black American population grew over the 20th century, so too did this perspective spread throughout it. By the late 1970s, homicide was the second leading cause of death among black American men.[24] By the mid-1990s, it was the number one cause.[25]

Prison reform of the 1960s didn't help matters. President John F. Kennedy, hoping to retain voting demographics, offered black American thought leaders crumbs of compassion. The bail process went through liberal reforms, sentencing for crime was reduced, parole policies became lax, and violent offenders were granted furlough.[26] This was certainly good news for hardcore criminals, but it only meant that they would be

21. "Screen Writer Bandit Killed," *Los Angeles Times* (June 17, 1925), p. 31.
22. Quoted in Edward L. Ayers, *Vengeance and Justice: Crime and Punishment in the 19th Century American South* (UK: Oxford University Press), p. 231.
23. Claire E. Sterk, *Fast Lives: Women who use Crack Cocaine* (PA: Temple University Press, 1999), p. 185.
24. John Godwin, *Murder U.S.A.: The Ways We Kill Each Other* (NY: Ballantine Books, 1978), p. 185.
25. D'Souza (1995), p. 7.
26. Godwin (1978), p. 189.

back on the streets terrorizing innocent people. While white American liberals celebrated their window-dressing progressivism over cocktails in the Rose Garden, hardworking, law-abiding black Americans suffered the most.

Murdering peasant farmers in Vietnam on order of a series of presidents, including Kennedy, didn't help the situation. Many war-distraught black American men came home with two things that would only bury their cultural morale deeper into despair: heroin addiction and firearms. Scores of smack and weaponry bled into black American neighborhoods.[27] If you recall the wave of inner-city drive-by shootings that scorched the 1980s and 1990s (discussed below), you might have wondered how those young men got their hands on firearms. *That's how.* Vets had just fought in Vietnam and yet returned to a country not as heroes, but as dupes. During an episode of the WABC-TV show *Like It Is* in 1980, legendary boxer Muhammad Ali famously articulated that hard truth about black Americans fighting in Vietnam: "My conscience won't let me go shoot my brother, or some darker people, or some poor, hungry people in the mud, for big, powerful America. . . . For what? They never called me n[***]er. They never lynched me. They never put no dogs on me. They never robbed me of my nationality, or raped and killed my mother and father."[28] Some of those weapons meant to shoot "hungry people in the mud" would find their way onto the streets and into the hands of children.

Culture of Lethal Retaliation

The constant abuse perpetrated by systemic white supremacy left some inner-city black American men in a somewhat emotionally and mentally fragile state. By the early 1970s, psychiatrist Alvin F. Poussaint could note: "A lot of black killings are struggles over self-esteem; who's going

27. Godwin (1978), p. 188.
28. This is often quoted as "No Viet Cong ever called me a N[***]er." See Stefan Fatsis, "No Viet Cong ever Called me N[***]er: The Story Behind the Famous Quote that Muhammad Ali Probably Never Said," *Slate* (June 08, 2016).

to have the last word, who put who down, that sort of thing."[29] For centuries, racists humiliated, disregarded, and emasculated black American men. They beat them in front of their children. They violated their wives mercilessly. They did everything they could to tear the Divine Masculine from their souls. This loss of the Divine Masculine can also be seen in white American men during the age of slavery and Jim Crow. The overwhelming majority of white Americans lived lowly and pitiful lives (despite what your JEDI master tells you). Having a lighter skin tone was all they had to hold onto for any sense of social respect. They bullied and lynched black Americans to give themselves some dismal sense of self-determination. Perhaps a culture of extreme sensitivity to manhood arises in certain segments of marginalized men? I cannot be certain, of course, but this hypothesis might offer some clues to help explain the surges of violence that occurred in the late 1970s, mid-1980s, and early 1990s, and the *reasons* for a lot of that violence.

We now must move beyond the kind of revenge cultures of earlier generations, when retribution was somewhat "justified" in the sense that the police didn't much care about violent crime in minority neighborhoods, and a certain amount of order had to be kept (for example, Nishikawa and Harris). Perhaps we see this lawless cultural trauma passed down in the generations of the 70s and 80s, when the slightest insult, or poke, or even friendly josh was seen as an affront worthy of lethal retaliation in no way that can be called justified. Consider the following (of countless) examples: in the late 70s, two friends were hauled up on barstools, debating who was to buy the next round of drinks. At some point, one called the other a "tightwad," perhaps in jest. The other man didn't find it so funny and shot him five times, right there in the bar. Two blocks away, on another night, a family sat down for a dinner party. During the usual course of table conversation, a father of four and mechanic told his brother-in-law that he didn't "know anything about cars."[30] His brother-in-law stabbed him in the eye (hitting his brain) with a carving knife. Melee ensued. By the time the fighting ended one man was dead, another suffered a fractured skull, and a young girl had knife lacerations across her face.

29. Quoted in Godwin (1978), p. 187.
30. Quoted in Godwin (1978), p. 187.

In her exposé of the Bloods and Crips, *Do or Die* (1991), Léon Bing records some of the reasons gang members murdered their peers: "cause of the way he walk," "cause I don't like him," "cause he said somethin' wrong," "cause he asked me where I was from," "cause he a disgrace," "cause he . . . took one of my French fries or somethin'," "cause he look at me funny," "for the fuck of it."[31] Truly troubling testimony comes to us from Bopete, one of the Bloods members interviewed by Bing. "When I'm mad I'm liable to shoot anybody . . . just for the fun of it," he says.[32] Even small disagreements, like whether or not a basketball went out of bounds, could—and did—lead to a murder.[33]

This shift from a "justified" culture of revenge to one of unjustified lethal retaliation bled into other areas of inner-city street culture. Lt. Hayden Finely of the Juvenile Bureau saw it himself. "There used to be a time when even the toughest gang kids had three strict 'no-nos.' First, never hurt a mother. Second, don't hurt little kids. Third, never kill a father figure, especially a very old man. But now they've got no rules. None at all," he says somberly.[34] Bopete also noticed this disregard of the three no-nos, "If I'm with a bunch of T.G.s [i.e., tiny gangsters],"[35] he recalls, "and they want to jack some old lady, I say, 'Fuck that, man—go for somebody else, like a man or somethin'.'"[36] One sixteen-year-old murderer disagreed with Bopete's ideas about leniency. Elderly people were fair game, he thought, because "[t]hey can't fight and they can't run, and some [are] even too scared to holler."[37] One of the more memorable aspects of *Do or Die* is the total nonchalance with which these young teenagers speak about murder, gang rape, friends and family members they know on death row, getting shot, stabbed, robbed, and/or beaten by rival gangs. Many of them were not but thirteen-years-old.

---

31. Quoted in Léon Bing, *Do or Die: For the First Time, Members of L.A.'s Most Notorious Teenage Gangs—Crips and Bloods—Speak for Themselves* (NY: HarperCollins Publishers, 1991), pp. 121–23.
32. Quoted in Bing (1991), p. 57.
33. Leovy (2014), p. 50.
34. Quoted in Godwin (1978), p. 205.
35. Tiny gangster refers to a younger gangster, those around ten years old.
36. Quoted in Bing (1991), p. 55.
37. Quoted in Godwin (1978), p. 200.

Mourning Again in America

This culture of lethal retaliation saw its most intense years towards the end of the 20th century. A new euphoriant, crack, had swept the United States in the mid-80s. In 1979, a Nicaraguan revolutionary outfit called the Sandinistas overthrew the regime of Anastasio Somoza Debayle (1925–1980). The Sandinistas leaned comfortably into Marxism, which soiled relations with the United States. The Nicaraguan Democratic Force (dubbed "Contras") rose in defiance of the Sandinistas, which the newly appointed Reagan administration moved to support when it took the White House in 1981. The Sandinistas had made a deal with Russia in March 1980, and the Reagan administration saw this move as detrimental to US interests during the Cold War. In response, the US would bankroll the Contras, while its allies in Argentina would offer combat training.

Congress quickly tried to freeze any US aid reaching the Contras through the First Boland Amendment in 1982 and the Second Boland Amendment in 1984. But loopholes in the legalese allowed Reagan to creatively work around the amendments by soliciting funds from third-parties aligned with America's foreign policy interests. By 1984 Oliver North of the National Security Council (NSA) secured $11 million through selling arms to Iran, ensuring that money and munitions would continue to flow into Nicaragua.[38] Within this lattice of shadowy government actions, journalist Gary Webb (1955–2004) birthed a CIA-cocaine-smuggling scheme through his "Dark Alliance" series published in the *San Jose Mercury News* (1996).

The conspiracy holds that the CIA secretly made a deal with some of the Contras, purchased their cocaine, and dispensed it in black American neighborhoods in an effort to maintain good relations with its Nicaraguan allies. The end result was the deadly wave of crack-related violence that exploded in America's inner cities. It also—so the conspiracy goes—provided the perfect excuse to peddle drugs to black Americans so that they could later be arrested for selling or using them. If Reagan couldn't legally enslave the people, he would find an alternative route through mass incarceration by turning a blind eye to the importation of China

38. "The Iran Contra Affairs."

White across the US border so long as it kept the Contras content.[39]

While a recent *Netflix* movie, *Crack* (2021), digs up this tired old conspiracy theory, the whole scenario doesn't make much historical sense. Vietnam, Loas, and Cambodia were still very fresh in the collective American mind; selling new anti-commie adventurism, in and of itself, would already prove an uphill battle. Even the slightest indication of drug-smuggling would have compromised the larger mission. Various agencies with the US government[40] took these smuggling allegations very seriously and commissioned an investigation headed by CIA Inspector General Frederick Hitz. Hitz was keen on the delicacy of the situation: "it was well known during this period that if the CIA was linked to any drug shipment, the political damage [to the Contra cause] would be irreparable. . . . They knew perfectly well because of past accusations in previous theaters that that would be the kiss of death," he said.[41] In fairness, not everything that happens in history appears in ink and paper. We cannot dismiss the very real possibility of individual bad actors within the CIA lining their pockets with smuggled cocaine money. However, these small exchanges of blow (should they have occurred) would have been nowhere near enough to have caused the great influx of that drug into inner cities. Hitz found "absolutely no evidence to indicate that the CIA as an organization or its employees were involved in any conspiracy to bring drugs into the United States."[42] As we'll see in a

39. Craig Delaval, "Cocaine, Conspiracy Theories, and the C.I.A. in Central America," *Drug Wars* (2014).
40. That is, the Drug Enforcement Agency (DEA), including the El Paso Intelligence Center; the Federal Bureau of Investigation (FBI); the Department of Justice (DOJ); the National Security Agency (NSA); the Defense Intelligence Agency (DIA); and the National Drug Intelligence Center. Also reviewed were "Congressional records, including relevant information compiled by the Kerry Committee and the intelligence oversight committees and [conversations] with individuals associated with the Joint Iran-Contra Investigating Committee and Office of Independent Counsel for Iran-Contra matters." To allege that the thousands of people working across these departments were all in cahoots strains credulity.
41. Quoted in Delaval (2014).
42. Statement of Frederick P. Hitz Inspector General Central Intelligence Agency before the Committee on Intelligence, United States House of Representatives, "Regarding Investigation of Allegations of Connections between the CIA and The Contras in Drug Trafficking to the United States, Vol I: The California Story," Congressional Hearings, Intelligence and Security (16 March 1998).

moment, the bulk of cocaine that crossed the US border came not from Nicaragua, but from Colombia.

While crack isn't typically considered a psychedelic, it is still very important to the story of psychedelic injustice, as the drug all but decimated many inner-city and rural black American neighborhoods at the end of the 20th century. And many myths—not least of which the Dark Alliance conspiracy—have formed since then causing misunderstandings in the psychedelic Renaissance today.

What was it exactly that led so many specifically black American kids down this path? Some of it had to do with the culture of lethal retaliation that they suffered daily. But that's only half the story. The other half had to do with two national themes of the 1980s: prosperity, and prosperity's regrettable offspring, decadence. A 1984 presidential campaign commercial for Ronald Reagan (1911–2004) had declared it "morning again in America." Considered "the most successful presidential ad campaign in history," the minute-long commercial offered hope to the "nearly 2,000 families . . . [that] will buy new homes, more than at any time in the past four years. [The] 6,500 young men and women [who] will be married, and with inflation at less than half of what it was just four years ago . . . can look forward with confidence to the future."[43] After two national recessions during the mid- and late 1970s and early 1980s,[44] this message resonated with the American public, and Reagan swept the '84 election. A new day of prosperity dawned from sea to shining sea.

For some, anyway.

Little over a decade before Reagan's campaign ad aired, General Augusto Pinochet had successfully usurped the democratically-elected Chilean government. He quickly broke-up the Chilean cocaine markets and instituted a merciless administration. The timing was paramount; Pinochet's dissolution of Chilean drug manufacturers and smugglers opened

---

43. " 'It's Morning Again in America . . .' and the Birth of Political Ads," *American Association of Advertising Agencies* (2023).
44. 1974 to 1975 and 1979 through 1982.

the cocaine market to the Colombians, who already had an impressive transportation and distribution network using airplanes to smuggle cannabis into the United States. Cocaine would prove far more lucrative than cannabis for a couple of reasons: first, unlike cannabis, cocaine is physiologically addicting, ensuring high-volume repeat customers. Second, cocaine sold at a much higher price than did cannabis. The Colombian cartel merely switched the cargo from cannabis to cocaine. Using the string of smaller islands just south of Florida, notably the Dominican Republic and the Bahamas, large amounts of cocaine flooded the underground Miami markets. And the operation was quite diverse! Massachusetts-born George Jung partnered with Colombia-born Carlos Lehder[45] and set up stop-off points for cocaine-carrying planes in the Bahamas guarded by German militants.[46]

Still there were problems. A high-end drug like cocaine can only flourish in healthy economies, and the mid-1970s US economy was anything but. The demand for cocaine hadn't waned but the denizens of the American underground could no longer afford it. What to do with the seemingly endless supply of processed white powder, the Colombians wondered.

Enter *basuco.*

Taken from the Spanish word for "garbage" (*basura*), *basuco*—a kind of cocaine paste—offered an inexpensive way for many downtrodden peoples in Latin America to get high. What's more, *basuco* proved easy enough to make: one only needed some raw coca leaves and a strong solvent like ether, and she could produce an economical, smokable cocaine gum. When *basuco* reached the Dominican Republic via the Colombian cartel (that wished to establish a market for it), the locals tinkered with the recipe. Raw coca leaves were swapped out for processed cocaine; ether was ditched in favor of baking soda; and the product would now be cooked instead of merely mixed. The end result?

Crack.[47]

45. Renamed Diego Delgado in the 2001 film *Blow.*

46. David Farber, *Crack: Rock Cocaine, Street Capitalism, and the Decade of Greed* (UK: Cambridge University Press, 2019), p. 34–5.

47. Farber (2019), p. 42.

When crack exploded in US markets in the mid-1980s, it offered marginalized peoples a chance to enjoy all the benefits of the free-market system. Manufacturing jobs that had enticed many black Americans to relocate to major cities during the Great Migration started moving overseas in search of thinning the bottom line. Tired of watching their parents struggle within a system that did not care for them, many youths decided to try their luck in the street economy, which was far more lucrative than any back-breaking and diminishing[48] factory jobs that would fire them at a moment's notice to cut costs. They preferred "puffin' away for the genie in the glass bottle," as one Philadelphia crack dealer opined.[49] A disciplined dealer could turn a few hundred dollars of cocaine into thousands of dollars of crack. Television showed inner-city black American youths a swanky and posh life that was simply out of reach for the majority of them. They too wanted their slice of the American dream; they too wanted to wake up in the new American morning. For the unrecognized entrepreneurial genius in many of these kids, selling large amounts of crack opened an avenue out of poverty otherwise unavailable to them.

Without all the deadly violence that came with the crack trade, some of these well-organized kingpins could have taught business classes in top universities. They weren't stupid; they were desperate. Barons looking for a market. Some of them did good with the money, handing out hundred-dollar bills to the poor in their neighborhoods and funding youth programs like the Boys and Girls Club of America and basketball leagues. But fat stacks inevitably lead to increased violence to protect one's assets.

Specifically within a larger culture of lethal retaliation.

The Culture of Silence

Homicide files and caseloads piled up on police department desks, resulting in deeper enforcement apathy. At one point, the LAPD was reporting one violent crime every eight minutes. One detective, Sal La Barbera, investigated five homicides in a single night.[50] In Los Angeles

48. Due to outsourcing that began in the early 1980s.
49. Quoted in Elijah Anderson, *Streetwise: Race, Class, and Change in an Urban Community* (IL: University of Chicago Press, 1995), p. 88.
50. Scott Gold and Andrew Blankstein, "It was a Terrifying Time," *Los Angeles Times*

between 1984 and 1993, over a hundred strawberries (i.e., women who traded sex for crack) turned up dead—the majority black American. Crack- and pizza-dealer Chester Turner, the so-called Southside Slayer, raped and murdered around a dozen women alone—one of whom, Regina Nadine Washington (1962–1989), was six-months pregnant.[51] These women were "lost in the crime wave."[52] The LAPD did little about it at the time. "Could you imagine—more than 100 women killed and nobody notices?" asked Margaret Prescod, founder of the Black Coalition Fighting Back Serial Murders. "Could you imagine it in Beverly Hills? Palos Verdes?"[53] Diana Ware, stepmother of Barbara Ware (1964–1987), upon hearing the news of her stepdaughter's murder, could only muster a heartbreaking truth, "At that time, it was just another young African American lady," she said. "It didn't get a lot of attention."[54] In 1984 alone, Los Angeles suffered 1,438 homicides.[55] The police investigated 757 of them.[56] This is not to suggest that the entire LAPD (or any PD) remained cold in the face of those slayings. Some officers truly cared about this meteoric rise in crime and relentlessly pursued the culprits. But they were up against a largely apathetic department and a dearth of officers.[57]

In some cases, even a determined investigator would be stonewalled by residents of the neighborhood in which the murder took place. The culture of lethal retaliation manifested a culture of silence born of a fear of snitching (which also accounted for the chasm between murders and arrests). In 1974, during a string of homicides in San Francisco that had the police baffled, a woman went fishing in the bay. Her attention left the gentle waves of the harbor when she heard a young lady screaming, trying to escape a man who followed close behind her. Catching up, the

(August 4, 2010).
51. John Spano, "L.A. Man Guilty of 11 Deaths" *Los Angeles Times* (May 1, 2007).
52. Gold and Blankstein (2010).
53. Quoted in Gold and Blankstein (2010).
54. Quoted in Gold and Blankstein (2010).
55. Los Angeles Department of Public Health, Injury and Violence Prevention Program, "Gang Homicides in Los Angeles County, 1980–2008," p. 2. Compiled from info from LA Sheriff Dept. LA Police Dept, LA Dept of Coroner, CA Dept of Health Services–Center for Health Statistics, Death Statistical Master File (April 21, 2011). Note: date on original reads "April 21, 1011." I speculate that the authors meant 2011.
56. Gold and Blankstein (2010).
57. Leovy (2014), p. 38.

man threw her into a van and sped away. The fisherwoman said nothing about the incident, despite witnessing it. Her story came out only later. One black American officer working those crimes mentioned in defeat, "I know we could break these murders, but the people won't come forward."[58] Additionally, many of the victims were themselves perpetrators of some other crime, which no doubt led them to keep quiet—even when questioned about incidents unrelated to anything they'd done.[59] In one case, LAPD officer Patrick Flaherty was tending to a gangster who had been shot. When asked if the victim knew the perpetrator, the dying man used his last breath to say "fuck you" before he passed.[60] Even as late as 2008, 108 homicides in Los Angeles went unsolved due to the culture of silence among witnesses.[61]

Finally, many black American journalists ignored the glaring homicide rates, fearing it would further deride black Americans as a whole.[62] Those journalists were correct; this issue concerned a very *small* subset of the larger black American population.

By the time of the great crack epidemic of the mid-80s, a lawless culture of lethal retaliation passed from parent to child. "I followed in my father's footsteps—except he was a Crip," said Bopete. "He twenty-nine now, been in jail for about ten years." He continues, "If I had a kid, years from now, I would kill him myself before I'd let another gang kill him."[63] Perhaps this is hyperbole; or perhaps it is the result of very deep cultural trauma. One crack addict recalls, "My old man was into cocaine. . . . About a year ago he started bringing it into the house. . . . He told me we would be partners."[64] The children of gangbangers would often seek revenge against rival gangs for murdering their parents.[65] This cyclical, generational violence would only beget future generational violence.

58. Quoted in Godwin (1978), p. 194.
59. Leovy (2014), p. 90.
60. Quoted in Leovy (2014), p. 66.
61. Leovy (2014), p. 74
62. Godwin (1978), p. 185.
63. Quoted in Bing (1991), p. 50.
64. Quoted in Sterk (1999), p. 39.
65. Leovy (2014), p. 92.

And it passed down through white American families too.[66] Women played a major behind-the-scenes role in many of these homicides, verbally emasculating men who refused to take vengeance on those who disrespected them.[67]

Even if the police cared about patrolling high-crime neighborhoods like the Bronx, the most violent area of New York City in the late 1970s and early 1980s, they were still outmatched. In 1978, the 41st Precinct (that patrolled South Bronx), had only 364 police officers, which worked out to one officer for every 469 citizens. The entire city had one officer for every 243 New Yorkers. Firefighters and other first responders would have both insults and bricks thrown at them while trying to put out a fire or save someone's life. Other times, they were shot at. These firefighters and other first responders were ethnically integrated.[68] It mattered not. Violent crime skyrocketed. One night in New York City, in July 1987, competing crack gangs opened fire on each other. Nine bystanders near the shootout were hit by stray bullets.[69]

Even those crack dealers who came from good, stable homes could become ensnared by the culture of lethal retaliation within the lucrative underworld drug markets. Kenneth "Supreme" McGriff, head of a major crack enterprise, the "Supreme Team," operating in South Jamaica, Queens, snubbed the comfortable, middle-class life his parents had worked hard to provide for him. New York City prosecutor Carolyn Pokorney claimed, "[W]hen Supreme gets in a fight with somebody . . . He hires a hit team to assassinate them, to blow them away, so that their moms can barely recognize them when they go down to the morgue."[70]

CHACRUNA INSTITUTE AND THE NEW JIM CROW

With the arrival of crack came an exponential growth in the black American prison population. Michelle Alexander argues in her bestselling *The New Jim Crow* (2012) that this rise in black American incarceration occurred because drug laws specifically targeted them through the

66. Godwin (1978), pp. 206 *ff.*
67. Leovy (2014), p. 40.
68. Godwin (1978), p. 198.
69. Faber (2019), p. 57.
70. Quoted in Farber (2019), p. 57.

formulation of the War on Drugs.[71] And yet, the 1970s—when Nixon launched the War on Drugs—saw a shrinking prison population.[72] By 1994 the Justice Department found that in the 75 "largest urban areas" black Americans "had a lower chance of prosecution following a felony than [did white Americans] and were less likely to be found guilty at trial."[73]

Alexander ignores a lot of variables (specifically, the violent crime attached to crack-dealing) that led to the rise in incarceration in the 1980s and 1990s. She also neglects to mention that this "rise" in the prison population was marked against a lack of incarcerated black Americans in the past. During the Jim Crow 1930s, 77% of all prison inmates were white American, compared to 22% black American.[74] The white American incarceration rate was much higher because police patrolled white American neighborhoods. By the 1960s, largely due to much-needed Civil Rights protests, the police had marginally begun to patrol black American neighborhoods, and the prison population saw an increase, which is not surprising.[75] Revenge culture was still very much the vogue in those areas, a traumatic holdover from the previous generations. All the violent crimes that had until then been ho-hummed by the police due to systemic racism began to be investigated, resulting in what seems to Alexander like a manufactured boom in the prison population. What Alexander is really describing in *The New Jim Crow* is not some artificial creation of drug laws to target black Americans, but rather the beginning of police departments addressing the lawless cultures of lethal retaliation and silence (which were exacerbated by the crack trade) in inner cities and other depressed areas.

Never far behind Michelle Alexander, affiliates of Chacruna Institute also push this questionable addition to the Racist Narrative. "Drug laws," Williams, Reed, and George tell us, "were never applied evenly across racial groups, with Black Americans targeted by law enforcement

71. Michelle Alexander, *The New Jim Crow: Mass Incarceration in the Age of Colorblindness* (NY: The New Press, 2012), p. 60.
72. Leovy (2014), p. 157.
73. Mac Donald (2017), p. 153.
74. Reilly (2019), p. 38.
75. Bruce Drake, "Incarceration Gap Widens between Whites and Blacks," Pew Research Center (September 6, 2013).

and receiving longer and harsher sentences for identical violations of the law as compared to White Americans. . . . the War on Drugs became a vehicle for the mass incarceration of Black Americans."[76] This is an academic abstraction. Drug *laws* were applied evenly. It was the violent crimes that came hand-in-hand with certain addictive drugs like crack that caused the recent ethnic imbalance in the prison population—violent crimes that Michelle Alexander and Chacruna Theorists ignore. What also doesn't get applied evenly is the number of prior arrests for offenders when factoring jail or prison sentences. A majority of black American drug dealers and kingpins had several prior arrests before receiving their long stretches for getting caught selling crack.[77]

Williams, Reed, and George continue, "Crack cocaine penalties were much more stringent than penalties for powdered cocaine use, the only difference being that Black people were more likely to use crack and White people were more likely to use cocaine."[78] There are several problems with this assessment: first, the majority of US states (37 out of 50) make no legal distinction between cocaine and crack.[79]

Second, penalties for methamphetamine use are identical with those of crack. And meth is more often used by white Americans than by either black or Latin Americans.[80] Back in 2006, 5,391 meth users were arrested. Of those, 54% were white American, and 2% were black American (39% were Latin American).[81] Chacruna Theorists says nothing about these "racist" meth laws that target white and Latin Americans.

Third, plenty of white Americans smoked crack during the mid-80s and early 90s; in some areas, they were the majority users.[82]

Fourth, while Chacruna affiliates are correct that crack-using black Americans receive harsher sentences than blow-snorting white Ameri-

---

76. Williams et al., "Culture and Psychedelic Psychotherapy . . ." (2020), p. 127.
77. See Bing (1991); Leovy (2014); Sterk (1999).
78. Williams et al. (2020), p. 127.
79. Mac Donald (2017), p. 155.
80. Christopher M. Jones, "Patterns and Characteristics of Methamphetamine Use Among Adults—United States, 2015–2018," *Centers for Disease Control and Prevention* (March 27, 2020); Sean Esteban McCabe et al., "Race/Ethnicity and Gender Differences in Drug Use and Abuse Among College Students," in *The Journal of Ethnicity and Substance Abuse* (May 13, 2008).
81. Mac Donald (2017), p. 155.
82. Farber (2019), p. 4.

cans, they omit that Latin Americans *also* receive lighter sentences for bumping cocaine than do both black and white Americans for smoking crack (in those states where the penalties between the two drugs are different). Prior arrests dependent, of course.

Fifth, the discrepancy in arrests between black and white Americans had far more to do with, broadly speaking (and for lack of a better term), the different crack behaviors between them. When white Americans drove to the inner city to score a rock or two, they didn't hang around waiting for fireworks. They bought their crack and drove far, far away.[83] This also meant that white Americans were less likely to be around crack addicts or cooks than were black Americans. The larger a kingpin's operation grows, and the more addicts and criminals know who the major players are, the more difficult it becomes to keep one's associates (both dealers and users) in line. One dealer tells how a "former cook lost control of her drug habit and shared business secrets with outsiders, including other high-level dealers and law enforcement officials."[84] This is all high-risk illegal behavior that was drenched in lethal retaliation.

White Americans were mostly—though certainly not completely—removed from all that. They weren't the main source of income for the crack empires in New York, Washington, DC, Chicago, Baltimore, Philadelphia, and Los Angeles. *Daily*, repeat customers provided the crack entrepreneur's bread and butter. Crack addicts operate on very different processing software than the sporadic recreational user. Crack addicts have been known to target innocent people to get their fix: the elderly, the defenseless, and especially the undocumented. One man from East Harlem revealed quite matter-of-factly, "Everybody be ripping off [Mexicans]; they easy prey 'cause they illegal most of them. . . . Mexicans be fucked."[85]

Crack addiction broke down families and rotted out neighborhoods. One high roller in St. Albans, Queens, Corey Pegues, recalls dealing with "fiends [who] were breaking into cars for stereos, breaking into neighbors' cribs for television and VCRs, stealing their mom's jewelry, their kid's record player, anything they could trade for crack."[86] Detroit crack

83. Farber (2019), p. 49.
84. Sterk (1999), p. 55.
85. Quoted in Farber (2019), p. 93.
86. Quoted in Farber (2019), p. 92.

dealer Larry Chambers described his usual clientele: "a crackhead comes to you and his woman is on his back, his babies don't have no Pampers, he hasn't eaten in two days, and he's about to spend his last five dollars on crack."[87] One cab driver in Philadelphia paints a grim scene: "I've had my share of run-ins with these women on crack.... One night a woman flagged me down ... and I could tell right away she wasn't right. She looked like a broomstick, and I knew she was a piper. But she had this little baby with her, so I felt sorry for her." The cabbie decided to pick up the woman and offered to drive her to a shelter. The woman instead wanted to be dropped off at a crack house. "No way I'm gonna give her money for drugs," he continued, "... That little baby stank like piss, and the Pampers hadn't been changed in a long time. All [crack addicts] care about is getting that pipe.... They don't have any feeling. And they'll do you in for money. But she looked so bad, dragging that little baby around."[88] Child neglect cases doubled from 1980 to 1994; 75% of those cases involved drug abuse. The majority drug abused: crack.[89]

When making the argument that the War on Drugs specifically targeted black Americans, Michelle Alexander and Chacruna Theorists turn a blind eye to the drive-by shootings, the gang rapes, the assaults, the murder of children, the armed robberies, and the cultures of lethal retaliation and silence that are all staples in the crack-using subdivision within the otherwise larger law-abiding black American population. Crack dealers brought a brutality to criminal activity simply not seen among recreational cocaine users with a straw up their nose. Michelle Alexander and Chacruna Institute Theorists' focus on the *drug* and not the *violent crimes tied to the drug* is an unhelpful sleight-of-hand trick that impedes understanding the true nature of the problem. Only we need to understand the problem if we are to develop solutions that will actually deter people from both prison and the morgue.

Sincere as they are, Chacruna affiliates nonetheless draw this same erro-

87. Quoted in William M. Adler, *Land of Opportunity: One Family's Quest for the American Dream in the Age of Crack* (Ann Arbor: University of Michigan Press, 2021), p. 118.
88. Quoted in Anderson (1995), p. 90.
89. Farber (2019), p. 96.

neous conclusion when they insist that black Americans are arrested for smoking cannabis more than white Americans, "despite similar patterns of use."[90] They are joined by David Bronner, a famous and successful soap entrepreneur who openly endorses psychedelic medicines. Admirable and genuine as Bronner is, his rhetoric unfortunately includes an acceptance of the Racist Narrative, as we see with one of his Instagram posts: ". . . [T]he war on drugs has . . . disproportionately affect[ed] Black people, who are 3.64x more likely to be arrested for cannabis, despite the fact that Black & White people use cannabis at similar rates. . . . Black people [are] . . . also sentenced more harshly. Sentences imposed on Black men are almost 20% longer than those imposed on White men convicted of similar crimes."[91]

Associates at Chacruna Institute and David Bronner are overlooking a key element. Those people sitting in jail for smoking "cannabis" were usually arrested for some other crime (gun possession, brawling, parole violations, etc.) and got the charges dropped to cannabis possession due to jail or prison overcrowding, plea bargains, or both.[92] They most certainly were *not* "convicted of similar crimes."

There aren't many people of any ethnicity in lockup for simple possession of cannabis these days, as the plant is now legal in 39 states. The United States has seen a steady decline in cannabis possession arrests over the last decade. For example, 2014 saw 2,172 cannabis arrests (with an average sentence of five months). That number dipped by nearly a quarter by 2019 (1,734 arrests), and by 2021, that number plummeted to 145. Almost 80% of those arrests (78.9) occurred in a single district in Arizona. The majority of all those arrests were not black or white Americans, but undocumented Mexicans. By 2022, the Federal Bureau of Prisons reported not a single cannabis simple possession case.[93] It seems that many draconian cannabis laws are well behind us in most places in North America.

---

90. Wendy Chapkis, "What Psychedelic Researchers and Activists can Learn from Medical Marijuana Legalization" (April 21, 2017).
91. David Bronner (2023).
92. See Mac Donald (2016); Leovy (2014).
93. Vera M. Kachnowski et al., "Weighing the Impact of Simple Possession of Marijuana: Trends and Sentencing in the Federal Justice System," *United States Sentencing Commission* (January 2023), pp. 2–3.

Chacruna affiliates mention how black Americans at the time were not interested in psychedelics because of the stigma attached to drugs. "There was little interest within the Black community for drugs as a means of expanding consciousness or personal growth," they say.[94] Notwithstanding that some crack dealers also dabbled in mescaline and LSD,[95] they largely ignored psychedelics because they are not addictive (so no daily, repeat customers) and inexpensive (so no high turnover on investment), and therefore did not offer a road to riches. Furthermore, due to unfair political and social circumstances beyond their control, it seems like many impoverished black American drug users (or really anyone of any ethnicity in such an unfair position) simply favored *escapes* from reality (as delivered by crack) over encounters with ultimate reality (as delivered by LSD, mushrooms, etc.).

Impoverished white American meth addiction is no different. It would go a long way if Chacruna Theorists could acknowledge that.

Additionally, psychedelics tend to leave psychenauts questioning the world of materialism. It isn't uncommon for a person who drinks ayahuasca or eats large quantities of mushrooms to "go native," if you'll pardon an expression that hasn't aged well. While psychedelics also got wrapped up with rock and roll in the late 1960s, and bands like The Beatles, Jefferson Airplane, and The Doors all enjoyed commercial success, "corporate" later became a "dirty word" among the post-hippie generation.[96] By the late 1970s, those who clung to hippiedom started communal farms or moved to more remote places to enjoy quiet and simple lives. Crack dealers, on the other paw, with their pimped-out rides, rims, fat stacks, designer clothes, and objectification of women, happily embraced the decadence of the decade—the result of those who also wanted to wake up in a new American morning but found themselves stonewalled due to the echoes of white supremacy.

Herbert Marcuse's hope of building a new "ghetto population" proletariat had failed masterfully! Black Americans didn't want to overthrow capitalism, they wanted to buy into it. And they did so through the few ways available to many of them. Crack created jobs. Thomas

94. Williams et al., "Culture and Psychedelic Psychotherapy . . ." (2020), p. 127.
95. Sterk (1999), p. 32; Farber (2019), p. 192, note 19.
96. Alex Blimes, "Jay-Z on his Music, Politics, and his Violent Past," *GQ Magazine* (June 28, 2017; original, 2005).

Mickens, a once well-known kingpin in Queens, New York, used the millions he made selling crack to open up a string of stores, creating jobs in low-income neighborhoods. Many of those stores bore the name Montana (e.g., "Montana Dry Cleaners, Montana Sporting Goods") in homage to Tony Montana, the infamous mobster from the movie *Scarface*, and a name which Mickens had adopted for himself.[97] Others like hip hop mogul Jay-Z invested his crack profits into Rock-A-Fella Records. Christopher Wallace (1972–1997), aka Biggie Smalls, turned the crack game into a short-lived successful music career until the culture of lethal retaliation cut him down too soon.

The whole situation hits me in a weird way. As someone who has also sold excessive amounts of substantia, I understand the need and desire of turning illegal money into legal money. Only with my operation, no one died. No one's life was ever ruined. No one ever robbed their family and/or friends to "score" some of my mushrooms. I never got greedy; I never engaged in any unethical or immoral practices as I curried pounds of cannabis and mushrooms, and a few ounces of MDMA, across various state lines. I would pick up ounces of cannabis in Nashville, Tennessee, and drop them off in Kansas City, Missouri; pick up ounces of mushrooms in Kansas City and drive them to New Orleans; grab more cannabis in New Orleans and drop it off in St. Louis; procure MDMA (from just outside St. Louis) and drive to . . . *wherever*. And so on and so forth. I did this zigzagging across the country, all under the cover of teaching roller derby clinics, which I did too. Roller derby gear became a code for plant medicines, measured out in ounces. If a league needed "three helmets," I knew that meant "three ounces of mushrooms." Cannabis was measured in elbow (*sativa*) and knee (*indica*) pads, while "disco roller skates" secretly represented MDMA.

But the game only lasts so long, and any wise purveyor needs to plan an exit strategy before the police or Jesus call us home. Jay-Z, reflecting on his time as a crack dealer, sums up this feeling perfectly: "I knew the first day I stood on the block the clock was going backwards. It was a

97. Farber (2019), p. 123.

countdown."[98] Due to his extraordinary lyrical talent and genius business acumen, Jay-Z made it out before the clock timed out at zero.

The majority didn't.

Contemporary conservatives might consider that earlier apathetic police forces worked rather hard to earn the distrust of our black American sisters and brothers. And this police indifference, coupled with both a lack of opportunity in the legal world and untold riches in the underworld, promoted a culture of brutal criminality, lethal retaliation, and silence in the face of it all. This is the real story of racist policing in the United States—not over-policing, but under-policing.

Psychedelic SJWs might consider that real white supremacists make up a pathetically small minority these days, mostly relegated to backwoods areas and the butt of jokes. They might also recognize that a cultural handoff occurred as the 20th century gave way to the 21st. Police officers *do* care about black American lives today in a way most of their predecessors objectively did not.

It's time for conservatives and psychedelic SJWs to update their browsers.

Towards the end of the 1970s and into the 1980s, high crime neighborhoods were more and more often patrolled by black American officers—notably the LAPD.[99] This immediately raises a series of questions. Which aspect of an officer's black American life matters? Does a black American's life suddenly cease to matter when she puts on her blue uniform? What about a cadet at a police academy? Does her life stop mattering once she graduates? What if a black American gangster and a black American cop both die during an altercation? Whose life matters in that situation? What about black American police officers who have children that died from gang violence?[100] Does the child's life matter while the father's sorrow and trauma doesn't? Or how about a plainclothes black American police officer? Shall Team CSJ institute a 3/5ths compromise on her life?

98. Quoted in Farber (2019), p. 117.
99. Leovy (2014), p. 54
100. See Leovy (2014).

Furthermore, when we consider that police precincts like those in Portland and Minnesota were told to stand down and let BLM rioters burn cities and towns to ashes, it seems safe to say that white supremacy is over. When forensic psychiatrist Aruna Khilanani can deliver a virtual presentation at Yale (during the Covid pandemic) and speak of "unloading a revolver into the head of any white person that got in my way . . . relatively guiltless, like I did the world a fucking favor," it seems clear that white supremacy in the United States is, thankfully, a thing of the past.[101] Or consider the rash of "hate crime hoaxes" that has swept college campuses in recent years.[102] Across the United States, self-absorbed activist attention-seekers faked one "hate crime" after the next to show the infection of racism in the student body. There is an obvious problem with this strategy: if one has to invent racism on college campuses to prove that racism is a problem on college campuses, then racism probably isn't a problem on college campuses.

And can you think of a single segment of American society that is not ethnically integrated? Even John McWhorter, whose stellar book on the religiosity of Wokeism, I feel, is mistaken when he tells white Americans, "Figures of authority are the same color as you. . . . You are not subject to steroetypes."[103] *Really*? Our political body is a sea of diversity—more so than any political body anywhere else on Earth. I have personally been pulled over by black American police officers, searched by black American police officers, and stood before a black American judge. So have millions of other white Americans. As for white American stereotypes, I turn McWhorter's attention to any DEI indoctrination script.

Are there still racists in the United States today? Yes. Sadly, there are and always will be racists all over the world, and they should be called out (and *in*) when occasion arises. But in the United States today, they are drowned out by a common liberalism that reaches across both sides of the political aisle—that unshakable, uniquely American belief that we are all—body, mind, and soul—born free.

101. Quoted in Murray (2022), p. 64.
102. See Reilly (2019).
103. McWhorter (2021), p. 31.

Those greater forces at work that landed me in a jail cell for giving a homeless man a dollar grew from the first concerted efforts to combat the excessive crimes in inner cities and impoverished neighborhoods that had seeded violent subcultures of lethal retaliation and silence. And it worked. Violent crime plummeted in the late 90s and early aughts.[104] That was until a young man was shot by a neighborhood watch coordinator in Sanford, Florida, prompting the origins of a movement called Black Lives Matter.

104. See Mac Donald (2017), pp. 231–32.

11

Marijuana-Crazed: Dr. Hart and Trayvon Martin

I'm a gangsta.[1]

—Trayvon Martin

I worry that vociferous misinformed moralists, masquerading as scientists, misrepresent the available data.

—Dr. Carl Hart, *Drug Use for Grown-Ups*

What we can't do is cherry pick data or use anecdotal evidence to drive policy or to feed political agendas.[2]

—President Barack Obama

Misinformed Moralists

The Racist Narrative has funneled down from larger society into the writings of truly influential people within the psychedelic Renaissance like Columbia psychiatrist, drug researcher, and bestselling author Dr.

1. Quoted in Michael Pearson and David Mattingly, "Gun, Drug Texts Feature in New Trayvon Martin Shooting Evidence," *CNN* (May 23, 2013).
2. Quoted in Mac Donald (2017), p. 70.

Carl Hart. While I find agreement with Dr. Hart on many issues (most specifically our need to "grow up" about the subject of drugs),[3] I would like to focus on an area where I believe Dr. Hart lost his otherwise laudable scientific objectivity and rested on the partiality of the Racist Narrative in a way that strikes this author as detrimental to healing race relations in the psychedelic Renaissance and beyond. Nowhere is this more evident than his myth of the "marijuana-crazed Negro" unpacked with confounding verse in chapter 7 of his bestselling book, *Drug Use for Grown-Ups* (2021).

Hart believes that certain police abuses of power only target black Americans, writing that "cops in [Southern] regions routinely cite the smell of cannabis as justification for stopping, searching, or detaining black people."[4]

I have no doubt that is true.

However, I have experienced the same thing in upstate New York. Driving home from Lake George back in the summer of 2002 (or 2003—I don't quite recall), my friend Gordon (also white American) and I were pulled over in a small, shithole town called Ravena, a two-and-a-half-hour drive north from Manhattan. Officer Fennel (yes, I still remember the bastard's name) told me that he smelled a cannabis odor coming from my car. *Liar*, I immediately thought. I *never* smoked in my car; I hadn't even smoked cannabis earlier that day. Nonetheless, Fennel placed Gordon in handcuffs and put him in the back seat of the cop car, which I was ordered to stand beside motionless. The day was a real scorcher, I was sweating bullets and dying of thirst; I could only imagine what Gordon was going through—handcuffed in a police car with the windows rolled up and no air conditioning. Despite the August heat, he had decided to dress extra metal that day, so his black jeans, black tee shirt, and aqua-green and black flannel only meant an additional burden. I could see the panic pouring out of him with each drop of sweat—a worrisome combination of fear and heat. He looked like he might pass out.

Fennel proceeded to tear my car apart. Mind you, we had just spent a weekend at a lake, so we had a number of bags, camping/hiking/fish-

3. Hart (2021), p. 1 *ff.*
4. Hart (2021), p. 158.

ing gear, and such. Fennell shred through all of it, scattering shirts and socks and books and fishing tackle and CDs and swim trunks and all the rest of it on the side of the road. He then went into my trunk, which was filled with various kinds of crap (e.g., extra sweaters for cold beach nights, CD jewel cases, magazines, and other kinds of things one would expect to find in the trunk of anyone in their early twenties at century's turn)—all of it, strewn across the road. At one point Fennel turned to me exasperated and screamed, "Just show me where the drugs are!"

"I don't have any drugs," I replied. And that was true. I didn't even have an empty baggy. The search continued. Fennel lost his mind and ripped up the carpeting from the floorboard and the trunk. Still *nothing*. Part of the upholstery on the back seat of my fifteen-year-old Caddy had some frayed threads (as one might expect from an old car whose owner does not care about automotive cosmetics). Fennel ripped open the backseat upholstery and tore into the cushion, effectively dropping my car's resale value from about $70 to $5. Frustrated and likely looking to save face, he cited me for speeding (which hadn't even been mentioned until that point) *and* gave both Gordon and me appearance summonses—we would have to drive back to that shithole town Ravena to stand before a judge for . . . *what exactly*? Gordon was released and Fennel drove off, leaving torn cushion, carpeting, and a mess of our belongings on the side of the road for us to clean.

Although it sucked at the time, looking back with the knowledge that twenty years of hindsight affords, I realize now that perhaps I got off easy. Not everyone does. Here, I draw your attention to Columbia, Missouri, on the night of 11 February 2010 when a SWAT team kicked down the door of Jonathan Whitworth's home, shooting his dogs, killing one of them, and severally injuring the other. The bullets could have just as easily hit Jonathan, his wife Brittany, or their seven-year-old son, P.M. What possible threat did the Whitworth family pose that could justify the SWAT team's use of deadly force? Were the Whitworths stockpiling arms? Running a sex-traffic ring? Plotting to kill the president?

Hardly.

Little over a week before the incident, the police had been snooping through the Whitworth's garbage due to a neighbor complaining about the smell of cannabis. And while they did not find even so much as a stem or a seed among the trash, they did come across a tiny amount of cannabis *residue*. Not a grow-operation. Not an arsenal. Not bomb-making equipment. Not blueprints to the White House. Not children locked in the basement. Not even a dime bag. Just *residue*. The SWAT team "stormed in screaming, swearing, and firing their weapons, and within seconds . . . they intentionally shot and killed the family pit bull." Even more disconcerting is the fact that Columbia had already decriminalized small amounts of cannabis for personal use.[5]

Jonathan Whitworth is white American. A man who did nothing wrong and had one of his family members murdered by incompetent and out of control, over-militarized police officers. Instead of the municipality coughing up some compensation for this callous violation of the family's civil rights—to say nothing of basic human decency—Whitworth received a $300 fine for possessing "drug paraphernalia" (i.e., a pipe). His family's lawsuit against the SWAT team for the vile and premeditated murder of their dog was thrown out of court. The threat Jonathan, Brittany, P.M., or their puppies posed to society remains unclear to this day.

Is it asking Dr. Hart too much to broaden his gaze and consider that police overreach is not confined to a single demographic (black Americans) in a specific region (the South)? As outlined in the last chapter, the real racism of policing through much of the 20th century was lack of policing—not enforcement overreach. Many people of various ethnic backgrounds have had their rights violated by power-hungry police officers in many areas of the United States.

None of us enjoy those interactions.

Flawed Numbers

Dr. Hart points to a handful of tragedies to demonstrate the awful reality of the "cannabis makes black people homicidal" (as he terms it) trope: Philando Castile (1983–2016), Michael Brown (1996–2014), Keith Lamont Scott (1973–2016), Ramarley Graham (1993–2012), Rumain Brisbon (c. 1980–2014), and Sandra Bland (1987–2015). Let's

5. Radley Balko, *Rise of the Warrior Cop: The Militarization of America's Police Forces* (NY: PublicAffairs, 2014), p. xiii.

go through each of them and see where there is room for both agreement and disagreement with Dr. Hart. For starters, we can agree that all of those instances (and many more) were terrible tragedies. But we would also have to agree that there is an issue with Dr. Hart's tally. In five of the six cases that he says were "initiated under the pretense of cannabis-use suspicion"—i.e., those involving Sandra Bland, Ramarley Graham, Michael Brown, Philando Castile, and Rumain Brisbon—cannabis played no role whatsoever in the initial police interactions.[6] Bland was pulled over for a minor traffic infraction and committed suicide in jail. Graham was believed to have a gun (he didn't). Castile was pulled over because he fit the description of a robbery suspect. And the sad incident with Brisbon did involve a drug, but that drug was oxycodone, not cannabis.[7] The only cannabis leaves on Michael Brown's person were embroidered on his socks.

Let's stay with Brisbon for a moment. Officer Mark Rine, the cop who shot him, was already on the scene due to a burglary call. While there, dispatch reported a drug deal in progress involving Brisbon. By law, Officer Rine *had* to respond. When he did, a chase and a scuffle between Rine and Brisbon ensued. Brisbon reached for something in his pocket, which Rine thought was a weapon. Sadly, after repeatedly failing to follow the instructions of Rine (who was scared for his own life) to not remove his hand from his pocket—lest he brandish a weapon—Brisbon was shot twice.[8] The story is dreadful. And perhaps the saddest part was it could have been prevented. As Maricopa County Attorney Bill Montgomery remarked, "The decedent's continued unwillingness to follow directions, while acting consistent with someone who possessed a weapon and not once communicating anything otherwise, placed the police officer in reasonable fear for his life."[9] While it is true that Brisbon did not have a weapon, he, for reasons unknown, did

6. Hart (2021), p. 158–159.
7. I wish to note here that Brisbon *did* have a prior cannabis conviction—(as well as a burglary conviction and DUIs)—perhaps that is to which Dr. Hart refers? In any event, cannabis played no role in his untimely death. See Megan Cassidy, "Unarmed Arizona Man Killed by Cop," *The Arizona Republic* (Dec. 4, 2024).
8. Cassidy (2024).
9. Quoted Megan Cassidy, "No Charges for Phoenix Officer who Shot Unarmed Man," *The Republic* (April 1, 2015).

everything within his power to obscure that fact while scuffling with Officer Rine. We cannot expect Rine to have waited to find out the hard way whether or not Brisbon had a deadly weapon and intended to use it.

And just as terrible, frenetic police officers like Fennel have no problem harassing white Americans like Gordon and me, they also do not have a problem killing white Americans under certain circumstances, such as when an officer believes her own life is in immediate danger. Just as former officer Richard Haste believed Ramarley Graham to have a weapon he did not possess (and killed him[10]), officers in Tuscaloosa, Alabama, thought a fifty-year-old white man named Jeffory Tavis had a gun and killed him. He was, in fact, holding a spoon "in a threatening manner."[11] We find plenty of similar analogues to Brisbon's case as well. One need only look to the case of William Lemmon, a twenty-one-year-old white American who had robbed a grocery store. During the police pursuit, officer (now sergeant) Brian Armstead ordered Lemmon to remove his hands from his waistband. When he refused to comply, Armstead, fearing for his own life, shot him.[12] Sergeant Armstead is black American.

What Dr. Hart does not seem to realize is that for every example he can offer of an unarmed black American needlessly dying by police hands, there is a white American counterpart who perished under comparable circumstances that didn't make national headlines. As we will see in the next chapter, when the police shoot an unarmed white American the legacy media will ignore it, which creates a false narrative of police shootings dastardly enough to fool even Ivy League professors.

As for the killing of Keith Lamont Scott, the case is far more nuanced than simply pointing to the myth of the marijuana-crazed black American man and racist policing. Like the Brisbon case, the officers were already in the area responding to a call that had nothing to do with Keith Lamont Scott. At some point, Scott drove up in his white SUV

10. We can agree that the shooting of Ramarley Graham might have been excessive and uncalled for. Sadly, there isn't enough evidence to say either way.

11. Ciara McCarthy "Alabama Man with Spoon Killed by Officer had a 'Mental Episode,' Police Say," *The Guardian* (August 24, 2015).

12. Jane Morice, "Akron Police Officer's Fatal Shooting of Accused Armed Robber Ruled Justified" (July 2, 2016).

and parked. The officers on the scene watched him empty a cigar; they watched him fill it with cannabis; they watched him fashion it into a blunt. They ignored him. The whole scene went south when the officers noticed Scott had a gun, as it is illegal to possess both a weapon and a "controlled substance" at the same time.[13] Whether we agree with the law or not—and I don't, by the way—the officers were required to uphold it. They repeatedly told Scott to drop his weapon. Scott refused. Officer Brentley Vinson, himself black American, ended up shooting Scott. I find it difficult to count this case in Dr. Hart's favor as it was less a cannabis case and more a gun case. Otherwise, the officers would have used their initial witnessing of Scott smoking a blunt as a reason to investigate. But they didn't. They were fine to ignore him as they dealt with other matters. They only intervened when they saw the gun.

During the riots that followed Scott's death, Rayquan Borum, a black American youth, shot Justin Carr, a fellow black American youth, in the head.[14] No outcry. No call to stop the riots. No marches for justice. Race hustlers nowhere to be found.

Justin Carr's black life mattered.

As for that terrible incident in Ferguson, Missouri, between Officer Darren Wilson and Michael Brown, Wilson didn't beat the charges because the courts proved that Brown was high on cannabis; he beat the charges because the forensic evidence and eyewitness testimony corroborated his story that Brown attacked him and reached for his gun. Brown and his friend Dorian Johnson were walking down the middle of the street, and Officer Wilson noticed the former holding a box of stolen cigarillos. Here is a small sample from the eyewitnesses: A biracial man called Brown a "threat" to Officer Wilson. An elderly black American man who observed the shooting remarked that he "would have fucking shot that boy too." And yet, he refused to cooperate with the police for fear of going against the "hands up, don't shoot" lie first uttered by Johnson. In fact, Johnson's blatant and destructive lie was so incredible that despite a black American witness who told the police that "the shooting was justified," he added that he would deny everything if he were called

13. 18 U.S. Code § 922 – "Unlawful Acts," *Office of the Law Revision Counsel United States Code*.

14. "Rayquan Borum Found Guilty of 2nd-Degree Murder in Fatal Shooting during Charlotte Riots," *WBTV* (March 8, 2019).

to confirm his statement.[15] Even though the grand-jury subpoenaed him, his fear of his neighbors if he betrayed the Racist Narrative, within a wider cultural context of lethal retaliation and silence, kept him from appearing. He'd rather go to jail.

Dorian Johnson was not the only person to lie about the incident. A woman in her early thirties claimed to have seen Officer Wilson shoot Brown in the back. After investigators brought her the autopsy report, which showed her story to be fallacious, she admitted to fabricating her account.[16]

But none of this explains how Wilson and Brown ended up colliding with each other. Since in his book Hart did not explore how the encounter began, we shall now. Wilson stopped Brown and Johnson as they walked down the middle of Canfield Drive. Minutes earlier, Brown had strong-arm robbed a convenience store, Ferguson Market and Liquor. Surveillance footage from the shop shows a towering shoplifter grabbing the shop owner, Andy Patel, by his throat and pushing him into a snack display. Brown *was* that violent shoplifter. We are not dealing with the "gentle giant" with which his family and popular culture wished to cloak his memory.[17] We are dealing with a young man who picked a fight with a police officer minutes after he forcefully shoved and robbed a small business owner. Attorney General Eric Holder reportedly tried to use his political privilege in an attempt to suppress the Ferguson Market and Liquor surveillance footage from ever seeing daylight, while Benjamin Crump, the Browns' personal attorney, refused to disclose whether Michael Brown had a juvenile record. Exactly what he didn't want us to know about this gentle giant is anyone's guess, but clearly there was more to Brown's character than many wanted us to know.

Despite Dr. Hart's claim that Michael Brown's death was initiated by cannabis, the unfortunate encounter began because Brown and Johnson were obstructing traffic minutes after Brown stole $50 worth of cigarillos from a convenience store; and ended after Brown attacked Officer Wilson and tried to grab his service weapon.

---

15. Quoted in Mac Donald (2017), pp. 23–4.
16. Mac Donald (2017), p. 24.
17. Ken Ashby (Letter to the Editor) "Michael Brown; Thug or Gentle Giant?," *The Dallas Morning News* (August 29, 2014).

This is not to say that there isn't room for agreement between Dr. Hart and me. For example, I recall yelling expletives at my computer screen as I watched Diamond Reynolds's video of the shooting of her boyfriend, Philando Castile (1983–2016), at the hand Jeronimo Yanez, then an officer of the St. Anthony Minnesota police. My invective was directed at Yanez, who, so far as I could see, had just murdered Castile in cold blood.

It wasn't a routine stop—Castile had fit the description of one of two black American men who had committed armed robbery a week earlier; *that*, not cannabis, was why Yanez pulled him over. Police dash-cam rolling, we watch Yanez approach the driver side window of a 1997 Oldsmobile 88 LS. He asks Castile for his ID. At this point, as any law-abiding civilian with a concealed carry permit (CCP) does, Castile informed Yanez that he had a gun in his car. Yanez instructed him not to reach for it and Castile—as any law-abiding, CCP holder would do—complied. Instead, Castile reached for his wallet to produce the very license Yanez had requested. Yanez proceeded to fire seven shots into the car, with five hitting Castile.[18] Reynolds quickly pulled out her phone and opened her camera app.

The next moments are dreadful.

We watch Castile die.

That Yanez was not thrown in prison for murdering an innocent man is a gross miscarriage of justice. You'd be hard-pressed to find anyone who knows the facts of the case and thinks the shooting justified.

Dr. Hart sees it differently.

He writes that 2nd Amendment advocates "were practically silent about this injustice."[19] While he is correct that the National Rifle Association (NRA) (as an organization) did not respond as strongly as it should have, he is wrong to paint all gun owners with a broad brush. There is more to the story. The NRA initially declined comment due to the ongoing investigation (smart!), promising a more extensive statement "once all the facts [we]re known." When the cannabis in Castile's car was made public knowledge, the NRA *couldn't* comment—like it or not (and I don't like it at all). The NRA cannot condone "illegal" behav-

18. Hart claims that all seven hit Castile; see Hart (2021), p. 159.
19. Hart (2021), p. 159.

ior, even if the very illegality of said behavior is positively ridiculous.

The gun club's members, however, were "furious" over the lack of support for Castile. "We don't want the NRA to just be for old white guys," a member remarked.[20] Another member of the group called the shooting a "travesty."[21] I personally spoke with other 2nd Amendment advocates about the shooting: NRA member Tim Goins insisted that the shooting "should have been another reason to get rid of qualified immunity." His wife Rebecca (not an NRA member herself, but a 2nd Amendment absolutist) stated emphatically, "I feel [the shooting] wasn't justified. [Castile] told [Yanez] he had a gun that he could legally carry. There was no reason to shoot Castile so many times either. . . . There are way better organizations that would have taken Castile's side. The NRA fucked themselves on that one."[22] A single, refreshingly nuanced headline from *The Washington Post* sums up the dichotomy: "Gun Owners are Outraged by the Philando Castile Case. The NRA is Silent."[23]

We might also consider that Dr. Hart overlooked two facts that I believe are somewhat relevant to the Racist Narrative; the first consideration is rather straightforward: Yanez is Latin American. The second is a little more nuanced. Dr. Hart lists the Castile shooting as initiating because of cannabis suspicion. That is *almost* correct; but does not offer a full picture of the events leading up to the shooting. Castile's car did smell of the Lord's plant. However, cannabis had nothing to do with Yanez's initial detaining of Castile and everything to do with the latter fitting the description of an armed felon detailed in an all-points bulletin (APB). In Yanez's official police statement, he admitted that he "wasn't going to say anything about the marijuana yet because I didn't want to scare him or have him react in a defensive manner." What concerned Yanez was the *gun*—not the cannabis.[24] And while it is true that Yanez tried to blame the smell of cannabis emitting from Castile's car as the

20. Quoted in Jazz Shaw, "Yes, the NRA (and all of us) Should be Speaking out on the Philando Castile Shooting," *Hot Air* (June 21, 2017).
21. Quoted in Avi Selk, "Gun Owners are Outraged by the Philando Castile Case. The NRA is Silent," *The Washington Post* (June 27, 2017).
22. Rebecca Goins, pers. comm.
23. Selk (2017).
24. SA Doug Henning and SA Christopher Olson, "Interview of Officer Jeronimo Yanez," *Minnesota Department of Public Safety Bureau of Criminal Apprehension Transcript* (July 6, 2016), p. 13.

reason he "feared for his life," there's hardly a rational person who believes him.[25] Cannabis didn't *really* have anything to do with the initial encounter. It merely provided *ex post facto* justification for a murdering imbecile who shouldn't be allowed to handle a butter knife, let alone a firearm. However, in the spirit of fraternity and out of respect for Dr. Hart, since cannabis *was* actually mentioned as part of the reason for the shooting (despite its questionable nature), I am willing to call this case a draw.

However, Dr. Hart's contention that people simply have no compassion for the illegal slaughter of black American men is unfounded and, quite frankly, insulting.[26] My own white American stomach turned as I watched Reynolds's video of Castile's murder; I haven't taken a formal survey, but I'm willing to bet millions of other white American stomachs turned too. This terrible tragedy represented a rare instance of compassion and righteous indignation that "managed to unite critics from opposite ends of the ideological spectrum."[27] This case was hardly split over color lines. To present it as such, as Dr. Hart does, only serves to divide us unnecessarily.

We've drunk the sacred vine, my fellow inner-travelers.

We should see beyond this.

Castile falls into that most horrible category of black American men murdered at the hands of incompetence at best and evil at worst. Though, such horrible encounters are what happen the *least*. As we will see in the next chapter, statistically speaking, more unarmed white American men are shot by the police every year, despite black American men having more confrontational interactions with law enforcement.

Let's now reassess Dr. Hart's claims in light of the aforementioned facts: Philando Castile was shot by a Latin American officer. Keith Lamont Scott was shot by a black American officer. Sandra Bland died at the hands of a black American woman—her own. Notwithstanding the murder of Ramarley Graham, of which I am truly at a loss to determine if it was justified (there isn't enough evidence), the two other cases he presents involving a white American officer shooting a black American

25. Christopher Ingraham, "Officer who Shot Philando Castile said Smell of Marijuana Made Him Fear for His Life," *The Washington Post* (June 21, 2017).
26. Hart (2021), p. 159.
27. Selk (2017).

suspect (i.e., Michael Brown and Rumain Brisbon) ignore the fact that both officers endured a physical attack before using deadly force.

Dr. Hart saves the bulk of his argument to discuss the unfortunate end of Trayvon Martin (1995–2012), a young man who lost his life back in 2012 after assaulting an armed neighborhood watch coordinator, George Zimmerman, who had been briefly following him, which ignited the Black Lives Matter Movement. Dr. Hart tells us that, due to Martin's age, this incident "hit home more acutely" than the other tragedies.[28] Here, he is following the President Barack Obama (and later, the New York Mayor Bill de Blasio) strategy of pretending that young black American men like Hart's own son are more threatened by the police than they are by other young black American men. Such blindness to the grim realities facing young inner-city black American men helps no one—especially young inner city black American men, whose lives matter.

Still, I'd like to find room for agreement. While some authors have pointed to the possibility that Trayvon Martin was a drug dealer, I agree with Dr. Hart that such a detail doesn't matter in the least. On the other paw, Dr. Hart makes a big to-do about whether or not Trayvon Martin had smoked cannabis before his terminable meeting with George Zimmerman—a much bigger to-do than Mark O' Mara, the lead defense attorney, ever did. While I do agree with Dr. Hart that whether or not Martin had ever smoked or sold cannabis is inconsequential to the facts of the case, in this instance, Dr. Hart is straw-manning the defense's strategy by over emphasizing the cannabis angle. The improbable stereotype of the "menacing cannabis smoker" is laughable. Still, I feel the need to address Hart's handling of the facts if for nothing more than to highlight a blind spot that seems to arise around these kinds of topics in even highly intelligent people. Dr. Hart points out that Martin's toxicology report showed a "mere 1.5 nanograms of THC per milliliter of blood in his body. This finding strongly suggests he had not ingested marijuana

28. Hart (2021), p. 159.

for at least twenty-four hours," he claims.[29]

Dr. Hart might have first checked with fellow Columbia professor, neurobiologist Dr. Margaret Haney, before drawing such conclusions. Dr. Haney is the Director of the Cannabis Research Laboratory at the university, and she has a *very* different idea about how cannabis can be measured in the body. Commenting on the difficulties police have testing cannabis levels in a detained motorist, Dr. Haney says, "It's really difficult to document drugged driving in a relevant way . . . [because of] the simple fact that THC is fat soluble. That makes it absorbed in a very different way and much more difficult to relate behavior to, say, [blood] levels of THC."[30] In other words, the amount of THC in Martin's blood cannot be used to determine how much cannabis was in his system. As Ziff Professor of Columbia's Department of Psychology, who has given "literally thousands of doses of marijuana and ha[s] completed multiple studies assessing the neurophysiological, psychological, and behavioral effects of the drug," perhaps Dr. Hart should have known that?[31]

Still, I'd like to underscore Dr. Hart's point and reinforce it: I would argue that Trayvon Martin could have been high as a kite on cannabis, and it still would not have mattered. To agree with Dr. Hart again, cannabis most certainly does *not* cause aggressive behavior, but rather "contentment, relaxation, sedation, euphoria, and (as we all know too well) increased hunger."[32] Zimmerman's defense team knew that. Of course they knew that! *Everyone knows that!* And that is why cannabis didn't merit much ink in the trial dossiers at all, despite Dr. Hart's claim contrariwise.[33] Whether or not Trayvon Martin was high on cannabis isn't the question.

---

29. Hart (2021), p. 161.
30. Quoted in Angus Chen, "Why is it So Hard to Test Whether Drivers are Stoned?" *NPR: Health News from NPR* (February 9, 2016).
31. Hart (2021), p. 160.
32. Hart (2021), p. 160
33. While I agree with Dr. Hart that cannabis does not make a person aggressive, it can make a person paranoid. Though, I do not believe that such paranoia can be blamed for the encounter between Martin and Zimmerman. The reason I think so is, well, personal: for those times that I have regrettably experienced paranoia caused by cannabis, never once did I decide to try and fight someone. In fact, such cannabis-induced paranoia rendered me quite terrified of even pleasant conversations with friends!

It's his *aggressiveness that evening* with which we must contend.

LAYERS OF TRAYVON

Unnoticed by Dr. Hart is a deeper level to this story found in Trayvon's toxicology report. Cannabis aside, Martin also dabbled in a drink called "lean" (or "purple drank" or "sizzurp"), a strong sedative and euphoriant. First concocted in Houston, Texas, around the local blues scene in the 1960s, lean is a hazardous mix of soda (usually Sprite or 7 Up); candy (like Jolly Ranchers, Nerds, or Skittles); and prescription, codeine-containing cough syrup (or over-the-counter brands like Robitussin). This drink, the ingredients of which are obtainable at any Walgreens, CVS, or local pharmacy, is a dangerous brew indeed. Around the turn of the century the drink moved into the hip hop community courtesy of songs like Three 6 Mafia's "Sippin' on Some Syrup" released in 2000. Houston-based DJ Robert Earl Davis Jr. (better known as DJ Screw), who championed the drink, died of a risky mix of lean, valium, and PCP (aka angel dust). Unlike smoking cannabis, drinking lean *does* cause aggressiveness.

Travyon Martin's use of lean is not speculation. Let's get back to his toxicology report, which makes a curious reference to a "patchy yellow discoloration" on Martin's liver—a telltale sign of lean usage.[34] Dr. Hart read the toxicology report—how did he overlook a damaged liver on an otherwise healthy seventeen-year-old? And while we don't know exactly when Martin started drinking lean, he did leave us a digital trail that begins a year prior to his tragic death. In July 2011 Martin began following the YouTube channel of Andy Milonakis, who, a month earlier (21 June 2011), had released a song titled "Red Lean, Purple Lean," featuring the Shakespearean lines:

Codeine ho clean off my dick
With your pretty red lips bitch, take off your lipstick
Put some purple syrup on it then suck my dipstick[35]

---

34. Office of the Medical Examiner Florida, Districts 7 & 24, "Medical Examiner Report" (February 27, 2012), p. 4.
35. Andy Milonakis, "Red Lean, Purple Lean" (June 20, 2011).

In a FaceBook message Trayvon sent to a person called Mackenzie DumbRyte Baksh, he spoke of having drunk a similar concoction and wanting to know where he could find more "codine . . . liquid." Mackenzie reminds Trayvon that he could just use Robitussin and soda to "make some fire ass lean."

Here is their conversation in full:

Trayvon: unow a connect for codine?
Mackenzie: why ni[**]a
Trayvon: to make *some more*[36]
Mackenzie: u tawkin bout the pill codeine
Trayvon: no the liquid its meds. *I had it b4*[37]
Mackenzie: hell naw u could just use some robitussin nd soda to make some fire ass lean
Trayvon: codine is a higher dose of [Dextromethorphan[38]]
Mackenzie: I feel u but need a prescription to get it[39]

Some have also pointed to what Trayvon Martin bought at 7-Eleven before his encounter with Zimmerman: Skittles and a drink. Those two items have been used to paint the picture of an innocent boy who only wanted to enjoy some candy and have a beverage to wash it down. Some defenders of Martin, like the hip hop duo G-Twinz, have called the beverage he bought "iced tea."[40] But that's not what it was. Trayvon had actually purchased AriZona Watermelon Fruit Juice Cocktail—not iced tea. This might seem inconsequential, but some critics of the shooting see that particular drink as telling, noting that, along with the Skittles, what Trayvon had actually bought was 2/3rds of the ingredients needed to make lean.[41]

Personally, I am not convinced. For all we know, Martin simply had a hankering for some fruit-flavored goodies on a rainy night. Nor do we know if he had any Robitussin at the condo. And anyway, isn't the

36. *Italics* mine.
37. *Ditto*
38. The active drug in Codeine.
39. Quoted in Cashill (2013), p. 150.
40. G-Twinz, "Skittles and Iced Tea" (August 13, 2013).
41. Adam Gussaw, "The Test: Rethinking Trayvon," *Southwest Review* Vol. 106, Issue 2, Southern Methodist University (Summer 2021).

usual liquid base for lean Sprite or 7 Up? Both are easily purchasable at any 7-Eleven. Regardless, the lean that he certainly had been using over the prior year had started to have a negative effect on his temperament. Overuse of codeine causes anxiety, depression, aggression, and impulsivity.[42]

The kinds of things that can cause a person to start a fight.

Lean aside, Dr. Hart also seems unaware of other particulars about Martin's life. Not long before his tragic end, an exchange Martin had on social media suggests he punched a bus driver.[43] He was also involved in what can be described as semi-organized underground street fighting where he both refereed some fights and participated in others. After one of his last fights, he told a friend via cell phone text that he was pissed because his opponent "aint b[l]eed nuff 4 me, only his nose . . . he gone hav 2 see me again." Often filming the fights, Martin would upload them to his YouTube channel. An anonymous female friend of Martin even noticed his change in behavior, texting him, "Bae y you always fighinqq . . . yuu needa stop fighting bae Forreal."[44]

Moreover, we also know that on his way to Green's condo after his suspension from school, Martin looked into buying a gun—a .380 specifically.[45] A photo on his cell phone indicates that at some point he might have gotten his hands on one.[46] However, just as attorney Benjamin Crump would refuse to reveal certain information about Michael Brown to the public after Darren Wilson shot him, he did the same for Trayvon Martin after George Zimmerman shot him. But enough of the real Trayvon Martin slipped through Crump's dragnet. By all accounts

42. David O' Reilly et al. "Cough, Codeine, and Confusion," *British Medical Association* (2015), p. 2.
43. "Trayvon Martin Shooting: New Details Emerge from Twitter Account, Witness Testimony," *The Cutline* (March 26, 2012).
44. Quoted in James Myburgh, "The Hunting of George Zimmerman," *Politicsweb* (August 14, 2013).
45. Lizette Alvarez, "Defense in Trayvon Martin Case Raises Questions about the Victim's Character," *The New York Times* (May 23, 2013).
46. I say "might have gotten" because the photo shows only a hand holding the gun. However, I think it would be naive to believe that it was anyone else's hand besides Trayvon's. Still, we can only speculate.

(including both Trayvon Martin's and his friends' own words), he was *violent.*

Very violent.

News outlets joined the cover-up by only reproducing earlier pictures of Martin when he was thirteen-years-old, despite the media standard, which is to use the most recent photos of suspects, victims, and arrestees.[47] In this case, however, the more recent photos of Martin showed him possibly holding a gun or giving the camera the middle finger in a quasi-tough guy pose. This last point—his quasi-tough guy pose—I personally couldn't care less about.

I mention it only as part of the cover-up.

Martin also favored a level of misogyny on par with Donald Trump's infamous "grab 'em by the pussy" comment; his now-deactivated Twitter account had this post: "fuck a bitch, any bitch, who you want? Take yo pick." And another crack at romantic poetry: "Hahaha Hoe u got USED fa yo loose ass pussy.! Tighten up.! #Literally."[48]

The Incident

How exactly did Martin and Zimmerman end up in a confrontation in the first place? Once again, Dr. Hart's handling of the case needs an overhaul. Let's review a sample of how he describes the encounter:

> But before [Martin] could safely arrive [home], he was scoped like game, stalked as if in the wild, and fatally shot by the neighborhood vigilante, George Zimmerman. The twenty-eight-year-old Zimmerman, who identifies as white, phoned the local police nonemergency number after merely spotting Trayvon en route to his father's place and claimed the teen looked like 'he's on drugs.' For no apparent reason, Zimmerman then chased the youngster, ignoring the dispatcher's directive to the contrary. 'We don't need you to do that,' the dispatcher admonished Zimmerman. Minutes later, he had drawn a 9 mm semiautomatic pistol and killed a child in cold blood.[49]

47. Alicia Shepard, "The Iconic Photos of Trayvon Martin & George Zimmerman & Why You May Not See the Others," *Poynter* (March 30, 2012).
48. "Trayvon Martin's 'NO_ LIMIT_ NI[**]A' Tweets," *The Daily Caller* (2024).
49. Hart (2021), pp. 159–60.

Notwithstanding three facts (all unimportant to the larger point), everything Dr. Hart thinks about this incident is incorrect. Before we unravel his narrative, let's see what he got right; first: Zimmerman did call the nonemergency number (instead of the emergency number). This would indicate to the careful observer that Zimmerman did not perceive Martin as a threat at first. Wouldn't a racist vigilante, as Dr. Hart imagines Zimmerman, call the emergency number?

Second: Zimmerman did tell the dispatcher, Sean Noffke, that Martin looked to be impaired.

Third: By the end of the confrontation, Trayvon Martin was dead. However, regarding all the *crucial* points—i.e., what led the two to come to fisticuffs in the first place—Dr. Hart is wrong on all counts. Let's take a look at the environment of the Retreat at Twin Lakes (heretofore referred to as "the Retreat" for ease), the condominium where Zimmerman lived, to gain some insight.

Construction on the Retreat in Sanford, Florida, had begun in 2004 with the intention of building a scenic middle-class complex. Investors bought condos hoping to flip them in the coming years. When the real estate market (and just about everything else in the United States) went belly-up in 2008 due in large part to predatory lending, the Retreat got swept in the undertow. Investors could no longer flip their condos, so instead resorted to renting them to just about anyone who came calling, ignoring basic background and credit checks.

The Retreat slowly deteriorated; violent crime spiked in 2010. One mother had three men break into her home. She barricaded herself and her baby son in a bedroom until the police showed up. Another resident was selling cocaine out of his mom's condo. Still another resident had two grills and a bicycle stolen from his porch. In just the first two months of 2012 leading up to Trayvon Martin's death on February 26th, residents of the Retreat called the police thirteen times—a mix of assaults, break-ins, and thievery. But those calls were only for *active* crimes. If we were to add *all* the calls made to the police (including crimes already committed), the number climbs to a staggering fifty-one! Fifty-one police calls in just under sixty days. Does your neighborhood look like that? If not, then it might be best to reserve judgment on the people who live in such surroundings. People like George Zimmermann and his neighbors.

As one can imagine, the residents of the Retreat made a fuss to the homeowner association. The result was a meeting headed by Sanford Police Department's volunteer coordinator Wendy Dorival. She urged the twenty-five (or so) residents who showed up to the meeting to pick a neighborhood watch coordinator. George Zimmerman seemed the obvious choice.[50]

Zimmerman had a good reputation in the community. A civil rights activist who had worked with the NAACP, Zimmerman had earlier campaigned to get a white American police lieutenant's son, Justin Collison, in legal trouble due to his unreported assault on a homeless black American man, Sherman Ware. And while the Sanford police were all too happy to sweep Ware's assault under the rug, it was Zimmerman who sought and won justice for him. Zimmerman also acted as "big brother" to two young black American youths via a program of the same name. The FBI took statements from thirty-five associates of Zimmerman—a mix of friends, coworkers, and neighbors—all of whom "had never seen Zimmerman display any prejudice or racial bias."[51] There is a reason the homeowner association turned to him.[52]

Dr. Hart is trying to paint the most extreme version of George Zimmerman possible: a trigger-happy, crazy, white American vigilante. And yet, he isn't any of those things. He isn't white American (he's ethnically mixed), isn't trigger-happy or crazy, and was, by definition, not a "vigilante." Vigilantes operate outside the law. Zimmerman was handed the community watch coordinator's handbook by Wendy Dorival (herself Latin American), director of the Sanford Police Department's volunteer program. I take no joy in what I am about to ask, but I'm curious what reason Dr. Hart had to call George Zimmerman a "white neighborhood

50. Cashill (2013), p. 40–1.

51. Quoted in Cashill (2013), p. 145.

52. Like all of us, Zimmerman was no angel. Issues with his former fiancée show that Zimmerman had his own demons with which to contend. While this fact is inconsequential to what happened on 26 February 2012, I mention it merely to present as full a picture of the man as possible. George Zimmerman is what we *all* are: complicated. See Cashill (2013), p. 145.

vigilante" who "identifies as white" if not to unnecessarily race-bait?[53] And the Retreat isn't very "white" either, but rather a multiracial community.

Zimmerman had good reason for thinking Trayvon Martin a criminal... because he *was* a criminal. A low-level criminal, for certain, but the facts remain. The following point will allow me to address not just Dr. Hart's mistaken assessment of the Zimmerman shooting, but also comments made by Marc Lamont Hill, host of *Black News Tonight*, during his refreshingly cordial conversation with Christopher Rufo, contributing editor of *The City Journal*. Lamont Hill laments that high school–aged black American kids are disciplined harsher than their white American peers.[54] Chacruna Institute board member, Dr. Monnica Williams, agrees, claiming "teachers racially profil[e] Black children starting in preschool."[55]

I ask Lamont Hill, Dr. Williams, and anyone else who holds such ideas to consider that studies have been conducted in this area. Back in 2012, the same year Martin met his unfortunate end, *The Philadelphia Enquirer* listed thirty thousand "violent incidents" in many minority government schools, including "robberies, rapes, and a pregnant teacher [getting] punched in the stomach." The very next year, the National Center for Education Statistics (NCES) listed its own numbers on violence in schools: countrywide, 12.8% of black American kids admitted to engaging in fistfights while at school compared to 6.4% of white American kids. So as to be scientific about these disparities, the NCES surveyed students a second time the following year. The numbers had barely moved: 12.6% of black American kids had a violent encounter with another student compared to 5.6% of white American kids. Students and teachers of 1,200 government schools (some majority black American, others majority white American) were once again surveyed in 2019, this time through the Fordham Institute. The researchers found that teachers working in low-income government schools admitted that

53. Hart (2021), p. 161.
54. "Marc Lamont Hill Interviews Key Opponent of Critical Race Theory," *Black News Tonight* (May 25, 2021).
55. Williams, "When Feminism . . .," in Labate and Cavnar (2021), p. 24.

"verbal disrespect was a daily occurrence." So were fistfights and battery against teachers. The study also found that, despite such high numbers, "underreporting of serious incidents was 'rampant.'" Such is the over-correction of equitable policing, as reporting violent crimes simply isn't fair and clearly a sign of white supremacy.

And while Lamont Hill and Dr. Williams can endlessly excuse that hard data, black American teachers are the ones suffering in the crossfire. In fact, those black American teachers surveyed stated that their black American students needed *more* discipline, not less; 60% of whom said that such violence *obviously* makes teaching and learning a Sisyphean task.[56] When we check all the available data about student suspensions that Lamont Hill and Dr. Williams disregarded, it becomes difficult to find some current, clandestine "white supremacy" angle to any of it.

Let's now see how these same equitable policies served Trayvon Martin. His use of lean and propensity for violence went unchecked. The equitable politic likely left him feeling entitled to do more or less whatever he wanted without suffering too harsh a penalty, receiving more passes and privileges for his behavior than I ever did at his age. He attended Dr. Martin M. Krop Senior High, a school within the Miami-Dade County Public Schools, one of few educational networks to have its own law enforcement, the Miami-Dade Schools Police Department (M-DSPD).

Former chief of the department, Charles Hurley, worried about the higher arrest rates for black American males and so practiced a very lenient, equitable system, urging his officers to "basically lie and falsify" police reports, as Sergeant William Tagle (himself Latin American) testified.[57] And who benefited the least from these dishonest practices? Tagle pulled no punches: "[Hurley] mentioned, in a statement, of changing the philosophy in our department, particular[ly to] young African American boys to avoid arrest. It alarms me that my Hispanic, white, Asian, and even Pakistani friends are at risk in the School District with Chief Hurley's philosophy," he testified.[58] Commander Deanna

56. Studies and quotations paraphrased from McWhorter (2021), pp. 99–101.
57. "Sworn Statement of Sergeant William Tagle," Miami-Dade Police Department (2012), p. 55.
58. "Sworn Statement of Sergeant William Tagle" (2012), p. 48.

Fox-Williams, a black American officer, also admitted that Hurley had directed her to fabricate police reports—so much so that a certain Major Gerald D. Kitchell admonished her to "start writing reports as is; don't omit anything."[59] In fact, Hurley would later come under fire, getting demoted for using such deceptive tactics "to manipulate the system and make himself look better."[60] He later resigned.

Let's take a moment and reflect on an interesting point that Lamont Hill, Dr. Williams, and affiliates at Chacruna Institute and Psymposia would prefer we ignored: according to sworn officer statements, Chief Hurley, who is white American, wanted to lie in police reports to keep the black American arrest statistics down, and black and Latin American officers disapproved of this practice.

But what did Hurley's equitable criminology look like in action? We need only look to Trayvon Martin to find out. Martin had been suspended from school twice on charges that, had I done such things, would have gotten me arrested. And here is where Hurley's clever fudging of the circumstances did not do the troubled Martin any good. When police officers found stolen items (a watch, women's jewelry) and burglary tools in Martin's backpack, they listed them as "found property."[61] Not *stolen* property—*found* property. To keep things equitable.[62] Moreover, the officers were to kick these kinds of cases back to the schools for discipline instead of processing perpetrators through the police department.

Due to the mishandling of Martin's criminal enterprises by the M-DSPD, his parents were never the wiser of how much their teenager was slipping. Since the police department was tied to the school, his records were sealed as "educational" during the trial instead of "criminal,"

---

59. "Sworn Statement of Deanna Fox-Williams," Miami-Dade Police Department (2012), pp. 10–11.

60. Christiana Lilly, "Charles Hurley, Miami-Dade Schools Police Chief, Won't Face FDLE Criminal Investigation," *The Huffington Post* (May 30, 2012).

61. "Sworn Statement of Sergeant William Tagle" (2012), p. 9.

62. Such equitable criminology isn't confined to Florida. In Arlington County, Virginia, attorney Parisa Dehghani-Tafti partnered with the Vera Institute of Justice to "find ways to reduce the incarceration of black people" along similar equitable justice practices. See, Rachel Weiner, "Arlington Prosecutor Promises Data-Driven Reduction in Racial Disparities," *The Washington Post* (April 24, 2021); Murray (2022), p. 150. In recent years, the Chicago Police Department has also begun volleying black American youth criminal activity back to their respective high schools; see Mac Donald (2017), p. 131.

which they were. Martin supporters objected that since he was a minor, his school records were protected under the Family Educational and Privacy Rights Act (FERPA). And this is certainly true. However, FERPA clearly states that this does not include "records maintained by the law enforcement unit of the educational agency or institution that were created by that law enforcement unit for the purpose of law enforcement."[63] In other words, sealing Trayvon's records was unethical. Perhaps even obstruction.

So Trayvon never ended up in the criminal justice system, which somewhat ironically, might have saved his life. And it wasn't a bad life. Martin was more a wanna-be gangster than any real threat to society. His parents were middle class—his mother a public housing official and his father a truck driver. They certainly earned enough income to provide stable and loving homes for Trayvon. It was the parental *guidance* that was missing.

Far from the poster-child of youthful innocence, Trayvon was tragically closer to a poster-child for demonstrating how equitable policing destroys young black American lives.

As for how Zimmerman and Martin came to blows, everything Dr. Hart says about it is mistaken. Zimmerman didn't stalk Martin "as if in the wild," as Dr. Hart suggests, but rather observed him lurking outside various condos in the rain, peeking through windows.[64] Given the crime wave that was running through the Retreat at the time and Zimmerman's position as watch coordinator, his neighbors counted on him to look out for suspicious behavior. Zimmerman didn't recognize Martin because, despite Dr. Hart's claim that Martin was headed to "his father's place," that isn't true;[65] he was heading to the home of Brandy Green, his father's girlfriend. Trayvon's mother, fed up with his behavior, had "kicked [him] out"—Martin's own words—of her home.[66] That is why Zimmerman initially made the nonemergency call—he didn't recognize Martin as a resident of the Retreat.

63. 20 U.S.C § 1232g (a) (4); "Sworn Statement of Deanna Fox-Williams" (2012), p. 51.
64. Hart (2021), p. 159.
65. Hart (2021), p. 160.
66. Quoted in Cashill (2013), p. 167.

Because Martin *wasn't* a resident of the Retreat.

And Zimmerman did not chase down Martin. The full conversation between Zimmerman and dispatch operator Noffke, which Dr. Hart only selectively sampled, tells the real story. While Dr. Hart is correct that Zimmerman *at first* followed Martin to keep a visual on him, that's only because Noffke asked him which way Martin was headed. For that reason, and only that reason, Zimmerman started to trail Martin. When Noffke told Zimmerman to stop following Martin, he did just that, and returned to his car—*which is why the confrontation took place near his car.* Had Zimmerman really been "stalking" Martin, the altercation would have happened closer to Green's condo.

Dr. Hart's assessment of the incident also ignores the fact that—according to the forensic evidence—Martin had four minutes to travel 100 yards to Green's home. A "walking time calculator" places the amount of time to travel the distance between where Zimmerman first saw Trayvon and Green's condo at about a minute and fifteen seconds. And that's at a *casual* pace—we happen to know that Martin *ran*, not walked, to the condo.[67] In fact, Martin had made it to Green's home safely, according to witness number 8, Rachel "Dee Dee" Jeantel, who was on the phone with him at the time of the incident.[68]

But at some point, he decided to turn around and confront Zimmerman.

The "defenseless black boy," as Dr. Hart imagines him, proceeded to sucker-punch Zimmerman, breaking his nose with that single blow.[69] He then got on top of Zimmerman "[Mixed Marital Arts]-style" and rained down hits to his head, as eye witness number 6, John Good, testified.[70] Then the defenseless boy grabbed Zimmerman's shirt collar and repeatedly pounded the back of his head onto the concrete dog walk. The last thing this helpless kid said to Zimmerman was "Your gonna die tonight, Mother F[uck]er" as he reached for the latter's gun *à la* Michael

67. Lizette Alvarez, "At Zimmerman Trial, Victim's Friend is Pressed on Her Story," *The New York Times* (June 27, 2013).
68. "Bernie de la Rionda Interview with Rachel 'Dee Dee' Jeantel," in Cashill (2013), p. 131.
69. Hart (2021), p. 161.
70. "John Good's Testimony" (March 20, 2012), p. 40.

Brown and Darren Wilson.[71] In that moment (his nose broken, his head bloody, verging on unconsciousness), Zimmerman had every reason to believe Martin's assertion. Unwilling to become another number in a violent crime statistic, Zimmerman pulled out his gun and fired.

Zimmerman hardly "scoped [Martin] like game" or murdered him in "cold blood." And his initial nonemergency call had nothing to do with race (which he didn't mention until Noffke asked) and everything to do with the recent crime wave occurring at the Retreat.

So what killed Trayvon Martin? The police department's focus on equitable policing. The school that excused his criminality. The specific kind of harmful drug culture in which he partook. The need to act tough to complement a specific kind of shallow, tough guy social media image. Capable, but inattentive, parents.

Trayvon Martin's killer was his *environment*.

George Zimmerman just so happened to be the unlucky bastard who pulled the trigger.

These are the real social issues that would benefit from the brilliant mind of someone like Dr. Carl Hart. His choice to focus on the Racist Narrative is unfortunate, as I think that if he opened his mind to other perspectives, he would be a boon to this kind of conversation in the psychedelic Renaissance. Until then, it's time we stopped pretending that race and/or gender dictate a person's insight into an issue (more on this in chapter 14). Mostly because we all know that we are pretending it does. Dr. Hart is black American and yet has not demonstrated even a novice's insight into black American crime or police shooting statistics, which we shall address now.

71. Quoted in Cashill (2013), p. 8.

12

Chacruna Institute and the New Psychedelic Racism

[T]he psychedelic community has the same biased beliefs that are found throughout society, including racist beliefs.

—Drs. Bia Labate and NiCole Buchanan, "Hate and Social Media in Psychedelic Spaces"

I am afraid that there is a certain class of race-problem solvers who don't want the patient to get well, because as long as the disease holds out they have not only an easy means of making a living, but also an easy medium through which to make themselves prominent before the public.

—Booker T. Washington, *My Larger Education*

Into the Fray

I'd heard of Chacruna Institute for a few years and mostly managed to ignore it.[1] But the Institute stepped on my turf in December 2021

1. Notwithstanding one time when I submitted an article to Chacruna's "Women in Psychedelics" series. When I was told that payment for my work would be "exposure," I

when editor of the *Chacruna Chronicles*, Osiris Sinuhé González Romero, demonstrated a stunning naïveté about Christian history and psychedelia. Romero, a graduate from Leiden University, made the amateur mistake of endorsing the so-called sacred mushroom conspiracy theory. For those of you who have never heard of this idea, I offer a brief rundown: the sacred mushroom conspiracy theory holds that a clandestine cabal of Christian elites throughout history *knew* that Jesus was really a metaphor for a psychedelic mushroom experience (or was a living person who used psychedelic mushrooms) and expressed this secret in art. Intriguing as the idea sounds, it is based in fantasy. Not a single legitimate scholar of the Old Testament or New buys it—nor do any reputable medievalists, art historians, or psychedelic historians. It lives solely in the domain of ignorance at best and hucksterism at worst.

If a Chacruna affiliate could be so wrong about this elementary issue, I wondered, what other ideas was the larger Institute pushing that actually matter? No one's life is at stake in light of the fact that the sacred mushroom conspiracy is total bunk. But Chacruna Institute isn't just pushing unfounded ideas like that one; much as its affiliates advance the Decolonize Narrative, so too they push the Racist Narrative with equal fervor. A Racist Narrative that has already divided the West. A Racist Narrative that will only serve to divide the psychedelic Renaissance.

In *Psychedelic Justice*, Drs. Bia Labate and NiCole Buchanan take issue with those who "attribut[e] racist incidents, specifically the high occurrence of police killing black people, to either rogue cops . . . or dysfunctional Black communities and Black culture."[2] David Nickels of Psymposia, who seems to prefer trite clichés in lieu of thoughtful discernment, mindlessly stumbles through critical social justice buzzwords when he calls the police "the state-sanctioned white supremacist enforcers of capitalism who murder Black, Brown, Indigenous, and poor people with impunity."[3] Provocative as such claims prove, the methods

---

declined the offer.

2. Labate and Buchanan, "Hate and Social Media . . .," in Labate and Cavnar (2021), p. 31.

3. Don't laugh. That is the best he can do. Nickels, "We Need to Talk about MAPS . . ."

for determining the true cause of black American homicide, coming from both Chacruna Institute and Psymposia, need a second look.

Black Lives Matter

Following the tragic death of Trayvon Martin in 2012 and subsequent acquittal of George Zimmerman, "trained Marxists" Alicia Garza, Opal Tometi, and Patrice Cullors formed Black Lives Matter in 2013.[4] According to BLM, we live in "a world where black lives are . . . systemically targeted for demise."[5] Only as we saw earlier, the true legacy of racist policing was more apathetic than proactive.

I think it necessary to separate the idea from the movement. I'm a big fan of the idea—*of course black lives matter*. I'm not as big a fan of the BLM movement, however. I understand that BLM grew out of a sincere belief that racist police officers were eagerly shooting unarmed black American men in the streets. I used to believe that myself, so I do not fault anyone who does. Our news media has manipulated all of us into believing it's true,[6] so I understand that some readers will initially dismiss what I have to say. I would have dismissed it too only a few years ago.

And yet, as mentioned in the last chapter, for most any example of an unarmed black American needlessly dying by police hands, there is a white American counterpart who perished under comparable circumstances that didn't make national headlines. The year 2020 ended with 1,020 police shootings, with the majority of those shot posing a deadly threat to the officer or a bystander. Of those shot, 457—just under half—were white American, and 243—just under a quarter—were black American. Of the 457 white Americans shot by police, 24 were unarmed; of the 243 black Americans shot by the police, 18 were unarmed.[7]

(2020).

4. Quoted in Joshua Rhett Miller, "BLM Site Removes Page on 'Nuclear Family Structure' amid NFL Vet's Criticism," *New York Post* (September 24, 2020).
5. Black Lives Matter, "About" (undated).
6. More on this in the next chapter.
7. "Number of People Shot to Death by the Police in the United States from 2017 to 2023, by Race," *Statista* (2023).

The biggest concern with drawing conclusions from legacy media outlets and special interest groups, as Chacruna Institute Theorists seem to do, is the way said channels mishandle statistics. They use broad population numbers to reach their conclusions. The faulty analysis, which you may have encountered yourself, looks like this: since the white American population is around 61%[8] and the black American population is around 13%, and roughly two white Americans are shot by an officer for every one black American shot by an officer, this means that black Americans are shot by the police at higher rates than white Americans; and the only possible conclusion is that they are being racially targeted. This kind of broad population metric finds favor within the NAACP, which claims that "the rate of fatal police shootings among Black Americans was much higher than that for any other ethnicity, standing at 35 fatal shootings *per million of the population* as of March 2021."[9] This same metric appears in the *American Journal of Preventative Medicine*, which also counts police shootings using numbers "relative to the U.S. population."[10] Among faltering news organizations, CNN takes its cues from researchers like Dr. James Buehler of Drexel University, whose "laughingly incomplete" study showing racial disparity in police shootings "measured death rates per total population size."[11]

But this is a misunderstanding of proper statistical analysis. The correct metric to use is not broad population numbers (as the NAACP, the *American Journal of Preventative Medicine*, BLM, Chacruna Institute, Psymposia, CNN, and may others employ) but rather the number of high-risk encounters between the police and civilians. The reason is obvious: right now, there are millions of both black and white Americans who are unlikely to see the business-end of a police officer's firearm—adolescent and teenage girls, and senior citizens, come to mind. They are all counted in the broad population number, yet they are unlikely to end

8. 61% identify as "white-only." Ethnically-mixed white Americans top out at 71%.
9. NAACP "The Origins of Modern Day Policing" (2024); *italics* mine.
10. Sara DeGue et al., "Deaths Due to Use of Lethal Force by Law Enforcement: Findings From the National Violent Death Reporting System," 17 U.S. States, 2009–2012" *American Journal of Preventative Medicine* (2016), p. S176.
11. Heather Mac Donald, "CNN Fans More Hatred of Cops, in Touting Flawed Study," Manhattan Institute (December 22, 2016); Jacqueline Howard, "Black Men Nearly 3 Times as Likely to Die from Police Use of Force, Study Says," *CNN* (December 20, 2016).

up in a violent encounter with police, making broad population numbers a flawed statistical benchmark.

To give you an idea of what this looks like, the 2021 tally for gun deaths among males eighteen-years-old and younger was 83%; among females the same age, the number was 17%.[12] Between 2009 and 2012, 91.6% of all police shootings involved men.[13] One can easily see that young *men* are more likely to end up in a violent encounter with the police than are young *women*. This isn't misandry on my part; it's just statistically true. The sample size gets even narrower when we factor in the elderly of both sexes, who are also highly unlikely to end up in a dangerous scuffle with the police.

The proper statistical metric for calculating police shootings should include only the percentage of those who end up in a violent confrontation with police. Political scientist Wilfred Reilly notes that the black American violent crime rate is roughly 2.5 times higher than for white Americans, meaning that the former has a 250% higher chance of ending up in a violent encounter with police officers "of all races" than does the latter. Reilly sums: "[T]he disproportion between the [black American] percentage of the U.S. population (13 percent) and the [black American] percentage of those shot by the police (23.5 percent) is wholly explained by the fact that the [black American] crime rate, violent crime rate, police encounter rate, and arrest rate are all at least 2 to 3 times the equivalent rates for [white Americans]. Adjusting for any single one of these rates—which essentially predict an individual's chance of a hostile encounter with police—eliminates any apparent racial disparity in the rates of police shootings."[14] When proper statistical controls that have been overlooked by Chacruna Theorists are allowed into the formulae, the BLM narrative collapses.

The Ferguson Effect

The rhetoric that police eagerly hunt black Americans in the streets has

12. John Gramlich, "Gun Deaths Among U.S. Children and Teens Rose 50% in Two Years," *Pew Research Center* (April 6, 2023).
13. DeGue (2016).
14. Reilly (2019), p. 43.

caused a phenomenon called the "Ferguson Effect,"[15] coined by St. Louis Police Chief Doyle Sam Dotson III. The Ferguson Effect sees the police backing away from patrolling high crime areas—exactly where they are needed the most—because they fear becoming the next media-circus "racist" exiled from society (as happened to Darren Wilson in Ferguson, Missouri). The Ferguson Effect has also led to thousands of officers returning their guns and shields—unwilling to put themselves in such potentially career- and life-ending situations.[16] This results in more murders in predominately black American neighborhoods.

Harvard economist Roland Fryer examined five US cities (Baltimore, MD; Chicago, Il; Riverside, CA; Cincinnati, OH; and Ferguson, MO), added up the estimates for homicide in each, and found, since the inception of BLM, an additional 893 homicides compared to previous years.[17] Immediately thinking the numbers too high, Fryer enlisted a second team to look at the data. Sure enough, the new team drew similar numbers as the old team. And these were just five cities. Data scientist Zac Kriegman "add[ed] . . . the estimates of murder from the different studies in various cities and time periods." He found "something in the neighborhood of 2,500 additional murders on the lo[w] end, but, possibly, well over 10,000 on the high end"—a staggering number of deaths on top of the roughly 8,000 black Americans murdered by criminals in a typical year—as a result of BLM rhetoric, trumpeted in mainstream media and by places like Chacruna Institute, that results in the Ferguson Effect.[18] For all of these victims there are thousands of their survivors thrown into a spiral of depression and trauma. JEDI mind tricks will only ensure that they remain in the trauma loop.

Ms. Carolyn Sweeper was a charming 93-year-old amputee who until

15. Also known as the "George Floyd Effect."

16. Rich Morin et al., "Behind the Badge," *Pew Research Center* (January 11, 2017).

17. Tanaya Devi and Roland G. Fryer, "Policing the Police: The Impact of 'Pattern-or-Practice'; Investigations on Crime," *National Bureau of Economic Research* (June 2020), p. 33.

18. Zac Kriegman, "BLM Spreads Falsehoods That Have Led to the Murders of Thousands of Black People in the Most Disadvantaged Communities," *Zac Kriegman* (Substack) (December 7, 2021).

recently lived in the Bronx, New York. She had to wait for the police to show up just to go to her mailbox; the hallways in her building were not safe for elderly, or even young, women of any ethnicity. The problem got so bad that Trespass Affidavit Program (TAP) officers were brought in to routinely patrol the stairwells, poorly lit corners, and basement areas of the building looking for crack dealers, who had been slinging rocks in the lobby for thirty years. Many women who live in this kind of environment become socially isolated. "I was afraid to leave my house. I love gardening, but I could get killed being out there pulling some weeds," one woman testified.[19] Others keep piles of trash in their apartments, fearing going curbside to drop it off.[20] I ask you, dear reader, do you live like that? I don't. Do you think anyone affiliated with Chacruna Institute lives like that? I doubt it. Carolyn Sweeper loved the police because she did live like that. "You can smell their stuff in the hallway; they're cussing and urinating. Then I don't want to come in because I'm scared. I'm scared just to stick my key in the door. . . . I wish we'd get our po-lice back. Puh-leez, Jesus, send them back!" she told Heather Mac Donald of the Manhattan Institute.[21]

Carolyn Sweeper doesn't fit the Racist Narrative, and so she is cast aside by the mainstream media; her voice silenced.

Carolyn Sweeper's black life mattered.

Also left in obscurity is Marcus Johnson. During one wave of BLM in 2015, Johnson was killed in a drive-by shooting. He was six.[22] His life mattered. And he is just *one* of the 26 children cut down that year due to gang violence.[23] I mean no disrespect to Dr. Labate or her colleagues at Chacruna Institute, but might they be a little too attached to their ideological narratives and a little too detached from the realities of certain inner-city subcultures to have any useful opinions that might actually help those most affected on the ground?

19. Quoted in Sterk (1999), pp. 188–89.
20. Godwin (1978), p. 99.
21. Quoted in Heather Mac Donald, "Courts v. Cops: The Legal War on the War on Crime," *City Journal* (Winter, 2013.
22. Denise Hollinshed, "Outing at St. Louis Park Turns to Tragedy as Bullets Fly, Killing 6-Year-Old Boy" (March 12, 2015).
23. Mac Donald (2017), pp. 80–1.

They also seem to misunderstand the nature of these crimes. Theorists like Jamilah R. George and Drs. Monnica Williams and Sara Reed state that "although Black Americans are 13% of the population, they comprise 35% of male inmates and 44% of female inmates."[24] However, they ignore that that 13% of the population perpetrates over 50% of the violent crimes in the United States (e.g., homicide, sexual assault, armed robbery).[25] The authors also make no mention that the overwhelming majority of people who file police reports against black Americans are other black Americans.[26] I find it difficult to imagine that these people have "internalized white supremacy," as one demeaning, half-baked, racist conspiracy theory might hold; they probably just want to feel safe walking down the streets at night. And anyway, crime reports *match* incarceration statistics—i.e., the incarcerated population directly correlates to crime reports.[27] Finally, Chacruna's Theorists also overlook that, when accounting for rates of violent crime, black Americans are *under*-represented in the prison population due to overcrowding, plea bargains, probation, and equity law.[28] Simply recall Jordan "Out by Sunday" Henry's actions up until his swan song. As we shall see in the next chapter, Henry is not alone.

Williams and company also assert, "The National Survey of American Life found that almost half of all African American women had been assaulted, which included 17% having been raped, 20% having been sexually assaulted, and 16% having been stalked."[29] The authors neglect to inform us that those violations against black American women are almost exclusively perpetrated by black American men.[30] They also ignore that these sexual assaults contribute to the later incarceration of black

24. Willaims et al., "Culture and Psychedelic Psychotherapy . . ." (2020) p. 128.
25. The real number of those committing violent crimes is even smaller than 13%. Women typically do not commit violence crimes and the majority of black Americans are law-abiding citizens.
26. Mac Donald (2017), p. 152.
27. Kriegman (2021); Reilly (2019), p. 44.
28. Mac Donald (2017), p. 215
29. Willaims et al., "Culture and Psychedelic Psychotherapy . . ." (2020) p. 128.
30. Carolyn M. West and Kamilah Johnson, "Sexual Violence in the Lives of African American Women: Risk, Response, and Resilience," *The National Online Resource Center on Violence Against Women, National Resource Center on Domestic Violence* (March 2013).

American women; of the 46%[31] of black American women in lockdown, 86% experienced some form of sexual assault in their lives.[32] While Chacruna Institute Theorists aren't alone in misrepresenting the statistics (though I do not believe they do so with malice of forethought—just ignorance), others knowingly juke the data. Recently, a professor of criminology at Florida State University, Eric Stewart, lost his position for "extreme negligence" in his data- and survey-based research. Stewart allegedly falsified data by making "racism seem more common than it is through his data and surveys that altered sample sizes."[33] I can only assume that when Stewart couldn't find racism, he ended up tweaking the data until it fit the Racist Narrative.

This is not really the fault of Chacruna's Theorists, who I believe are acting in good faith. They are being lied to every bit as much as you and me from organizations like Black Lives Matter, various academic journals, race-hucksters like Michelle Alexander, Eric Stewart, Robin DiAngelo, and a medley of dishonest legacy media outlets of which to speak. Only since the lie conforms to their biases, there is little incentive to check the record.

The Racist Narrative is effective because it tugs at our heartstrings. Drs. Labate and Buchanan write of "the police killings of . . . countless . . . Black [American] children."[34] Here, they are echoing the BLM chant heard in Chicago back in 2016, "CDP, KKK, how many children did you kill today?" And yet, during the time Chicagoans were marching to this chant, two dozen children (twelve years of age and younger) were killed due to street violence, notwithstanding a three-year-old boy who survived a bullet but will remain paralyzed (and no doubt traumatized) for the rest of his life.[35]

---

31. As opposed to Williams, Reed, and George's 44%. I do not find the numerical discrepancy to be of any statistical significance.
32. National Black Women's Justice Institute, "Black Women, Sexual Assault, and Criminalization" (April 11, 2023).
33. Scott Jaschik, "Florida State Fires Professor Over 'Extreme Negligence' in His Research," *Inside Higher Ed.* (July 20, 2023).
34. Labate and Buchanan, "Hate and Social Media . . .," in Labate and Cavnar (2021), p. 29.
35. Quoted in Mac Donald (2017), p. VII.

In fairness to Drs. Labate and Buchanan, the horrible reality is that sometimes children are shot by the police. We feel the weight of it in every cell of our body when it happens. Unfashionable as it certainly may be to entertain (because we are talking about children), the cases are far more nuanced than pointing towards an all-pervasive white supremacist police force. One might consider Ma'Khia Bryant, as *ABC News* does, a sixteen-year-old black American girl who was shot by Officer Nicholas Rearden. *ABC News* makes brief mention of "a fight and an attempted stabbing."[36] What the reporter doesn't tell us is that Bryant was the one brandishing the knife, trying to stab two women. Either Officer Reardon was going to allow Bryant to kill those women, or (as is his sworn duty) he was going to protect them. Other times, the shooting victims are white American kids.[37] Sometimes the officer is white American;[38] sometimes the officer is black American.[39]

Other cases are far less nuanced and inexcusable, showing clear negligence on the part of law enforcement. The death of seven-year-old black American Aiyana Stanley-Jones comes to mind.[40] The door of her home was kicked down; a swarm of officers entered under cover of a flash grenade. Detroit's Special Response Team pushed its way into the apartment complex looking for a homicide suspect (who lived a floor above the Stanley-Jones family). Only one shot was fired. Aiyanna's story is tragic—a horrible accident—and perhaps perfectly exemplifies what can happen when overzealous or otherwise undertrained officers

36. Kiara Alfonseca, "Police Have Killed More Than 100 Children Since 2015 in US, Data Shows," *ABC News* (April 28, 2021).
37. Jeremy Mardis was shot by a black American officer, Derrick Staford; see, "Officer Convicted of Manslaughter in Shooting Death of Boy, 6," *CBS News* (March, 2017); Stavian Rodriguez was shot by 5 white American officers; see Jared Formanek and Ray Sanchez, "Charges Dropped Against 5 Oklahoma City Officers who Fatally Shot 15-Year-Old," *CNN* (July, 2023); Kameron Rodriguez was shot by 5 officers whose ethnicities have not been released; see Guillermo Contreras, "Family of 6-Year-Old Boy Shot and Killed by Bexar Deputies in 2017 Files Lawsuit," *San Antonio Express-News* (December 2019); among others.
38. "Fired San Antonio Police Officer Indicted for Shooting Teen as he Ate Hamburger in McDonald's Parking Lot," *CBS News* (December 2, 2022).
39. Staff Writer, "Family Sues Akron Police for Killing Unarmed Man William Lemmon they Suspected of Robbery," *Akron Beacon Journal* (September 26, 2016).
40. Charlie Leduff, "What Killed Aiyana Stanley-Jones?" *Mother Jones* (Nov.-Dec. 2010).

enter dangerous situations looking for homicide suspects.[41]

The person who killed Stanely-Jones, Officer Joseph Weekley, is white American; his commanding officer, Sergent Anthony Potts, is black American. The people who killed Jeremey Nardis, Officer Derrick Stafford and Norris Greenhouse, Jr., are black American. A third person on the scene whose bodycam recorded the shooting, Sgt. Kenneth Parnell, is a white American. It becomes difficult to find a law enforcement stereotype. Tragedies involving children jab at our emotions in an especial way. But it gets difficult to boil them all down to "white American cop kills black American child because *racism*," once a full understanding of the situation is confronted.

White American children face similar police incompetence. Six-year-old Jeremey Nardis was killed while strapped in his father's car when law enforcements officers unloaded 18 bullets at the vehicle following a short chase.[42]

According to Pew Research, black American children were "roughly five times as likely as their [white American] counterparts to die from gunfire in 2021." Overall that year, 46% of all gun deaths among teenagers involved a black American victim and 32% involved white American kids. However, of the 32% of white Americans killed by gun violence, 66% were suicides and 24% (still no small number) were homicides. As for the 46% of gun deaths among black American kids, 84% were homicides, and 9% were suicides.[43] High crime areas inevitably mean more police presence. More police presence means a higher probability that an innocent child will be tragically killed in urban crossfire (consider Stanely-Jones's tragic end). It also means that the police need more—not less—training to deal with deadly and confusing situations where one has only a moment to react. And might these disproportionate numbers in homicides among black American teenagers as opposed to other demographics have anything to do with the culture of lethal retaliation disrupting the inner cities? Might said culture of lethal retaliation account for the ethnic disparities in prison populations? Might

41. Elisha Anderson, "Police Sergeant Fights Tears in Describing Girl's Death," *USA Today* (June 5, 2013).
42. Associated Press, "Slain Boy's Father Says Officers Shot Them Without Warning," *NBC News* (March 21, 2017).
43. Gramlich (2023).

more children get accidentally killed when police step into that kind of environment? Such possibilities have seemingly never occurred to anyone at Chacruna Institute or Psymposia.

Considering differences between black and white American homicide rates among men, the numbers going all the way back to 2017 tell the same story. In six and a half years (at the time of this writing), the police have shot 1,376 black Americans, the majority of whom posed a serious danger to the officer or a bystander. This figure is doubled by the number of white Americans shot by the police during that same timeframe, totaling 2,545.[44] The majority of those white American men were also presenting a deadly threat to the officer or another person.

During just *one* of those six years, 2020, the body count of black-on-black American homicide reached an unprecedented 9,753.[45] The number of black Americans shot by the police that same year: 243. Only 18 were unarmed, meaning 225 were armed, dangerous, and a threat to public safety.

But even the term "unarmed" here—especially as employed by *The Washington Post*—obfuscates the truth. For example, one instance *The Washington Post* records as an unarmed elderly black American man wrongfully killed by the police occurred during a shootout with an armed suspect who was firing his gun at the officers. The elderly man, unfortunately, was struck by a stray bullet when the police returned fire. According to *The Washington Post*, that tragic accident counts as a racist police shooting of an unarmed black American. In another case, a towering suspect was beating an officer senseless, having broken several of

44. "Number of People Shot to Death by the Police in the United States from 2017 to 2023, by Race," *Statista*; (2017)—458 white Americans shot by the police; 222 black Americans shot by the police. (2018)—459 white Americans shot by the police; 228 black Americans shot by the police. (2019)—424 white Americans shot by the police; 251 black Americans by the police. (2020)—457 white Americans shot by the police; 243 black Americans shot by the police. (2021)—302 white Americans shot by the police; 177 black Americans shot by the police. (2022)—389 white Americans shot by the police; 225 black Americans shot by the police. (2023; as of April of that year), 56 white Americans shot by the police; 30 black Americans shot by the police. Note: Statista also measures police shootings by broad population numbers (i.e., "per million of the population") instead of the more accurate metric—likelihood of ending up in a violent encounter with the police.

45. Peggy Lowe, "Missouri has the Highest Black Homicide Rate in America—and Some of the Loosest Gun Laws," *KCUR* (April 26, 2023).

his bones. Before going unconscious, the officer pulled his gun and fired (much like George Zimmerman's lethal reaction to Trayvon Martin's attack). Keep in mind that beatings of this kind are the third highest cause of homicide in the United States. Once again, our friends at *The Washington Post* count that as a racist police killing of an unarmed black American too. There are hundreds, perhaps even thousands, more cases just like those two—all supposedly listed as racist police shootings of black Americans, when they clearly are not.[46]

As a result of such dishonest practices, good-hearted liberals have been dupped into believing that the number is way higher due to selective reporting of these incidents by major media outlets. A 2021 Skeptic Research Center study revealed that 22% of white Americans who identify as "very liberal" believe the tally of police shootings of unarmed black American men to be 10,000 or more a year, while nearly 40% of liberals believed police killed at least 1,000 unarmed black American men that year.[47] The real number of police shootings of unarmed black Americans in 2021 was ten.[48] Perhaps more eye-opening, police are statistically more often shot by black Americans then the other way around.[49]

Between 2014 and 2020, Missouri's black-on-black American homicide rate increased 46% (including a 29% increase from 2019 to 2020).[50] The vast majority of those killed (90%) were killed by other young black American men. And it all happened at the height of BLM's calls to "defund the police." The numbers, both historically and currently, show that defunding the police leads to *more* deaths of young black American men. If Chacruna's Theorists are correct, and police are really the cause of the majority of black American murder today, why did we see an increase in black American homicide after the police stopped patrolling high-crime areas? How will Drs. Labate, Buchanan, Williams, or anyone else at Chacruna Institute or Psymposia explain that?

We saw earlier how structural racism created the environment of lethal retaliation, and a lack of opportunities fueled deadly underground

46. Mac Donald (2016), p. 77.
47. Skeptic Research Center, "How Informed Are Americans about Race and Policing?," CUPES007 (2021).
48. Murray (2022), p. 27.
49. Mac Donald (2017), p. 79.
50. Lowe (2023).

crack markets. But numbers do not lie. If white supremacy played a role in the 1,376 deaths of black Americans shot by the police between 2017 and spring 2023, then it also played a role in the deaths of 2,545 white Americans shot by the police during that same period—the majority of whom posed a threat to another human life at the time they lost theirs. And what of those people of all ethnicities who were legit victims of police brutality?

I say all of their lives mattered.

What do you say?

We need to come together as a unified psychedelic Renaissance and stand up for cultural reform as one voice. We need to bring these medicines into both the inner cities and the police departments—arguably the two most culturally traumatized segments of our society. For certain, while Roland Fryer found the BLM narrative about racial bias in police shootings to be fallacious, he did confirm that officers are statistically more aggressive with black American men than they are with those of other ethnicities.[51] This, too, must be addressed. Suppose that biased reaction comes from trauma? Would this not be a good litmus test for our claims about the healing powers of psychedelic medicines?

Buy Large Mansions

And of BLM as a movement, here's how much they care about our black American sisters and brothers who are real victims of police brutality. Rev. Jerry McAfee, a pastor at New Salem Missionary Baptist Church, comments: "[BLM] collected some $30 million off of the death of George Floyd. . . . And they've put not one dollar in our community."[52] He is echoed by Rev. T. Sheri Dickerson, who says, "The families are feeling exploited, their pain exploited, and that's not something that I ever want to be affiliated with."[53]

Patrisse Cullors, a co-founder of Black Lives Matter, stepped down from her more-privileged-than-I'll-ever-be position in May 2021 amid

51. See Devi and Fryer (2020).
52. Quoted in Kristine Frazao, "The Black Lives Matter Movement Brought in Millions. So Where Is That Money Now?" *KATV ABC News 7* (February 21, 2033).
53. Quoted in Aaron Morrison, "BLM's Patrisse Cullors to Step Down from Movement Foundation," *AP News* (May 27, 2021).

questions about the foundation and her personal finances.[54] She ran away to one of her several mansions, which she bought with the good-intentioned dollars sent by people who thought their money was going to victims of police violence. Cullors' actions fly in the face of Drs. Labate and Buchanan's claims that BLM is not "opportunistic, and/or masking ulterior, sinister political motives."[55]

Turns out, that is *exactly* what BLM is doing.

As outlined in chapter 9, I fully recognize the role that structural racism played in creating this mess in black American neighborhoods. But that mess had nothing to do with police killing black Americans in cold blood. The mess formed when a deadly mix of police indifference to black American crime met a culture of lethal retaliation (specifically around crack dealing) in the mid-1980s. If one positive outcome can be detected in any of this disaster, the crack epidemic at least brought the plight of the black American neighborhood center stage, *forcing* police departments to actually start caring about the problem.

But is that the only issue?

Numerous black American intellectuals, President Obama, and even the smartest man in the world, former CNN anchor Don Lemon, have all stated at one time or another that the problem stems, at least in part, from absentee fathers, which hovers around 72% among black Americans.[56] Fatherless homes come with a constellation of social problems. As just a few examples: children (especially boys) without fathers are more likely to drop out of school, more likely to commit violent crimes, are more depressed and anxious, have more behavioral problems, have less overall happiness and well-being, are more likely to end up in prison, and are more likely to become absentee fathers themselves.[57] Interestingly, in the 1940s, during the age of Jim Crow and real structural racism,

54. Stella Chan, "Black Lives Matter Co-Founder Stepping Down from Organization," *CNN* (May 28, 2021).
55. Labate and Buchanan, "Hate and Social Meda . . .," in Labate and Cavnar (2021), p. 32.
56. Jesse Washington, "Blacks Struggle with 72 Percent Unwed Mothers Rate," *NBC News* (November 7, 2010).
57. "Statistics Tell the Story: Fathers Matter," National Fatherhood Initiative (2024).

the single motherhood rate among black Americans was around 19%.[58] When it increased to 20% by 1960 and 24% by 1965—that was seen as cause for alarm.[59] We should all agree that structural racism does not force any man, of any ethnicity, to impregnate a woman and then leave her—otherwise the above percentages of single motherhood in the black American community would be reversed (i.e., we would have seen this issue intensified during the age of Jim Crow).

And this is a problem with white Americans too, whose illegitimacy rate rests around 24%. For younger, low income white Americans, it rises to 40%.[60] This crisis isn't about ethnicity; it is about fathers who abandon their children. It is an absence of the Divine Masculine, the provider and protector (more on this in the final chapter). Children—especially young boys—need fathers. What are we to make of BLM's efforts to break up the black American family—the first and last line of defense between a child and prison or the morgue?[61]

I have no reason to believe that Dr. Labate, or anyone else affiliated with Chacruna Institute, is purposefully misrepresenting the data the way CNN, *The Washington Post* and other legacy media outlets, BLM, NAACP, and countless institutions do without a thought for the social damage they are causing. I believe that Dr. Labate and her colleagues truly care about these issues and want to be of good service to them. However, all available evidence shows that they have misdiagnosed the *current* reasons we are not seeing equal outcomes. What's more, that misdiagnosis causes real harm in the world.

Compassion and Accountability

Since a broader understanding of history and statistics shows the cur-

58. George A. Akerlof and Janet L. Yellen, "An Analysis of Out-of-Wedlock Births in the United States," *Brookings Institute* (August 1, 1996); Robert Clegg, "Percentage of Births to Unmarried Women," *Center for Equal Opportunity* (February 26, 2020); others place the number at 14%; see also Reilly (2019), p. 30.
59. Reilly (2019), p. 38; Akerlof and Yellen (1996).
60. Reilly (2019), p. 28.
61. Miller, (2020). BLM has since taken down their anti-family stance from their website, no doubt due to backlash against this truly terrible idea. Though, as "trained Marxists," it's highly unlikely that that philosophy isn't still found among the BLM constituency.

rent, divisive Racist Narrative to be far more nuanced than those at Chacruna Institute or Psymposia acknowledges, should we really allow it to tear the psychedelic Renaissance apart? As thought leaders of the psychedelic Renaissance, Chacruna Institute's associates ought to be concerned with truth if they are to use their connections, social privileges, and resources in meaningful ways. And the truth is that we cannot help kids struggling in America's inner cities—the most marginalized victims still reverberating in the echoes of past white supremacy—if we are asking the wrong questions, ignoring the real problems, and chasing phantoms of a bygone era. Facilitating psychedelic medicine and education about it, within a victim framework, so as to reinforce a defeatist mindset with JEDI mind tricks, is, in my opinion, not a good strategy. Allowing Pachamama[62] and the Mushroom Goddess to show black American youths that their potential is limitless—that they can create any life they want—I think, has a better chance for a more positive lasting outcome. To use psychedelics to indoctrinate other flimsy narrative-driven perspectives keeps us all down.

Psychenauts need to be able to admit that past white supremacy created the theater of violence and that destructive aspects of modern street culture (i.e., lethal retaliation and silence) have continued the cycle. However, screaming "white supremacy" in the streets today is not a solution; prostrating oneself before the altar of white guilt has never solved a single problem. Land acknowledgments give land back to no one. Likewise, teaching divisive rhetoric and an ever-oppressive narrative like that found in JEDI, implicit bias, and microaggression trainings is not a solution either. Neither can we adopt the far right's "slavery ended over a century ago—get over it!" stance.

And so we find ourselves at a strange and momentous historical intersection. Systemic racism is gone, but it lingers on through cultural trauma reinforced by the Racist Narrative, which is itself exacerbated through JEDI training. The solution to our current division in the psychedelic Renaissance seems clear. We need to have compassion about the past while not misrepresenting the present. We must give historically marginalized communities opportunities without infantilizing them. Above all, we must stop misrepresenting racial issues in the United

62. That is, ayahuasca.

States until anyone affiliated with Chacruna Institute, Psymposia, Dr. Carl Hart, or any psychedelic SJW can offer any evidence that anything I've stated about the Racist Narrative is factually mistaken. Should they prove successful, I will do what I've done a million times over the course of my life—admit I was wrong and change my mind.

Pretending that everything is racist is an excellent way to stop potential allies from talking to each other. How will spouting all these divisive narratives amount to what our civilization really needs right now?

A unified psychedelic Renaissance.

13

This, Psymposia Calls "Journalism": How to Discredit Yourself

When millions of people are terrified of threats that do not exist, there is strong evidence that someone is deliberately trying to scare them.

—Wilfred Reilly, *Hate Crime Hoax*

American Media

On 17 August 2009, a man identified at the time only as "Chris" stood outside a rally in Phoenix, Arizona, where President Barack Obama would speak on the topic of healthcare.[1] Chris was armed with an AR-15 slung over his right shoulder and a handgun fastened to his left hip. Contessa Brewer of MSNBC painted the scene, "there are questions about whether this has ... racial overtones. I mean, here you have a man of color in the presidency and white people showing up with guns strapped to their waists."

As she speaks, our attention is diverted from Brewer in the studio

1. Stephen Lemons, "Christopher Broughton's Pastor Steven Anderson Prays for President Obama's Death," *Phoenix New Times* (August 26, 2009); Mike Stuckey, "Guns near Obama Fuel 'Open-Carry' Debate," *NBC News* (August 24, 2009).

to the Obama rally in Phoenix where an MSNBC camera operator fixes her lens on the holstered firearms. The message from MSNBC is obvious: despite Obama's lofty position as president of the United States, Chris's white privilege superseded even that most high of offices, allowing him to attend the rally fully strapped with no consequences.

There was only one problem with MSNBC's narrative.

Chris is black American.

While the whole scene was a publicity stunt, Chris Broughton's politics were very real: he viewed the Obama administration as "the most corrupt Mafioso on the face of the Earth."[2] Despite having no plans to unholster his peacemakers, Chris does not fit the Racist Narrative. Could that be why MSNBC's camera operator carefully shielded his face and hands from our view? Did Brewer simply assume he was white, or did she knowingly lie to her viewers to serve the Racist Narrative? Either way, following the prescription from critical social justice to see racism everywhere (regardless of context or basic facts), Brewer *created racism* where racism did not exist. But it wasn't just MSNBC. Other large media outlets that covered the story made no mention of this detail about Chris.[3] He was not politically useful, so his identity could be erased. Some local presses were more interested in the truth—the *Phoenix New Times* both acknowledging Chris's race and admitting that such a fact is "bound to reduce the tone of criticism in the media."[4]

When I first started researching crime and police shooting statistics for this book in 2019, I noticed something odd. The databases I was looking at did not match what I was seeing on both social and national media platforms. Perhaps you've noticed it too. Story after story excluded mentioning race of both perpetrator and victim when the violence was intraracial (i.e., white-on-white American or black-on-black American). With interracial violence (i.e., white-on-black American or black-on-

2. AZ BlueMeanie, "Update on Protestor with Assault Rifle at Obama Event in Phoenix," *Blog for Arizona* (August 22, 2009).
3. Daniel Stone, "Guns at Obama Rallies: Where's the Outrage?" *Newsweek* (August 18, 2009).
4. Ray Stern, "Guns at Obama Protest Scare Folks, but Cops Say no Laws were Broken," *Phoenix New Times* (August 17, 2009).

white American), mention of ethnicity depends on the skin tones of the perpetrator and/or victim. If the perp is white American and victim black American, you will certainly hear about race. If the roles are reversed, you will not hear about race—or at least race won't be a focus.

Consider the attempted robbery of a liquor store in Riverside, California, in July 2022. Craig Cope (d. 2022) was working late in his store when a black SUV pulled up. Through his security camera, he watched two men get out of the car, one holding a machine gun. Thankfully, Cope got to his shotgun as the perpetrators entered the shop and fired a single round, hitting one of them in the arm. They quickly retreated, dove into their SUV, and sped away. News stories about the attack did not mention the races of either perpetrators or victim.[5] Why? Likely because all the robbers are black American and Craig Cope was white American. Only by digging into the Riverside Sheriff Department's mug shots could I find this fact.[6] Let's try a thought experiment: take a moment and imagine a car full of white American kids attempting to rob a liquor store owned by a black American man; your social media feeds and preferred legacy media outlets would detail little else except the ethnicities of the known parties.

I soon discovered that should both victim and perpetrator be black American, the races will also often go unmentioned. Outside a McDonald's in the Bedford-Stuyvesant neighborhood of Brooklyn, New York, on 1 August 2022, Michael Morgan shot an unnamed employee over soggy french-fries. Several news outlets covered the homicide but mention only "a man" accused of shooting the fast-food employee.[7] Another story, this one from *Eyewitness News*, reports on a murderer described as "a woman's 20-year-old son."[8] It took searching the *later* arrest photos to find out that man's ethnicity. Incidentally, Morgan was also charged with

5. "80-Year-Old California Store Owner who Shot Robbers Dies," *Associated Press* (December 27, 2022); Joshua Rhett Miller, "Store Owner Craig Cope, 80, Who Shot Robber Armed with AR-15 Rifle Says it was 'Him or Me,'" *New York Post* (August 2, 2022).

6. Riverside County, "[Archived] Attempted Armed Commercial Robbery–Update," Riverside County Sheriff (August 4, 2022).

7. "Man Charged in Shooting of McDonald's Worker over French Fries also Charged in 2020 Murder," *Eyewitness News, ABC7* (August 3, 2022).

8. Mark Crudele and Crystal Cranmore, "McDonald's Worker Shot in Neck during Dispute in Brooklyn," *Eyewitness News, ABC7* (August 2, 2022).

an additional murder that took place in 2020. He had, in fact, thirteen prior arrests before he killed someone over moist french-fries. But even though the courts are biased against black Americans, as Chacruna Institute Theorists maintain, he remained free to commit further violent crimes before finally serving a long stretch.

Reports of a stabbing incident that took place at another McDonald's in East Harlem gives us only these details about the assailant: "male, 5'11" or 6'0" tall, wearing a black and green jacket."[9] *Spectrum News* disclosed even less of a report, content on mustering an amorphous "person" to describe the assailant.[10] (Not to be confused with all those horses that have recently been stabbing people.)

Burger King similarly featured in a murder in East Harlem in March 2022—right around the block from the very McDonald's just mentioned. Here, Winston Glynn pistol-whipped and shot a 19-year-old employee, Kristal Bayron-Nieves, during an attempted robbery. *Eyewitness News* was once again there to report as little as possible. Glynn was described only as a "30-year-old."[11] It is only through looking at arrest photos, courtroom photos, and (sadly) the memorial photos that we get any indication as to the ethnicity of both perp and victim. Bayron-Nieves was a young Puerto Rican woman. Glynn is a black American man. Had Glynn been white American, Bayron-Nieves's life would have mattered to the legacy media. But her death does not fit the Racist Narrative.

Glynn had seven priors. Now on his eighth arrest he played the victim, claiming that his persecution was on par with "Nelson Mandela and Jesus Christ." He boasted that he was only guilty of being a "leader," and that his peers were "jealous" of him. During his trial he blamed lack of slavery reparations as the reason for his actions. Certainly a possibility. It's also possible that the crack he regularly smoked severely affected his judgment, leading him to murder an innocent woman. It remains a mystery. Although, we must admit a moment of honesty relayed by Glynn

9. "McDonald's Worker Stabbed while Defending Coworkers in East Harlem," *Eyewitness News, ABC7* (March 9, 2022).
10. Spectrum News Staff, "NYPD: McDonald's Worker Stabbed while Defending Coworker in East Harlem," *Spectrum News NY1* (March 9, 2022).
11. "Man Who Shot, Killed 19-Year-Old Burger King Worker in Harlem Indicted for Murder," *Eyewitness News, ABC7* (March 3, 2022).

during his trial when he stated: "These people don't want crime to stop, as long as it's not affecting them."[12] I can't think of a better description of both elite leftist journalists and the Democratic Party than that.[13]

Let's leave the wild world of East Harlem fast-food bloodshed, back ourselves up several years to 4 August 2007, and move across the state line that separates New York from New Jersey. On that terrible night in Newark, an MS-13 gang member, Jose Carranza, and five of his associates, murdered "execution style" three black American college students, Terrance Aeriel, Iofemi Hightower, and Dashon Harvey. A fourth, Natasha (Terrance's sister), despite Carranza sexually assaulting her and another attacker slashing her throat with a machete, miraculously managed to escape the fate of the others.[14]

No one in the legacy media cared. The story didn't fit the Racist Narrative. Since Carranza is Peruvian and a member of a particularly violent and vicious gang, the three black American lives that he heartlessly ended could be overlooked. Popular Los Angeles radio host Terry Anderson articulated this point better than anyone at the time, remarking: "If you make one simple change, and change Jose Carranza to a white man, I will guarantee you that [Al Sharpton and Jesse Jackson] would be screaming and marching in the streets."[15]

Anderson understood the Racist Narrative.

The same holds true in the case of police shootings of white Americans. On 2 October 2022, a Dallas cop shot a 17-year-old kid outside a McDonald's as he ate his hamburger. No mention of either the cop's or the kid's ethnicity in local or legacy news stories because both are white American.[16] Likewise, should a police shooting involve a black American officer and either a black or white American victim, these details will also be left off the table. Go through any major news organization's database and you'll reach the same conclusion: ethnicity will rarely (if

12. Matthew Sedacca and Georgia Worell, "Accused Burger King Killer Winston Glynn Compares himself to Jesus and Mandela," *New York Post* (November 26, 2022).
13. This is not to say that I am a republican (I'm not). It is to say that republicans care about crime in a way that I do not see democrats matching.
14. Quoted in Bill Wichert, "Newark Schoolyard Killings: Jose Carranza loses Bid to Overturn Conviction" (Oct 22, 2014).
15. Steven Malanga, "The Rainbow Coalition Evaporates," *City Journal* (Winter 2008).
16. "Fired San Antonio Police Officer . . ." (2022).

ever) be mentioned for black-on-black American crime, black-on-white American crime, black-on-Latin American crime, or white-on-white American crime; it will typically only be addressed if the perpetrator is white American and the victim is black American, creating an obvious imbalance that only serves to further divide us along ethnic lines on the street level.

Consider these two headlines:

1. "Family Sues Akron Police for Killing Unarmed Man William Lemmon They Suspected of Robbery."[17]
2. "The Story of How a White Phoenix Cop Killed an Unarmed Black Man."[18]

In the first case from Akron, the deceased was an unarmed white American and the shooting officer was a black American (thus no mention of race in the headline). The second case from Phoenix fit the Racist Narrative, so there is no mystery why race features prominently in the headline about that case.

I can do this hundreds of times over.

With a simple search of any modern news archive, so can you.

Other stories are outright ignored should they run counter to the Racist Narrative. On the rare occasion that a white American perpetrates a crime against a black American (specifically a police shooting), your Instagram, Facebook, and Twitter (now X) feeds will descend into firestorms of chaos with the usual "ist" epithets thrown across the larger political aisle. There will be days of faux-mourning and virtue-signaling from the legacy talking heads; and, of course, we can expect a healthy turn of mostly peaceful riots and the insistence that white Americans take the time to reflect on their role in the tragedy and how they personally perpetuate white supremacy. Then, in answer to our prayers, celebrities will descend from Heaven and stumble their way through unintelligi-

17. Staff Writer, "Family Sues Akron . . ." (2016).
18. Terrence McCoy, "The Story of How a White Phoenix Cop Killed an Unarmed Black Man," *The Washington Post* (December 5, 2014).

ble points about how we must all "do better" (before returning to their crime-free neighborhoods). And yet, white-on-black American crime happens far *less* than the other way around. Interracial crime is rare in the United States relative to intraracial crime. Uncommon as it is among all crime, roughly 80% of all interracial crime is black-on-white American.[19]

One could easily fill a multi-volume anthology of such examples. The Racist Narrative would have us believing that white-on-black American violence happens the most, and so media outlets will usually withhold the ethnicities of the parties involved unless said ethnicities support the Racist Narrative. Even if all available statistics and crime reports tell a different story. Perhaps it is no surprise that between "81 to 94 percent of the 'U.S. media elite'" veer to the left.[20] And for the critical social justice left—especially journalists—stirring grievances often takes precedent over telling the truth.

Enter Sandmann

Because the Racist Narrative is pre-factual it tends to misfire if enough evidence emerges showing a fuller story after the masses have already rushed to judgment. We saw such an instance in 2019 when Nicholas Sandmann (who was sixteen at the time) and other teenagers from Covington Catholic High School (located in Covington, Kentucky) were immediately demonized after their encounter with Nathan Phillips, an indigenous elder of the Omaha Tribe, during their visit to Washington, DC. The teenagers had gathered on the National Mall to attend March for Life, an anti-choice rally; Phillips was there for an Indigenous Peoples' March that day. Media outlets quickly released a snippet of the encounter, recorded with a cell phone. The narrative they spun led their readers and viewers to believe that the Covington kids had somehow surrounded Phillips in an effort to belittle and harass him.

We all saw the same initial short clip: Phillips beating his drum as Sandmann stands face to face with him and the mostly white American kids in the crowd clap along and chant. Sandmann's milky-white face, red "Make America Great Again" hat, and blue hoodie contrasted with

19. Reilly (2019), p. xvi.
20. Reilly (2019), p. 44.

Phillips's tan skin, drum, and chant, kicking the Racist Narrative into action: Sandmann *must* be a white supremacist while Phillips *must* be the oppressed "noble savage." Large media companies and your batty leftist aunt unfairly slandered Sandmann (and the rest of the group) in all the usual critical social justice gibberish: "bigot," "racist," "white supremacist." We were to make our determination based on nothing more than white American kid vs. indigenous American elder—the white supremacist and the noble savage. Context didn't matter.

But when longer videos of the encounter surfaced, the truth emerged. The cell phone camera follows Phillips as he walks around the crowd. He eventually stops in front of Sandmann and begins to hit his drum and chant in the boy's face. It was Phillips and his crew who approached the Covington teenagers, not the other way around (as we were instructed to believe). Sandmann keeps his cool; though, unsure of what to do in such an awkward situation, resorts to standing there smiling at the indigenous American elder. Not yelling or saying derogatory or racist remarks; just smiling. The longer footage also unveils another interesting detail. As it turns out, there *were* racists and homophobes at the Lincoln Memorial that day, but they didn't come from Kentucky. A black supremacist group called the Black Hebrew Israelites (BHI) led by Chief Ephraim Israel was also in the capital that day. Chief Ephraim and the other BHIs derided both groups of marchers: Phillips's group and the Covington kids, who they called "a bunch of [faggots] made out of incest."[21] Few news outlets covered it. They already had their villain. The *perfect* villain: a white American kid wearing a MAGA hat.

In media interviews after the short video came out, Phillips made a number of inconsistent and false statements, claiming he was the victim (*of course*).[22] After the longer video came out, showing him to be the aggressor, few asked him about his earlier misstatements. No one pushed the BHI story. The Omaha elder and the black supremacists do not fit the Racist Narrative. We are to excuse them. To its credit, a *Time* article did its job, reminding its readers that they are often "ill-equipped to deal

21. Quoted in Ben Feuerherd and Bruce Golding, "This 'Black Israelite' from Brooklyn Sparked the Covington Controversy," *New York Post* (January 22, 2019).
22. "Native American Elder Nathan Phillips on Confrontation: 'I Forgive Him,'" *Today* (January 29, 2019).

with online disinformation."[23] The incident should have been a revelation about the shortsightedness of rushing to judgment. Instead, we were reminded that white supremacy is still a problem.

Moreover, how do we square the total cover up of Trayvon Martin's and Michael Brown's sordid past with what happened to Nick Sandmann? The rush to judgment for Sandmann was so swift and decisive that even one conservative author and podcaster fell for the original lie.[24] How is having your name unfairly dragged through the mud, as Sandmann experienced, a privilege? How is having your distasteful past almost completely scrapped from public record, as Trayvon Martin and Michael Brown enjoyed postmortem, not a privilege? Two violent, entitled kids were paraded as "civil rights martyr[s]" while the innocent Sandmann became the face of all that is evil in the world.[25]

None of this is meant to discount the violence black Americans have historically endured in the face of white supremacy. The past injustices of slavery and Jim Crow cast a looming and pernicious shadow over innocent peoples, particularly those living in low-income neighborhoods. I am merely trying to bring some balance and nuance to these conversations within the psychedelic Renaissance. We are *all* being played by a dishonest media that uses selective reporting of these tragedies to create a bogus Racist Narrative so that we will stay divided and clicking on their bullshit articles.

It's also great for getting votes.

The Notorious Dr. Ball

Psymposia's staff mimics this biased approach found in the larger American media. In 2021, Psymposia fixed its crosshairs on author, lecturer, visionary artist, musician, and former 5-MeO DMT facilitator, Dr. Martin Ball. For those of you not familiar with this soul-revealing compound, 5-MeO DMT is the strongest psychedelic medicine on the planet. In fact, to even call it "psychedelic" does not do justice to the experience. It was Dr. Ball himself who coined the phrase "The God Molecule" to de-

23. Katie Reilly, "The Viral Lincoln Memorial Confrontation Shows We're Ill-Equipped to Deal with Online Disinformation," *Time* (January 23, 2019).
24. Ben Shapiro made posts on Twitter about the incident that have since been deleted.
25. Mac Donald (2017), p. 40.

scribe the entheogen. 5-MeO DMT can be produced synthetically and can also be extracted from the Sonora desert toad, which it secretes when threatened. Most facilitators prefer the synthetic form of the medicine for two reasons: first, because it is easier to gauge dosage; second, cute little toads don't get hurt in the extraction process. With 5-MeO DMT, it is better to have your friendly neighborhood underground alchemist create it with good intentions than have the medicine derive from the fear the toad is experiencing as you massage its glands to extract the God Molecule.

Dr. Ball was an active thought leader in psychedelic spaces, most renowned for his theories on non-dualism (i.e., "we are all one"). He hosted the Exploring Psychedelics Conference and his podcast, *Entheogenic Evolution*, remains the longest running podcast devoted to psychedelics. As a 5-MeO DMT facilitator, his tactics were certainly uncommon, if not downright controversial to polite society. He has been known to vomit on his clients, touch their genitals, and once pressed his tongue against the tongue of an elderly woman to resuscitate her after noticing that she'd stopped breathing. Yes, these practices might make you squeamish. I certainly wouldn't want to be vomited on while under the influence of 5-MeO DMT (or really any other time). But these unusual methods were the very reasons his clients sought him out over other 5-MeO DMT facilitators in the area.

Humanity is a rich tapestry.

In 2016, Dr. Ball gave a two-and-a-half hour lecture on his practices for the Los Angeles Medicinal Psychedelics Society (LAMPS) at the University of California, Los Angeles (UCLA). LAMPS organizers filmed the event and posted it on their YouTube channel. The video has more views than any other on LAMPS's channel. Reading the comments, one finds a majority of support for Dr. Ball and his unique approach to psychedelic medicine work. As part of a larger power struggle within the psychedelic Renaissance, which we will discuss in a moment, Psymposia set out to investigate and cancel Dr. Ball for what they saw as his wholly inapproriate methods and behavior.

Their attacks on Dr. Ball began when a writer at Psymposia, Russell Hausfeld, created a short edit of Dr. Ball's LAMPS talk at UCLA that highlighted the sections that he presumably found most objectionable or problematic. Hausfeld also employed a series of audio/visual alterations in his edit, including slowing down Dr. Ball's voice and zooming-in to various parts of his body in an effort to make him seem as ridiculous as possible. Before informing Dr. Ball of the edited video, which would be shared on Psymposia's YouTube channel, Hausfeld reached out to Dr. Ball via email, asking for some clarifications about statements made in the LAMPS lecture. Dr. Ball obliged, even sending Hausfeld the PDF document he shares with any potential clients. Says Dr. Ball of this exchange:

> My intent was to show [Psymposia] that I fully disclosed how I worked with every potential client prior to arranging a session so that I knew that [the client] was fully informed. . . . I would then spend an hour reviewing all these materials with each client before ever beginning a session. I shared this, along with sections of my 2017 book that covered much of the same material, in order to provide Psymposia with context and clear evidence that people who came to work with me knew what to expect and were informed, consenting adults. I also shared the PDF with the instructions that it was not for publication or public dissemination and that I was providing it as a professional courtesy.[26]

Psymposia used this material to create another video—this time, a roundtable discussion among their associates, which concluded that Dr. Ball was "a sexual deviant, a rapist, an abuser, and a groomer, who coaxed people into working with him so that he could fulfill his perverted desires upon them." Dr. Ball reached out to Hausfeld, asking if he wanted to sort this all out on either his podcast or that of Psymposia. The response read in part: "We will not be joining you on your platform and will not be having you on ours."

The blowback was quick. Messages poured into Dr. Ball's inbox from all over the world, calling him a host of names like "psychopath," "rapist," and "abuser." Other messages spoke of having Dr. Ball thrown in jail and registered as a sex offender. Others implied that he was a pedophile—no doubt inspired by Psymposia writer Neşe Devenot, who spewed such

26. Dr. Martin Ball, "My Scarlet Letter" (transcript of podcast sent to author). Following quotes from that source unless otherwise indicated.

slanders during the roundtable discussion. Still others wished death upon him. His house was vandalized, and soon he started receiving dis-invitations from public forums at which he had been scheduled to speak. And yet, try as they might, Psymposia couldn't find a single victim of the notorious Dr. Ball.

Thankfully, not everyone in the psychedelic Renaissance bought Psymposia's narrative. Dr. Ball was defended not only by those who knew Psymposia wasn't acting in good faith but also by his former clients who began to speak up and confirm that he had not abused them, sexually assaulted them, or relieved any perversion upon them. Dr. Ball's practices might indeed turn a person off. But they do not turn off the many people who swear by his techniques. Psymposia supporters gaslit these consenting adults, claiming they suffered from Stockholm Syndrome. The very clients to which Dr. Ball speaks in his original LAMPS talk even reached out to Psymposia defending him. Psymposia told them to "fuck off." According to Dr. Ball's clients, dealing with Psymposia's managing editor was like talking to "a sociopath who was immune to evidence, reason, or rational discussion."

At the time of this writing, it has been several years since the "scandal" broke. Despite his exoneration in the psychedelic Renaissance's court of public opinion, and the adamant defense of his clients insisting he had not abused them, Dr. Ball still remains on the margins of the movement for crimes he never committed.

This, Psymposia calls "journalism."

The Wonderful Dr. Gerry

Dr. Gerry Sandoval (or "Dr. Gerry," as he is known in psychedelic circles), a Mexican-born medicine man, has achieved a fair amount of fame due to his appearance on Vice TV's show *Hamilton's Pharmacopeia*, and is recognized as the person who first gave heavyweight champion Iron Mike Tyson 5-MeO DMT. That's his public face. His private face, known by those in the psychedelic Renaissance who've dealt with him, is a different matter altogether. There *are* victims. There *are* testimonies. In this world, Dr. Gerry is seen as a *known* abuser. His former partner, Slovenia, charges that he "drugged her with an unknown substance and then raped her."[27] Two women disclosed anonymously that Dr. Gerry "was aggressively sexual with them, including keeping them drugged and basically held hostage until he decided they wouldn't reciprocate his advances, not allowing them to leave."[28] One victim claims to have suffered "suicidal depression" years after her encounter with Dr. Gerry.[29]

I should say that Dr. Gerry has not been tried in any court of law, so his misdeeds remain allegations. But the list of accusations against him is quite long, and the consensus of victims who do not know each other telling of similar abuses has raised some eyebrows: sexual assault, drugging people against their will, thievery,[30] fraud, and kidnapping. Other charges include planting drugs on people before crossing national borders. As one commentor put it, "you name it, [Dr. Gerry is] accused of it."[31]

Perhaps everyone is wrong, and Dr. Gerry is not dangerous at all.

But wouldn't you want to know first?

That's why some of us were surprised when we saw his name on the roster to speak at a fall 2022 conference (via Zoom—he isn't currently allowed in the United States) hosted by the Detroit Psychedelic Society (DPS), a majority black American-run nonprofit psychedelic organization. I asked on the conference Facebook event page if any of the organizers had an issue with the abuse allegations made against Dr. Gerry. I was met with silence. I then reached out by phone to one of the head organizers. The organizer was well aware of Dr. Gerry's sordid past and reputation. But there was a problem—Dr. Gerry often sent newbies to the DPS to participate in their mushroom growing classes, for which they might shell out a few hundred dollars. Without Dr. Gerry's participation, DPS's bottom line would be at risk. A most pernicious heist with a psychedelic twist.

27. "Open Letter Concerning Abuses by Octavio Rettig and Gerry Sandoval," DMT-Nexus (2019).

28. Martin Ball, pers. comm. In fairness to Dr. Gerry, anonymous accusations do stand on shaky ground. But there are also those like Slovenia who are willing to identify themselves and speak up.

29. "Open Letter . . .," DMT-Nexus (2019).

30. I personally know someone who let Dr. Gerry stay in her house; he used it as an opportunity to lift a few items.

31. Yann with Ayahuasca, "An Open Letter to Octavio Rettig and Gerry Sandoval—Here It Is" (April 16, 2019).

Getting nowhere with DPS, I reached out to the president of the Portland Psychedelic Society—the same fellow who wanted me to take an implicit bias course. Considering this young man headed up one of the largest psychedelic societies in the world, I asked if he wanted to make a public statement against Dr. Gerry's invitation to the DPS conference. Due to the ethnicities of those involved (Mexican and majority black American, respectively), the PPS president wanted nothing to do with the issue. I then reached out to Psymposia's Politics and Ecology Editor, Brian Pace, to see if Psymposia—considering their stance on outing "abusers" (real or imagined)—might produce some exposé. Pace had not been aware that Dr. Gerry would speak at the DPS conference and agreed that it wasn't a good idea to platform him.

I did not participate in the conference, so I have no idea who attended or what was said. Today, it is impossible to find any evidence online that Dr. Gerry spoke at the 2022 conference.[32] Either the concerns of those who stood against his participation were heard and he was disinvited, or DPS has scrubbed any hint of his presence at the conference from the Internet. As far as I am aware, DPS has made no public comment one way or another, and Psymposia has never produced a video investigating the many serious allegations againt Dr. Gerry.

It simply does not fit the Racist Narrative.

MAPS Canada

Dr. Ball was just a pawn in a larger struggle to insert ever greater levels of critical social justice ideology into the psychedelic movement. As a key part of this effort, Psymposia set its sights on then Executive Director of MAPS Canada, Mark Haden. In 2020, he was approached by two women, Keeno Ahmed-Jones and Ava Daeipour, asking him if they might establish a Volunteer Diversity Committee within the MAPS Canada organization. Haden agreed that such a committee should exist and deputized these junior members of MAPS Canada with the task of creating one.

32. Regardless, Dr. Gerry did speak at the DPS conference in 2020, a year after allegations against him were well-known.

Ahmed-Jones and Daeipour had become incensed over the "racist vitriol" that the staff at a Quebec hospital allegedly spewed at Joyce Echaquan, an Atikamekw woman, shortly before her death.[33] Listening to the recording of the incident shows very demeaning and terrible treatment by the staff, no doubt; however, it does not reveal any racist comments at all. Even the headline of the news article to which the letter links, which surely would have called attention to any actual racial epithets slung at Echaquan, mentions only "slurs." The hospital staff—rude, uncaring, and unprofessional as they proved—said nothing of Echaquan's indigeneity, but rather commented on her "bad life choices."[34]

Like many who have been captured by critical social justice ideology, Ahmed-Jones and Daeipour were making a terrible incident—in this case, Joyce Echaquan's death—all about race and then asking why racism is seemingly everywhere. It's like seeding a garden and then wondering why vegetables are growing in your backyard.

Roughly a month after giving the volunteers the greenlight to form the Volunteer Diversity Committee, Haden invited them to dinner to see how things had progressed. Ahmed-Jones and Daeipour showed up with a list of demands—demands well out of the range of MAPS Canada's abilities, resources, and legal limits. They wanted MAPS Canada to fix all the "wrongs of colonialism since the dawn of time."[35] Despite sharing a name with its older, well-established parent in the United States—MAPS—the Canadian branch operates on a much smaller scale with a much smaller budget.

But there was another problem: all nonprofits file an Articles of Incorporation with their state governments, which outlines what social or cultural issues the organization wishes to address. For example, a non-

33. Keeno Ahmed-Jones and Ava Daeipour, "An Open Letter and Call to Action for MAPS Canada" (October 21, 2020).
34. Benjamin Shingler, "Investigations Launched after Atikamekw Woman Records Quebec Hospital Staff Uttering Slurs Before Her Death," *CBC News* (September 30, 2020).
35. Trevor Millar, pers. comm. (8 August 2023). All quotes from here unless otherwise indicated.

profit like Black Lives Matter cannot suddenly decide that it wants to divert funds towards legalizing psychedelics, because such ambitions presumably do not appear in the BLM Articles of Incorporation. All nonprofits are required by law to uphold only those goals originally outlined in their Articles of Incorporation. MAPS is not allowed to step outside the bounds of its Articles of Incorporation, which, presumably, do not hold the organization responsible for fixing colonialism. Haden replied by way of analogy: "MAPS supports Green Peace, but we are not about to go out and try to save the whales." Because doing so would be illegal. MAPS Canada's Articles of Incorporation only sets them up for *one* task: legalizing psychedelic medicines for therapeutic uses. So even if Haden wanted to and could somehow correct all injustices in the past, he is legally prevented from doing so. Perhaps it's a bad law. Haden is stuck with it. These provisions tie the hands of all nonprofits, regardless of the melanin level of the executive director.

Ahmed-Jones and Daeipour also complained that the board of directors was staffed mostly by white Canadian men (no surprise, as white Canadian men make up a large section of the Canadian population)[36] and their solution was to put someone on the board who would implement Chacruna Institute's JEDI strategy. They also lamented the lack of public support MAPS Canada showed the BLM movement.

Haden found a compromise: he asked Ahmed-Jones and Daeipour to draft an official statement for MAPS Canada showing its support of BLM. The two got right to work. They finalized a draft, which they then forwarded to Haden. However, there were some nonprofit law problems with the statement that Haden edited in good faith. But for Ahmed-Jones and Daeipour, his edits were apparently unacceptable. They published part of their original statement with Haden's edits on Psymposia's website.

Original: "We stand in solidarity with the Black Lives Matter movement and condemn the police brutality against the Black/Brown/Indigenous communities in the US and Canada. We pledge to do the necessary work [*do the work*!] to both spread awareness and actively oppose the inherently racist systems that perpetuate violence against BIPOC."

Haden's edits: "We support the Black Lives Matter movement and

36. Roughly 49.64%.

condemn the police brutality against Black, Brown and Indigenous communities. MAPS Canada is an organization which is dedicated to healing and healing on many levels is urgently needed now."[37]

There are a few noticeable differences. Haden changed the word "solidarity" to "support," along with cutting out "in the US and Canan-da," and the entire last sentence.

Legally, he had little choice. First, MAPS's Articles of Incorporation, filed in 1986, say nothing about the aims of BLM (how could it? BLM didn't exist yet).[38] Revisions made in 2019 also do not mention BLM.[39] Second, nonprofits are severely limited in what they can do or say politically. Complete solidarity with anyone—Green Peace or otherwise—could mean a forfeiture of nonprofit status. Nor can nonprofits "actively oppose" anything politically motivated, whether its saving whales or police brutality. Haden was most certainly knowledgeable of these laws. After giving Ahmed-Jones and Daeipour's statement a careful read, he *had to* excise those words and phrases from the original draft or risk toppling his organization.

As another compromise to their demands, Haden would place a member of MAPS Canada's Board of Directors on the Volunteer Diversity Committee to see if they could find some satisfactory middle ground. The member placed on the committee was chair of the MAPS Canada board, Trevor Millar, an iboga facilitator familiar with serving the underserved in East Vancouver. For those unfamiliar with this medicine, iboga comes from the African basswali tree and has proved highly effective in treating addictions like alcoholism, hard drug use, and anorexia/bulimia.[40] To that end, Millar worked with all kinds of people: indigenous, French-Canadian, and especially the Muslim-Canadian community. Millar seemed the right man for the job. He met with Ahmed-Jones and Daeipour to discuss how best to meet in the middle. He believed a good way to show his support for the committee was to give them carte blanche: "Do what you can to increase diversity," he told them. "We'd love that!"

37. Quoted in Ahmed-Jones and Daeipour (2020).
38. "Articles of Incorporation of Multidisciplinary Association for Psychedelic Studies, Inc."
39. MAPS "Article Three: Revisions adopted October 17, 2019."
40. Karen O'Neel (iboga facilitator), pers. comm.

Unfortunately, this strategy did not address how a small, under-resourced organization like MAPS Canada would right all the wrongs of history.[41] Ahmed-Jones and Daeipour, perhaps unsurprisingly, had no solutions either. The problem with Millar was not his friendly disposition or his record of assisting marginalized peoples; the problem was Millar is a white Canadian man. And so, Millar stopped receiving invitations to Volunteer Diversity Committee meetings until, as he was told, he "took a long look in the mirror." Wondering what was going on with the committee (which was his job as chair of the board), Millar reached out to its representatives and was finally able to join a Zoom call over these issues.

As bad luck would have it, a few days before the Zoom meeting, Millar found himself in an argument on Facebook (always a bad idea!) about a topic unrelated to psychedelia. A friend of his, Bradley Foster, founder of the Toronto Psychedelic Association, joined the conversation thread telling Millar that he needed to "stick to [his] knitting." Not sure of what Foster meant by that, Millar took to idiom.com to find out. As it turns out, "stick to your knitting" is a colloquial way of saying "stay in your lane," or "focus on your specialty." Millar is a psychedelics guy—whatever the Facebook argument in which he was embroiled had nothing to do with psychedelics, and Foster was merely reminding him of that in a friendly way.

Back to our Diversity Committee Zoom call. Millar told the committee members the story of how Foster had told him to "stick to my knitting . . . and that's what MAPS Canada has to do. [We] have to stay in our lane and focus on legalizing psychedelics. MAPS Canada can't be all things to all people. MAPS Canada needs to stick to its knitting." Ahmed-Jones and Daeipour decontextualized Millar's words in an "Open Letter," published on Psymposia's website, and made it seem as though he was telling them—two women—to "stick to knitting," which, without context, does

41. Nor did it address the bountiful human rights violations of First Nations peoples, Africans, or Middle Easterners.

reek of misogyny. They write: "Millar—while discussing work we were doing for the committee with Haden's assistant—told him we should 'stick to *our* knitting'—a misogynistic, belittling comment revealing his true mindset, and a stark contrast to the support he had given us in public settings."[42] The larger stereotype of women knitting gets funneled into the narrative so it can be weaponized by bad faith actors—even though that was not what Millar was saying. He wasn't talking about Ahmed-Jones and Daeipour (or anyone on the committee) when he used the knitting colloquialism; he was taking about MAPS Canada. These are the word games of the victim-minded. Psymposia's writers didn't bother to check or verify any of it. The quote could be weaponized against Trevor Miller, and that was all they wanted.

This, Psymposia calls "journalism."

Which brings us back to the notorious Dr. Ball. Mark Haden had contacted Dr. Ball to design the cover art for his upcoming book, *Manual for Psychedelic Guides* (2020). His use by Psymposia was nothing more than a cheap maneuver in a larger plan to discredit Haden through association with Dr. Ball. Sadly, it worked. Mark Haden and Trevor Millar both stepped down from MAPS Canada. MAPS Canada's website now features a "Commitment to Antiracism and Reconciliation" section that reads exactly like what it sounds: an embarrassing, self-flagellating barrage of CSJ word salad: "We recognize the roots of oppression embedded in patriarchy and colonialism. We recognize the use of coercive and discriminatory policies and laws as a tool to continue the oppression of marginalized groups. . . . [W]e also acknowledge the challenges for those facing other inequalities including women, persons with disabilities, queer, trans, and two-spirit people"—just to cover all grounds.[43] And, of course, such challenges and inequalities are never defined.

We are to take them on faith.

Dr. Ball is still, at the time of this writing, *persona non grata* in the psychedelic Renaissance. Meanwhile, high-profile psychedelic organiza-

42. Trevor Millar; *italics* mine; Ahmed-Jones and Daeipour, "An Open Letter"; *italics* mine.
43. MAPS Canada, "Policies."

tions refuse to criticize Dr. Gerry, while others excuse his questionable past for financial gain. Psymposia, aware of at least some of the story, remains silent.

That innocent people like Dr. Ball, Trevor Millar, and Dr. Mark Haden can be cast as every "ist" CSJ psychedelia has to offer, while credibly accused abusers like Dr. Gerry, bad-faith actors like Ahmed-Jones and Daeipour, and assorted enablers remain unscathed, I believe, is not good for the psychedelic community. *Quod erat demonstrandum*, we see how the biased standards of our larger American media infiltrate the psychedelic Renaissance and rot it out from within.

At the beginning of this book, I mentioned that I would do my best to not make abstractions. I hope I have stood by my word thus far and would like to add to it. Not everyone from Psymposia strikes me as having questionable motives. Brian Pace, who I mentioned earlier, is a good example. Misguided, no doubt—but in the very least leading with the heart. This is my ultimate gripe. The ideology captures *good* people.

And there certainly is a need for community watchdogs like Psymposia. Abuses do happen, and Psymposia's reporters have it within themselves to use their powers for good by exposing predators, disingenuous actors, and others—no matter the color of their skin. Additionally, so far as disingenuous actors are concerned, Psymposia might start with a little house-cleaning of their own. When the larger Psymposia organization purposely contributes to the Racist Narrative by unapologetically broadcasting misinformation, it severely undermines both its own credibility and the very problems it is trying to solve.

Part IV

The Gender Narrative

14

Stunning. Brave. The Most Important Topic in the World

In general, you know, [transitioners] want this, but they don't want this, but they want this, but they don't want this from a hormone, and I'm like, well, you know, you might not be binary, but hormones are binary . . . that doesn't work very well.[1]

—WPATH doctor

The Gender Narrative

You will have immediately noticed that this third and final section of the book is thinner than the former two. The reason is that I don't have much to say about the Gender Narrative that hasn't already been said by others better equipped to navigate such choppy waters. Mostly because the discussion veers too deeply into psychology, of which I have no formal training.

I find that my views on the recent gender hubbub are aligned with

1. "WPATH Video Quotes: From WPATH's 'Identity Evolution Workshop held on May 6, 2022,'" *Environmental Progress* (2024).

most liberal thinkers: informed and consenting adults should be allowed to have any surgery they want and think about themselves any way they like. It is common courtesy to use the pronouns of their preference (she/her or he/him) to complement their outward appearance, which many of us (me included) are happy to oblige. I find that it is a natural right for mature adults to live a life in a way that feels the most comfortable and authentic for them; I highly question (and often snicker at) supposed "freedom-loving" Americans who tend to think that only their preferences count as "freedom." Notwithstanding transwomen playing sports against women, I am diametrically opposed to anyone who wishes to exclude trans people from pursuing a life of liberty and happiness.

Then there is the Gender Narrative, which is less a way of being than it is an ideology that I find promotes dogmas detrimental to both the psychedelic Renaissance and society at large. In no particular order they are: the authoritarian attack on free speech and thought, the erasing of women and homosexuals, the curious desire to be considered "oppressed," and (most concerning) the mutilation, and psychological and emotional abuse of children.

Like the Decolonization and Racist Narratives, the Gender Narrative holds kernels of truth. Since the rise of Christianity, heterosexuality has been seen as the unshakable norm, with any deviations from it considered sinful among theologians and disordered among psychologists. This prompted social discriminations, misunderstandings, bullying, and at times, murder. The Gender Narrative deserves praise for adding a much-needed correction to such a myopic view of human sexuality. In fact, I believe the Gender Narrative represents the end result of a society that is far too anal about human sexuality. I also believe that wondering, even wanting, to experience what it might be like to live as the opposite sex is a natural human compulsion for some people.

But like most endeavors that seek a more just course of action for society in the face of historical wrongs, the Gender Narrative has at times over-corrected the issue by adopting too many incoherent postmodern principles into this otherwise serious discussion. The most obvious affronts come from Michel Foucault's ideas of power/knowledge, which we briefly addressed in an earlier chapter. To recap: according to Foucault objective truth is not obtainable through inquiry and experiment, but rather created by the consensus of those who hold cultural power in society. Consider equitable math, which we also covered earlier. Within Foucault's power/knowledge principle, 2 + 2 only equals 4 because shadowy tastemakers working behind the scenes have fooled us all into believing it. Had our overlords decided that 2 + 2 equals 7, we would all believe that instead (despite the obvious shortcomings of such a view). And, of course, to Foucault all knowledge serves as a political statement.

Foucault's ideas opened the door to the possibility that gender itself is both detached from biology and a "social construct." To prove it, the gender ideologue will rightfully point out that social mores and trends change over time. As just one of countless examples, consider the standard colors used for baby clothing these days: pink for little girls, light blue for little boys. And yet, during the late 1920s, pink was seen as the more masculine color, while blue was considered softer and more feminine.[2] Such a drastic changing of a social norm within less than a century provides all the proof the gender ideologue needs to claim that biological sex isn't real, but rather just another social construct.

TRENDSGENDER

We've heard various terms for this neo-gender phenomenon, the most popular is "social contagion." A fine term, no doubt, but I think it only represents a euphemism for a more accurate term: *fashion trend.* Gender ideology strikes me as a fashion trend, no different from powdered wigs and bellbottom jeans. Now, that does not mean that there aren't *real* trans people. I believe there are and always have been. What I'm referring to when I say "fashion trend" is the explosion of chicanery we have endured since the late 20-teens in the form of "nonbinary" and other "neo-genders" (as I call them), and the obsession with preferred pronouns. While some might say that the reason for this rapid growth has to do with society becoming more tolerant, the fashion trend markers of trendsgenderism are quite obvious: firstly, trendsgenderism didn't exist until only a few years ago; and I predict, will be nothing but a memory in five to ten years (although, there will always be hangers-on). Secondly, a large predictor of whether a kid decides she's trans is whether or not

2. Jo B. Paoletti, *Pink and Blue: Telling the Boys from the Girls in America* (IN: Indiana University Press, 2012), pp. 90–1.

her friends are trans. (Reread that last sentence and replace the word "trans" with either the word "punk" or "goth.") Kids are impressionable and want to fit in. They also go through awkward phases in puberty of which the majority (85%) outgrow.[3] How stunting the physical, emotional, and mental development of a confused child helps her in any way remains a mystery. Finally, countries like Sweden have had very progressive, warm, and accepting policies and social attitudes around the trans issue for half a century's time. Sweden was the first European country to legalize transgender surgery back in 1972. Still, Sweden has seen a boom in transgenderism since the late 20-teens.[4] This is not the result of a society becoming more accepting (of which Sweden already has a long-standing record); it is the result of a fashion trend.

Cognitive Liberty

One of the issues with the broader Gender Narrative is the way it tries to limit free speech through intimidation and harassment, which is counterintuitive to cognitive liberty, cultural progress, and personal healing. Transmuting thought into speech calms the central nervous system; feeling scared or even threatened to speak suffocates. It feels like a central part of our vitality is being sucked out of us, harvested for the comfort of the emotionally dysregulated. We feel captured in a dystopian chokehold. And so we shut ourselves down for fear of our friends and peers shunning, unloving, ostracizing, attacking, and/or otherwise hating us. I can think of no soil more fertile for developing superficial relationships than that.

Where does this attack on free speech come from? What is its origin point? Sexologist Ray Blanchard advanced the idea that transgenderism stems from autogynephilic roots. Autogynephilia is a paraphilia wherein a person is sexually aroused by seeing her or himself as the opposite sex.

3. Donna M., "Yes, Your Kid's Trans Thing is a Phase," *New Discourses* (September 18, 2021); Devita Singh, Susan J. Bradley, Kenneth J. Zucker, "A Follow-Up Study of Boys with Gender Identity Disorder," *Frontiers in Psychiatry*, Vol. 12 (March 28, 2021).
4. Betsy Reed, "Sweden Passes Law Lowering Age to Legally Change Gender from 18 to 16," *The Gurdian* (April 17, 2024).

While this theory has certainly met criticism,[5] studies conducted in the area give weight to it.[6] According to Blanchard, the hostility stems from "envy of women and resentment at not being accepted by women as one of them."[7]

Author Michael Bailey is one of many people who found himself in the transactivist crosshairs for disclosing the autogynephilia angle in his book *The Man Who Would Be Queen* (2003). The backlash came quickly. Online hate and harassment poured in; even his children were attacked. One transactivist, Andrea James, put pictures of Bailey's children online with captions such as: "there are two types of children in the Bailey household: [those] who have been sodomized by their father [and those] who have not." James further inquired if Bailey's daughter was a "cock-starved exhibitionist, or a paraphiliac who just gets off on the idea of it."[8]

Admittedly, I do not know enough about psychology and endocrinology to make an informed decision on the extent to which autogynephilia plays a role in transgenderism. But I do know something about basic human decency. And James' attack on Bailey's family, and his cognitive liberty, was nothing but indecent.

Although we might also consider that Andrea James's protest raises a question: why does an autogynephilic foundation for transgenderism cheapen it? Are we so culturally censorious that even the thought of a sexual origin for certain behaviors is somehow wrong or unreasonable? And if Andrea James really believes herself a woman, why does she care what anyone else thinks? Why does she need everyone else to believe it too? In what other aspect of Western life is such a forced and rigid suspension of disbelief required by nonbelievers on a societal scale??

To answer those questions, some have pointed to the higher numbers of narcissistic personality disorders among trans people. In 2008, Dr. Anne Lawrence, herself a transwoman, published a paper wherein she argued that among trans people narcissistic personality traits like

5. Alex Sharpe, "Review of Helen Joyce's *Trans: When Ideology Meets Reality . . .*; and Katherine Stock's *Material Girls: Why Reality Matters for Feminism . . .*," *Critical Legal Thinking* (October 8, 2021).
6. Helen Joyce, *Trans: When Ideology Meets Reality* (London: Oneworld Publications, 2022), p. 40.
7. Quoted in Joyce (2022), p. 49.
8. Dishonorably quoted in Joyce (2022), pp. 46–7.

feelings of entitlement, a concerning lack of empathy, and claims of grandiosity abound.[9] We can see a noticeable example in the way some trans people expect all of society to bend to their narrative. But it is only *some*. I do not believe that all trans people suffer from narcissistic personality disorders. My trans friends are some of the kindest, most openminded, and compassionate people I know.

Perhaps there is room for an alternative explanation. What if this sudden rise in what many call "narcissistic" is being used far too broadly to describe what is really an extreme form of self-centeredness created by modern amenities? What if—and here's where my inner old fart emerges—the egotism isn't a trans thing but instead a generational thing? And the Gender Narrative is nothing more than a byproduct of a worrisome combination of social media addiction and feelings of purposelessness? There is evidence to back this up. For example, while Millennials and Zoomers are "convinced of their own greatness," they also struggle with self-esteem, forming a very concerning cognitive dissonance.[10] From the shallows of social media to participation trophies, to bulldozer parenting strategies, and a host of other pedagogical misfires, is it really so surprising that kids are less concerned with finding objective truth ("research") and more obsessed with their own story ("mesearch") these days?

But is it really all their fault? I don't think so. It isn't hard to imagine some kids stuck in very rurally conservative areas with nothing to do who want to explore the range of human sexual expression, but feel stifled in doing so; to escape, they create whole new lives for themselves on the Internet. They can separate their daily life from their Internet life, so as to keep the whole thing a secret if they must. Still, if the Internet life is better than real life, it can become easy to detach from the latter altogether. And as we all know, Internet algorithms cater to our specific desires, pulling us further and further away from reality. This certainly can help partially explain the rise of the Gender Narrative in recent years.

Hardcore conservative parents who reject their kids' growth phases and styles, I believe, exacerbate the problem. If they could just ease off their kids, who are going through all the same confusion and worry that

9. Anne Lawrence, "Shame and Narcissistic Personality Disorder in Autogynephilic Transexuals," *Archives of Sexual Behavior*, 37 (April 23, 2008): 457–61.
10. Time Staff, "Millennials: The Me Me Me Generation," *Time* (May 20, 2013).

we all went through at their age, perhaps the phase can pass with fewer headaches and shouting matches at the dinner table. It isn't very complicated: a kid wants to experiment outside heteronormativity (either due to natural orientation or to follow the fashion trend), parents flip out, kid sinks deeper into despair; she doesn't stop the behavior, she just gets more clandestine. The Internet will provide all the cover she needs. The lack of love and understanding only leads to secrecy and, eventually, radicalization. And radicalization tends to lead to mob mentality. Soon, she is lost in the abstraction.

This issue puts me in an unenviable position. While I believe strongly in compassion for anyone struggling with gender dysphoria, I also fear that we are witnessing the demonization of common sense. And many live in fear. Fear that they—like Michael Bailey and countless others—will be labeled bigots simply for not agreeing with *everything* the Gender Narrative demands—even outlandish requests to reclassify the word "woman" as hate speech.[11]

The Sacred Feminine

While I do not believe that all trans *people* are misogynists, there are some noticeable markers that put the *Gender Narrative's* misogyny on full display. Lately we've been hearing about "birthing persons" and "womb bearers" but not a peep about "sperm carriers" and "fart providers."

Language is the realm of the trans ideologue because language is subjective. But there exist certain biological and chemical truths beyond any subjectivity, even granting that humans invented the word "chemistry" and all subsequent words found on the periodic table of elements, like, say, "magnesium" (and 117 others). But we could have just as easily swapped out the word "magnesium" for the word "elephant," and all the underlying scientific truths of magnesium and elephant, now traded linguistically, would remain. Elephant would still be good for sleep, digestion, and stress management; a magnesium would still have a long trunk, large floppy ears, and tusks (provided she was an African magnesium and not an Asian magnesium).

The attempted erasure of women should disturb us all, both in the

11. "Woman Billboard was Transphobic and Dangerous," *BBC* (September 26, 2018).

material and spiritual realms. Materially, women require reproductive autonomy—whether you agree with me about a woman's right to choose doesn't matter—it has nothing to do with transwomen. Spiritually, there is an aspect to extreme gender ideology that reinforces the patriarchy of the Abrahamic religions through tearing down the Sacred Feminine. By pretending that the very representatives of the Sacred Feminine on Earth (women) are a mere cultural construct, the ideology debases the Goddess along with all womankind.

Some of us (and I include myself in this company) employ entheogens as ways to access the creative forces of the Sacred Feminine. Certain psilocybin mushrooms, like Golden Teachers, have a feminine presence to them. Likewise, there is a reason ayahuasca is referred to as Pachamama ("Earth Mother").

Not Earth Father.

Not Earth Xyr.

Not Earth Them.

Not Earth Creating Person.

Earth *Mother.*

Like Golden Teachers, Momma Aya has a feminine resonance about Her. My dear friend Flamy calls Her "Mom." I call her Gaia. Others call her Pachamama. We're all talking about the same thing (although I have no doubt that we receive the messages through culturally-bound symbols that we understand on individual bases).[12]

The cosmic polarities between the Sacred Feminine and the Divine Masculine have been recognized in religious symbolism since the days of the pre-Sumerian Ur Civilization in the form of the Sacred Marriage of Inanna and Dumuzi.[13] Yahweh once had a wife named Asherah.[14] Even Christianity needs Mary, mother of Jesus. Other symbols of the Sacred Feminine have all but been forgotten. Abandoning the Sacred Feminine

12. Although, that is not always the case. A friend of mine once heard an entity speak a word to her during a deep DMT experience. She had never heard the word before, but after her dive Googled it anyway. It turned out to be an ancient Sanskrit word that means "oneness." Much as I love my friend, she is not an ancient language scholar. And yet, she received a message from an outside source telling her of something that existed of which she knew nothing about at that time.

13. Hatsis (2018), pp. 50–1.

14. Bennett (2023), p. 32.

simply because someone's sense of identity feels threatened by it doesn't work for me.

The sex binary isn't only quite obviously biologically real, whether we are talking about elephants (or magnesiums if you prefer) or any other family of lifeform, it is also a part of the sacred blueprint of life on Earth—from insects to God-fearing apes. Looking deeper, we find it in the ethereal realms of plant medicines (the Sacred Feminine in ayahuasca and Golden Teachers, and the Divine Masculine in iboga and peyote).[15] Perhaps beneath the façade of the Gender Narrative there exists a very deep psychic wound between women and men that has yet to be healed. I can understand that.

But is denying that women exist the correct solution?

The Trans Genocide

No one can deny that trans people face daily difficulties and harassment that others do not. But in recent years there has been a kind of oppression pilfering by some gender activists from other groups who have been historically abused to extreme degrees. Let's briefly explore how the appropriation of real systemic oppression once faced by black Americans is currently exploited by modern gender activists. The funnel from black American to trans has its origins in the Black Lives Matter movement. BLM was based on the idea that black American *men* (specifically) were unfairly targeted by white American police officers for slaughter. Woke as such a message was, it wasn't Woke enough. Soon we started seeing flags and placards declaring "Black Trans Lives Matter."

The Black Trans Lives Matter movement began in 2014 by Cherno Biko. One of the cases that stands out to Biko involved Deonna Mason, a black American transwoman, who was killed by a police officer.[16] Anthony Williams, of the Afrikan Black Coalition, also responded to the death by drafting an article where he demands justice for Deonna.

15. Both respectively referred to as "Grandfather."
16. Lauren N. Williams, "Trans Activist Speaking up for Victims of Violence and Transgender Women of Color," *Time* (2024).

"We cannot claim to be pro-Black if our fight for Black lives does not include transwomen," he says. For Williams, Deonna was just one "of over 20" black American transwomen killed in 2015 (including India Clarke and Mya Hill, which he offers as two other examples).[17] Only India Clarke wasn't killed by the police. She was shot by Keith Lamayne Gaillard. Mya Hill was shot by guards during a "violent confrontation" after she crashed through the gates of the National Security Agency headquarters.[18] She was allegedly zonked out of her mind on some kind of drug(s)—the specifics have not been released—and ran towards the officers. Mya refused any lawful orders to stop. Believing they were under attack, the guards opened fire. No one who shot her knew that she was a transwoman at that time. As for Deonna Mason, she was hit by a car as she illegally tried to cross a major interstate on foot at night. That it was a police car that hit her was merely a coincidence.

That is not to say that Cherno Biko and I can't meet for tea and a bong hit. I agree with her that transwomen can be uniquely targeted for murder; but it simply isn't the police doing it. For example, Jimmy LaShawn Williams shot 17-year-old Ariyanna Mitchell (d. 2022) simply because she was a transwoman.[19] A lot of these women are sex-workers killed by johns scared of exposure. Because such deeds happen in secret, the murders happen in secret too.[20] Sadly, the majority of trans murders (of any ethnicity) are not solved for that reason. We *do* know that the majority of these transwomen are not killed by the police. Between 2017 and 2021, police officers shot and killed five trans people in the United States. And all five of them posed an armed threat to the officers. Most sadly, common throughout all these cases (save one) were unaddressed mental health issues.[21]

---

17. Anthony Williams, "#JusticeforPrissy, or How We've Failed Our Trans Sisters," *TransMusePlanet* (January 7, 2016).
18. "Driver Killed at NSA Identified as Transgender Sex Worker, Friend Says," *Chicago Tribune* (June 22, 2019).
19. Aesia Toliver, "Court Docs: Suspect Asked, 'Are You a Boy or a Girl?' Before Fatal Hampton Shooting," *Wavy* (April 15, 2022).
20. Examples include Ali Forney, Tanya Moore, and Tina Rodriguez, among others.
21. Matt Drange, "They Called 911 for Assistance. Then the Police Used Lethal Force," *Business Insider* (November 22, 2022).

From there, it was just a short step to claiming some kind of "trans genocide" was taking place in the United States. In 2023, 320 trans people were killed globally, the majority in Central and South America (numbering 236). In North America, the number topped out at 33.[22] When trans people are shot by the police there are usually mitigating circumstances (like with Deonna Mason and Mya Hill). As unfortunate as all those deaths were (no matter the cause), none of this amounts to an actual genocide.

And certainly not one involving the police.

In the Nature of Things

Undoubtedly, the most grotesque aspect of the Gender Narrative is the systemic medical abuse of the most vulnerable amongst us, children.

The idea that a child could choose her gender was based on the discredited ideas of sexologist Dr. John Money (1921–2006) of Johns Hopkins University. While Dr. Money did not invent the Gender Narrative, our current obsession with it stems from his theories, as he was the first person to remove "gender" from language and apply it to people (by coining terms like "gender role" and "gender identity"). Money also had a knack for acting inappropriately with his patients. One young man with a rare endocrine disorder had come to see Dr. Money, who proceeded to ask that patient if he had ever indulged in a "golden shower."[23] The reason for asking such a question, which confused the young man (who had not heard of such an act), was never specified. Dr. Money also believed that pederastic relationships could be beneficial to children. "If I were to see the case of a boy aged ten or twelve," Money told the journal *Paidika*, "who's intensely attracted toward a man in his twenties or thirties, and the relationship is totally mutual, then I would not call it pathological in any way. . . . It's very important once a relationship has been established on such positive and affectionate grounds that it should not be broken up precipitously."[24]

---

22. 31 in the United States; 2 in Canada. Anna-Jayne Metcalfe et al., "Trans Murder Monitoring Update" (30 September 2023), p. 1.
23. Quoted in John Colapinto, *As Nature Made Him: The Boy who was Raised as a Girl* (NY: HarperCollins, 2001), p. 28.
24. Quoted in Colapinto (2001), p. 30.

Most important for our story, Dr. John Money believed that gender boiled down to social constructs; a child's gender was malleable up until the first two and a half to three months of life, a window that he called the "gender identity gate."[25] A biological boy raised as a girl before the gate closed wouldn't know that he was really a boy so long as everyone in his life system convinced him otherwise.

And so it happened that Janet and Ron Reimer had welcomed their first two children, twin boys, Bruce (1965–2004) and Brian (1965–2002), into their family. When it came time to circumcise the boys, Dr. Jean-Marie Huot opted to use not a scalpel but a cautery instrument. She put the cauterizer to Bruce's foreskin. A sudden whiff of barbeque in the air informed the doctors that something had gone terribly wrong. Dr. Huot had accidently seared little Bruce's penis. The decision was quickly made to not attempt a circumcision on Brian.

After living for nearly a year in the face of this awful tragedy, Janet and Ron happened to catch an episode of *This Hour Has Seven Days*, which featured an interview with Dr. John Money. Janet and Ron were not aware of any of Money's idiosyncrasies. What they saw on television that night was a charming (if somewhat bawdy), intelligent sexologist affiliated with a major research university—and one who just so happened to hold the answer to their desperate prayers. The Reimers wrote to Dr. Money and soon the family boarded a plane to take them from their hometown of Winnipeg, Canada, to Johns Hopkins University in Baltimore, Maryland. Money explained that the best course of action was to give Bruce sex reassignment surgery and raise him as a girl. Janet recalls how Money pushed them towards this decision, accusing them of "procrastinating" when they were acting with caution.[26] Money also outright lied about the possibilities of such surgery, telling Janet and Ron that vaginoplasty could create an orifice "adequate for sexual intercourse and for sexual pleasure, including orgasm."[27]

While Dr. Money was a rising star in the sexology world, not every-

25. Colapinto (2001), p. 51.
26. Quoted in Colapinto (2001), p. 51.
27. Quoted in Colapinto (2001), p. 50.

one was charmed by him. One biologist, Dr. Milton Diamond (1934–2024), drafted a response to Dr. Money's Johns Hopkins team titled "A Critical Evaluation of the Ontogeny of Human Sexual Behavior," wherein he trounced all over the idea that humans are "completely divested of their evolutionary heritage."[28] As if to anticipate the praxis of modern gender activism, instead of debating Dr. Diamond, Dr. Money simply punched him while both attended a conference. Child psychiatrist Dr. Bernard Zuger (1905–1998) also called Dr. Money's ideas into question by reexamining the sixty-five cases cited by the latter as evidence that social constructs superseded biological reality. In all but four cases (each with its own mitigating and highly questionable circumstances), Dr. Money's claims proved baseless. Dr. Zuger quickly penned his findings, which would be published in the 1970 issue of *Psychosomatic Medicine.* Dr. Money received an advanced copy of the critique and ignored Zuger's discerning points.[29]

But the true depths of Dr. Money's twisted perversions only surfaced when he found himself alone with the twins, Brian and Bruce (the latter renamed "Brenda" to match the child's outward appearance). Sometimes he would ask them inappropriate questions about their genitalia (e.g., asking six-year-old Brian "do you ever get an erection?") or show them pictures of naked children or adult pornography.[30] Other times he would have them disrobe and inspect each other's nether regions. David (the name Brenda chose for himself after later detransitioning) recalls the abuse: "[Dr. Money] told me to take my clothes off . . . and I just did not do it. I just stood there. And he screamed '*Now!*' . . . I thought he was going to give me a whupping. So I took my clothes off and stood there shaking."[31] Dr. Money also had the twins simulate sexual acts upon each other when they were six-years-old. He ordered Brenda to assume doggy-style position while Brian repeatedly rammed his groin into her backside. Other times, Brenda was to lay on her back spread-eagle and accept (with poise, one imagines) her brother's thrusts. Most disturbing, on at least one known occasion, Dr. Money took pictures of the twins imitating sex acts on each other. Considering his passive view on pedo-

28. Quoted in Colapinto (2001), p. 44.
29. Colapinto (2001), p. 74.
30. Quoted in Colapinto (2001), p. 86.
31. Quoted in Colapinto (2001), p. 87.

philia, one can only guess (and perhaps tremble over) what he did with those photos. He also told Janet and Ron that they should allow Brian and Brenda to see them naked; in fact, that it would greatly benefit the children to watch their parents engage in sexual intercourse.

By the time she reached adolescence, Brenda knew something was different about her. Finally learning the truth about her biological reality, Brenda immediately began the detransition process, adopting the name David, hoping to cobble something of a normal life for himself from the remains of such a barbaric ordeal. Sadly, it would all be for naught. David eventually killed himself, the end result of the traumatic abuse perpetrated upon him by Dr. John Money's gender fantasies. Brian died of an overdose.

However one feels about the modern Gender Narrative, that was how it all began. It is an origin besieged with lies, battery, slander, abuse, sexual misconduct, pedophilia, an egotistical drive for fame and fortune, and the tragic deaths of the founding guinea pigs of those contemptable experiments. The episode brings us to the heart of the Gender Narrative: that gender is a social construct, unfettered from biological reality. Only Dr. Money's experiments proved the opposite. While Money lied profusely that Brenda's "behavior as a little girl [was] in remarkable contrast to the little-boy behavior of her identical twin brother," nothing could be further from the truth.[32] Brenda was a very rough-and-tumble child, more boyish in fact than Brian. Joan Nibbs of the Child Guidance Clinic recalls, "[Brenda] always just been fighting with the kids and playing in the dirt.... She didn't want to sit down with a book. She'd rather play knock-'em-down-shoot-'em-up cop games." Brian, of course, also noticed that Brenda was not like other girls—"[n]ot at all," he remembers. The twins' kindergarten teacher, Audrey McGregor, sums, "She was more a *boy* . . . in the *nature* of things."[33]

And Dr. Money knew it. When Brenda was only seven-years-old, "she" already fantasized her future self as a man, as evidenced by her

32. John Money and Anke A. Ehrhardt, *Man and Woman, Boy and Girl: The Differentiation and Dimorphism of Gender Identity from Conception to Maturity* (MD: Johns Hopkins University Press, 1972), p. 162.
33. Quoted in Colapinto (2001), pp. 60–3; *italics* in original.

response to the Draw-A-Person test given to her by Dr. John Money himself. In a letter he sent to the Reimers' lawyer, Dr. Money was very clear about the "psychological hazards" that can come from "affirming" a child's confused notions of gender.[34] Psychological hazards that he never once mentioned publicly.

The Reimers certainly provided a unique case that demonstrated rather unequivocally that womanhood and manhood are not social constructs. Still, Bruce, or Brenda, or David's situation addresses our current fixation with gender affirmation, i.e., the practice both in therapy and regular life of convincing, say, an adolescent girl, that she isn't really a girl when she is going through all the insecurities that most adolescent girls endure. Again, my lack of psychological knowledge prevents me from saying much about this. As such, I will let the gender affirmation doctors speak for themselves.

Child Abuse

Recently, journalist Michael Shellenberger exposed gender affirmation care as what he terms "the worst medical scandal in history" among the affiliates of the World Professional Association for Transgender Health, or WPATH.[35] Although, WPATH isn't necessarily staffed solely with physicians, but also has a large contingent of activists within its ranks, meaning that individuals lacking in any medical knowledge whatsoever are influencing the organization's decisions (not that the doctors are doing much better). "The WPATH Files prove that gender medicine is comprised of unregulated and pseudoscientific experiments on children, adolescents, and vulnerable adults," says Shellenberger. Digging deep into the files of WPATH reveals that the doctors pushing gender affirmation therapy know that it comes with many problems, including "sterilization, loss of sexual function, liver tumors, and death."[36]

The WPATH documents also reveal that this butchering of childhood innocence is being done without informed consent. As one en-

34. Quoted in Colapinto (2001), p. 79.
35. Michael Shellenberger, "The WPATH Files: A New Report Exposing Dangerously Pseudoscientific Surgical and Hormonal Experiments on Children, Adolescents, and Adults" (March 5, 2024), p. 3.
36. Shellenberger (2024), p. 3.

docrinologist, Dan Metzger, stated: "I think the thing you have to remember about kids is that we're often explaining these sorts of things to people who haven't even had biology in high school yet."[37] Informed consent by a child who does not understand basic biology simply isn't possible. Perhaps moving forward, we need less affirmation and more information? The doctors pushing children into this know it's wrong. They know it is harmful. They know it's deadly. They know that most kids who are not affirmed grow out of their trans phase, and usually mature into healthy, well-adjusted homosexuals. But the all-mighty dollar and an inflated sense of self-righteousness that would make even Jesus blush keeps these doctors in the business of perpetrating this harm on children.

In 2019, a large dataset on transgenderism was released from the Karolinska Institutet in Sweden and the Yale School of Public Health. The study found that "gender-affirming" care "improved mental health outcomes."[38] Only the study was so flawed that the authors were pushed to reevaluate the numbers a year later. Once proper controls were added to the stats, "the results demonstrated no advantage of surgery in relation to subsequent mood or anxiety disorder-related health care visits or prescriptions or hospitalizations following suicide attempts in that comparison."[39] The findings are conclusive: the overwhelming majority of those experiencing gender dysphoria who opted for sex-reassignment surgeries did not experience the mental health benefits they were promised. In fact, the study revealed that those who underwent such surgeries were more prone to develop anxiety disorders. But that finding was muted in the original report. The authors only fessed up and issued a correction after receiving a deluge of criticism.

In fairness, when my trans friends tell me that affirmation care and surgery saved their lives, I believe them. I can see the positive changes in them. It's obvious. And when detransitioners tell me that the "cascade

37. Quoted in Shellenberger (2024), p. 6.
38. "Correction of a Key Study: No Evidence of 'Gender-Affirming' Surgeries Improving Mental Health," *Society for Evidence Based Gender Medicine* (August 30, 2020).
39. "Correction to Bränström and Pachankis," *The American Journal of Psychiatry*, Vol. 177, Issue 8 (August 1, 2001), p. 734.

of interventions"[40] caused more isolation, pain, and distress in their lives, I believe them too. It's obvious. How can we know who affirmation and surgery will help and who affirmation and surgery will harm? The factor that I've noticed the most is *age.* My healthy, well-adjusted trans friends are all roughly around my age (i.e., Gen X and older Millennials) and made the decision for themselves as adults with complete understanding of the risks and rewards that come with gender surgery. Children, at least according to WPATH (and I believe them), are in no such position to understand the risks and rewards. And what are we to make of the fact that the majority of effeminate boys and masculine girls grow up to be gay men and lesbian woman?[41] Should they also be affirmed that they are the opposite sex, or should we let the phase run its course and spit them out as mentally healthy lesbian and gay adults? Dr. Jill Simons, executive director of the American College of Pediatricians, states "we have serious concerns about the physical and mental health effects of the current protocols promoted for the care of children and adolescents in the United States who express discomfort with their biological sex." She pleads to her colleagues to "immediately stop the promotion of social affirmation, puberty blockers, cross-sex hormones, and surgeries for children and adolescents who experience distress over their biological sex."[42]

Perhaps it's best to wait until a child has reached a degree of maturity before filling her head with ideologies that are too complicated for her to fully understand—and certainly before any permanent surgical changes are made. Otherwise, gender activists might very well be engaging (even if inadvertently) in the largest gay conversion therapy endeavor the West has ever seen.

As for consenting adults who understand the full breadth of the risks and rewards that come with affirmation care and surgery? I hope they do whatever helps them live a happy and healthy life.

Doc Marie's

Nestled in Southeast Portland one will find Doc Marie's, a "lesbian bar

40. Joyce (2022), p. 75.
41. Joyce (2022), p. 71.
42. "American College of Pediatricians Statement on Gender," *Toronto Sun* (June 10, 2024).

for everyone," owned by Olga Bichko and Nikki Ferry. The bar is named for Marie Equi (1872–1952), a famous Portland physician and feminist. Doc Marie's was set to open to much fanfare, as there hadn't been a lesbian bar in Portland since the Egyptian Club closed in 2010 (I know, I couldn't believe it either!). Their opening night on 21 May 2022 looked very promising, with a line of eager patrons wrapped around the block. Only once they were allowed inside and the shots started to pour, melee ensued. The bar for everyone, it turns out, was somehow not inclusive enough. One patron, Twi, who somehow "does not feel safe as a queer person" in queer-friendly Portland, was "nervous about invading a space" that was so freely inclusive.[43] According to some patrons, the African art on the walls had been "appropriated" by the white American owners. Someone got slapped and a racist remark was allegedly hurled. And despite Covid being over, Doc Marie's was accused of ableism for ignoring vestigial mandates that had already been lifted. The two bar managers quit the following day and the bar closed a week later. The rest of the staff had mutinied, formed an *ad hoc* union (the Marie Equi Workers Collective), and turned their grievance to social media. They felt "misled about the space being safe and welcoming," an Instagram post read. They accused the "unsafe" owners of "enable[ing] an openly racist aggressor."[44]

Finally, the Workers Collective, which had not invested one cent into the bar, demanded that Bichko and Ferry hand Doc Marie's over to them. "Our vision is a queer worker owned cooperative [run] democratically, [that] provides mutual aid, and hosts free opportunities for education to our community," they stated. Doc Marie's would become an "actively antiracist space," the staff "committed to ongoing racial bias training." Perhaps most importantly, Doc Marie's was to "cente[r] trans people." Otherwise, it is a "bullshit white supremacist institution," as one critic, Danger Dallas, comically spouted.[45] And, of course, a series of "threats and online harassment" to Bichko and Ferry soon followed.[46]

43. Quoted in Kat Leon, "Queer Community Reacts to Portland's New Lesbian Bar," *PSU Vanguard* (May 4, 2022).
44. Danger. Dallas, "PSA: The Instagram for the Workers is marie_equi_workers_collective" (July 5, 2022).
45. Danger. Dallas (2022).
46. Janey Wong, "Lesbian Bar Doc Marie's is Reopening Following its Troubled Start," *PDX Eater* (August 12, 2022).

Bichko relented. "We hear you and we are taking steps to ensure that we can carry out our mission of being a proud, safe and inclusive space for our community," she wrote in a since-deleted social media post.[47]

Doc Marie's is open again. And why shouldn't it be? The owners aren't responsible for critical social justice insanity, even if they invited it through their doors. However, Bichko and Ferry could have lost everything for creating a space so inclusive that people somehow felt excluded.

Bichko and Ferry were not the only Portlanders to feel the brunt of the gender mob, only the latest. In the glistening summer of 2015, Emily Stutzman also tried to create a space for anyone who was not a straight man. While that certainly doesn't sound inclusive to me, we can empathize with Stutzman. Lots of women can feel unsafe around straight guys and they deserve spaces where they can chill without worrying about some drunk asshole riding up on them on the dance floor.

So Stutzman started an event, The Fantasy Softball League, which organized monthly group outings at a bar called Vendetta in North Portland. Her ad sounded very inviting: "Hey ladies . . . Cool girls, drinking cool drinks in a cool bar, talking about cool stuff."[48]

During one of the meet-ups, a stranger aggressively approached Stutzman. "The person was hostile, and wanting to pick a fight. . . . This person was offended and said they would tell their friends that we were a group of people that were non-inclusive and not respectful of their gender," remembers Stutzman.

Stutzman was confused (and probably a little embarrassed). As she looked around Vendetta, she saw a rich medley of queer-identifying people. What had she done wrong? Turns out, the antagonist who confronted her did not use she/her pronouns and was offended that Stutzman's promo for The Fantasy Softball League only referenced "ladies."

"What we wanted to say is, if you're a straight dude, don't come to this event. . . . Everyone else was fine," says Stutzman.

She quickly caved and changed The Fantasy Softball League to "an

---

47. Shane Dixon Kavanaugh, "How a Portland 'Lesbian Bar for Everyone' Closed After One Day" (August 10, 2022).
48. Following quotes from Ellena Rosenthal, "Who Crushed the Lesbian Bars? A New Minefield of Identity Politics," *Willamette Week* (November 30, 2016).

event for queer women." More trouble followed. "Everything I tried, someone was offended," remembers Stutzman. "It got weird and political, and I wanted it to be a fun thing."

Stutzman eventually gave up and handed the meet-up to an associate, Alissa Young, who rebranded the queer event for women to Gal Pal's. Unfortunately, Young had learned nothing from Stutzman. Her use of the word "Gal" caused much harm to self-centered gender activists.

Gal Pal's is gone.

Most extreme, the Temporary Lesbian's Bar was accused of engaging in "trans women exterminationism." Besides the blood-curdling horror of having the word "lesbian" in the event title, the organizers had looked to the labrys—a two-sided axe of ancient Greece, symbolic of women's strength and virtue—as their logo. The logo caused great distress to Viridian Sylvae, who somehow felt that the labrys symbolized "violence against trans women." Therefore, the organizers were guilty of genocide.

But genocide is a real thing. It is a long and arduous horrific spectacle of all the worse angels of human nature and involves things like concentration camps and firing squads and forced labor and sterilization, starvation, and gas chambers. This near-obsession to be seen as oppressed to reap the social benefits of such a label, partially contributes to the view of trans people as narcissistic—even though I think that such a label is overused. Nonetheless, we are perhaps seeing the first time in history when some people live such privileged and misguided lives that they find nothing wrong with faking their own extermination.

Favorite Delusions

Conservative commentator Ben Shapiro once referred to transgenderism as "mainstreaming delusion."[49] If that is true, I find that an atheist can say the same thing about his religion, Orthodox Judaism. And both Shapiro and atheists feel the same way about my religion, no doubt. And those gender ideologues who wish to erase women *really* don't like my religion! I couldn't care less about what any detractors of my beliefs have to say, and I imagine Shapiro feels similarly about Orthodox Ju-

49. Daniel J. Solomon, "WATCH: That Time Ben Shapiro Called Transgender People Delusional," *Forward* (December 7, 2016).

daism. I suppose we all have our favorite delusions to some extent. If a man simply wants to live his life as if he were a woman, I have no issue with it—any more than I have an issue with a person who believes in Yahweh. The concerns arise when it comes to proselytizing. Shapiro and I may enjoy our favorite delusions, but Jewish people (rather famously) aren't interested in converting anyone to their faith, while my religion is comprised of a congregation of *one*. Neither of us push our religious beliefs on anyone. We should all be happy that there isn't really a trans genocide taking place. But if it is your favorite delusion to believe such things, have at it.

Just never forget that, as thinking apes, none of us is required to believe anything that cuts against our own common sense.

15

Queering Psychedelia: Questioning the Identity Perspective

Scientific theories that don't correspond with reality can't benefit marginalized people, or anyone.

—Helen Pluckrose and James Lindsay, *Cynical Theories*

Gender Math from Left Field

Just over an hour before Francine Douglas claimed that psilocybin mushrooms revealed to her that children were buried under Kamloops Indian Residential School at the 2022 Spirit Plant Medicine Conference, another speaker, Dr. Phillipe Lucas, discussed the results of the Canadian Psychedelic Survey. It was "the largest and most comprehensive" psychedelic study in that country, featuring 2,393 participants answering 650 questions. Dr. Lucas, among other very impressive accolades, is also a founding member of MAPS Canada. Those achievements were put aside for the moment, as Dr. Lucas announced to the crowd that he was a "cis male." Dr. Lucas then took us through a constellation of criteria, statistical measurements, and findings. The Canadian Psychedelic Survey found that the main reasons people used substantia were "healing, forming more meaningful relationships with others, facilitating creativity and spirituality, coping or healing from the problematic use of non-psychedelic drugs," among other positive outcomes.[1] I listened with rapt attention, hoping there would be time for a Q and A. I had a question about Dr. Lucas's possible findings of any overlaps between two of the categories he'd mentioned, therapeutic use and spiritual use. Unfortunately, there wouldn't be time.

After his speech I approached him in the lobby area and introduced myself. He was quite the friendly chap. I asked him my question about any overlaps between the therapeutic and spiritual categories, and we spoke for a moment about the Canadian Psychedelic Survey. I then told him that while I did not want to come off as rude, I had to ask why he made his "cis male" comment at the beginning of his speech.

"I wanted people to know that my perspective comes from a place of privilege," he replied.

"Sure," I said, "but what does that have to do with the Canadian Psychedelic Survey?"

"To let people know that I am coming from a place of privilege," he responded.

"Yes, but yours was a statistical analysis—a mathematical calculation, correct?"

"Yes," he said.

"And what does your gender identity have to do with math?"

"Because I am coming from a perspective of privilege," he said again.

I sighed. "Dr. Lucas, you just delivered a fine, intelligent presentation that involved a statistical analysis meant to gauge a variety of psychedelic experiences, medicine preferences, and other overlapping drug behavior patterns. Statistics are based in math; math is based in numbers. Those numbers were tallied based on how 2,393 volunteers answered the 650-question survey provided by MAPS Canada and the Canadian Association of Psychedelics. Are you telling me that the numbers would be different if you were a Middle Eastern woman? That your gender identity somehow breaks the laws of mathematics and must therefore be divulged in order for us to decide if your research has statistical validity? Is the concept of *2* not really *2* through a Middle Eastern woman's perspective? Is your study viable, or isn't it?"

1. Dr. Phillippe Lucas, "Psychedelic Use in Canada: Results of the Canadian Psychedelic Survey," Spirit Plant Medicine Conference (2022).

Dr. Lucas stared at me awkwardly.

Then he smiled, said it was nice to meet me, shook my hand, and walked away.

Canadians . . . amIright?

Dr. Lucas had given a fine speech. I suppose that is why his nod to his gender identity felt so out of left field. He is clearly a very kind, intelligent, cis-gender (he'd want me to say that), considerate man who knows how to captivate an audience with a thoughtful presentation. For him to feel the need to express his gender identity on stage during a talk that has nothing to do with gender identity[2] can really be boiled down to a single word: *fear.* This was his virtue-signal to the crowd. His way of psychically pleading to the audience not to cancel him, as happened to his colleagues Dr. Mark Haden and Trevor Millar a year earlier. I have no problem with adults believing whatever they want about themselves.

But what does it have to do with math?

The shame is that Dr. Phillipe Lucas is a really good guy. He shouldn't have to live in fear simply because of his immutable characteristics.

Identity Perspectives

On the other side of the gender coin we meet Dr. Angela Carter, who among other things is a naturopathic physician and member of the Oregon Health Authority. Most importantly, Dr. Carter advised on Measure 110 in Oregon back in 2020, which decriminalized all drugs in the state (more on this in the next chapter). While Measure 110 didn't create the mental health and addictive drug issues Portland currently faces, it is difficult to argue that it didn't exacerbate them. That is not the fault of Dr. Carter; we are in full agreement that drug laws need a *serious* overhaul. Measure 110 was a noble experiment, of which Eden and I voted in favor. We also campaigned for it in an unofficial way: talking about it at parties and social gatherings and supporting and networking with friends and colleagues more involved with the political side of the movement. We were true believers. But due to a lack of implementation of services by the municipalities, 110 just didn't garner the real-world results for which we had all hoped.

2. Besides 4% of participants questioned.

The philosophical underpinnings that best reveal the crossroads where Dr. Carter and I part company can be found in something as simple as a speaker biography, the kind of thing you'd read in a program for a conference or other public forum. Most speaker bios mention what a researcher has done in the field, books and/or articles she's written, television and podcast appearances, yadda yadda. Dr. Carter's speaker bio in the 2022 *Horizons Northwest: Perspectives on Psychedelics* program begins: "white, queer/genderqueer/neuroqueer, intersex transformative justice activist."[3]

For lack of a better word, I call these intersectional identity markers "taglines." Taglines are very important in the psychedelic Renaissance, serving several functions. Most imperative, they let us know right away who has good ideas and who does not. The more taglines a person can claim, the better are her ideas (so the theory goes).

Taglines also serve as a necessary virtue-signal. For example, Dr. Carter's mention of being white American. One might think that such an admission in the new CSJ psychedelia would work against Dr. Carter, but it isn't so. "White," in this case, is an admission of guilt in the unobtainable pursuit of unalloyed allyship—much like Dr. Lucas's comment from left field. The rest of Dr. Carter's tagline train—and I mean no disrespect by this—is little more than trendsgender wordplay. Albeit very powerful trendsgender wordplay.

Naming your gender—whether Dr. Lucas or Dr. Carter—is not science or criminal law reform; it's a *strategy*. Dr. Lucas (with some amount of justification) is almost certainly scared of being cancelled like his colleagues Dr. Mark Haden and Trevor Millar, while Dr. Carter sets up both a human shield and a verbal spear. Each tagline serves as a plate of armor, culled from the finest scales of the most benevolent mermaids of identity politics. Since Dr. Carter is a good person (and I mean that), any criticism to the ideas can be brushed aside as "phobic" in some way—indeed, we have plenty of minefields to trip over. Is the good doctor a neurointersex queer or a transformative gender activist?

I already forgot.

So did you.

Taglines also serve another purpose. We *must* listen to what Dr. Car-

3. "Horizons Northwest: Perspectives on Psychedelics" (2022), p. 15.

ter has to say—good ideas, bad ideas, no ideas—it doesn't matter. I'm not saying that Dr. Carter has bad ideas (indeed, we are in full agreement on amending drug laws). And I'm not saying that Dr. Carter has good ideas (for the same reason). I'm saying that Dr. Carter's ideas unfortunately come secondary. First and foremost is ensuring that everyone sees psychedelia though the perspective of a white, queer, genderqueer, neuroqueer, intersex transformative justice activist.

Relatable things like that.

In some way that remains unclear, these intersectional identity perspectives matter to questions of science, mathematics, and law. One such identity perspective that I am told exists is the "white-male perspective" (more or less what Dr. Phillippe Lucas was talking about in truncated form). It is, in fact, the only identity perspective that is supposed to come with a social apology. But we immediately encounter problems. I have only lived as a white American male and yet I have no idea what such a perspective entails. Does that mean that I feel a different sadness when a loved one passes away than how a black American transwoman would feel? And which of my perspectives are we talking about exactly? My perspective on sports (further broken down into my perspectives on baseball versus hockey versus roller derby)? My perspectives on food? My perspectives on movies? Books? Music? Psychedelics? Throughout my life I have held (and changed) a variety of perspectives on countless topics, of which people from a diversity of backgrounds have both agreed and disagreed. Or just consider Dr. Lucas and me. We are both white males, and yet have totally different perspectives on whether or not our white-maleness has any relevance to conducting a statistical analysis. The identity perspective eats itself.

Like Dr. Lucas, Dr. Carter's need to self-identify a questionable guilt couched in trendsgender neologisms doesn't really forward any cause for positive changes in psychedelic science and law. And it's a bummer; I find both Dr. Lucas and Dr. Carter to be highly intelligent, kind, charming, indefatigable supporters of the psychedelic Renaissance. And that has nothing to do with their gender perspectives or taglines and everything to do with the goodness in their hearts.

Curse of the Cis

A rising voice in the queering psychedelia crowd is Yale psychology professor Dr. Alexander Belser. Like others in the movement, Dr. Belser laments that the majority of psychedelic researchers are "White straight cis gender male[s]."[4] Putting aside that Dr. Belser checks off *three* of those *four* boxes, he overlooks a key consideration: while women outnumber men by about three million in the United States, the latter hold the majority of positions in the hard sciences, where there is always something new to learn about psychedelics.[5] During the heyday of psychedelic research in the 1950s, the majority of scientists in the United States were white American men. But as current research has shown, white American, Canadian, and European women have played a far more integral role in early psychedelic therapy than previously recognized.[6] There was sexism, no doubt, but it was more nuanced than simply excluding women: women weren't absent in early LSD research; they were just overlooked for their contributions until quite recently.[7] And here, Chacruna Institute deserves the most praise; its "Women in Psychedelics" series has brought many of these unsung heroes out of the murky depths of the past and into historical purview. More to the point, though, we might also consider that during the 1950s and 1960s, no one was trying to "hetero" psychedelia. The doctors working with LSD were just trying to help people as best they knew how at the time.

And it's hard to find a specifically "white" patriarchal foundation for any of it; the majority of psychedelic researchers in Iraq during the 1950s were Middle Eastern men. First Nations men dominated psychedelia—to the exclusion of women until only very recently. If psychedelic research suddenly started to take China by storm, the bulk of researchers would no doubt be Chinese men.

4. Alexander Belser, "10 Calls to Action: Toward an LGBTQ-Affirmative Psychedelic Therapy," in Labate and Cavnar (2021), p. 123.
5. Recall Georgetown University's Center on Education and the Workforce study on university majors broken down between the sexes (p. 59 of this book).
6. Ericka Dyck "What About Mrs. Psychedelia?" presented at Breaking Convention (2019).
7. See Erika Dyck et al. (eds.), *Women and Psychedelics: Uncovering Invisible Voices* (NM: Synergetic Press, 2024).

Like Drs. Phillipe Lucas and Angela Carter (and the majority of psychedelic SJWs), I believe Dr. Belser is acting in good faith. I also feel that a voice as smart and compassionate as his would go a long way towards unifying the rifts in the psychedelic Renaissance if he factored all this additional history into his assessment.

Regrettably, Dr. Belser also inadvertently touches upon one of the more shortsighted traits of the Gender Narrative—the belief that anything that doesn't fully accommodate Team Gender must be eliminated from practice. In this case, Dr. Belser refers to the "male/female dyad" among psychedelic therapists, who sometimes work in a pair with a single client, which he would like to see "retire[d]" due its "gender essentializing" nature.[8] Dr. Belser and I find agreement in the fact that some people will inevitably gravitate towards a therapist who has shared similar life experiences (a veteran tending to another veteran, for example). But does that mean that a female/male dyad is inherently wrong? What about those like San Francisco–based ketamine therapist Veronika Gold, who "directly experienced the potential value of the male-female co-therapy team from a participant perspective," during her involvement in the MAPS MDMA trials? She continues, "I cherished the emerging balance that their collective presence provided. Receiving the full, undivided attention of the male and female energies and being witnessed, non-judgmentally supported, and cared for was for me healing in itself."[9]

I suppose I'm left wondering why we have to *retire* the female/male dyad when we can simply *add* "gender neutral dyads" (as Dr. Belser suggests) to any psychedelic therapy program.[10] Why does a model that works for some people have to be dismantled simply because it doesn't work for everyone? Developing newer models and more choices, I feel is a better strategy than overturning protocols that benefit good folks like Veronika Gold. Dr. Belser might have checked with fellow *Psychedelic Justice* contributors Katherine Costello and Marca Cassity, who write, "Any discourse that privileges a singular narrative runs the risk of being oppressive since it inherently delegitimizes other narratives."[11] Putting

8. Belser, "Ten Calls to Action . . .," in Labate and Cavnar (2021), p. 123.
9. Gold, "Reflections on Personal Experiences . . ." (2019).
10. Belser, "Ten Calls to Action . . .," in Labate and Cavnar (2021), p. 123.
11. Katherine M. Costello and Marca Cassity, "Why Oneness is Not Incompatible with Identity Politics," in Labate and Cavnar (2021), p. 128.

aside that that is a complete misuse of the word "oppressive," I think Costello and Cassity are correct. Dr. Belser might consider that retiring the female/male dyad in favor of a gender-neutral dyad results in the very delegitimizing outcomes that Costello, Cassity, and I—and no doubt Dr. Belser himself—are trying to avoid.

Ego Loss and the Death/Rebirth Experience

One of the more well-known kinds of psychedelic experience is the achievement of ego loss, or a sense of unity with the cosmos. A person might speak of feeling like she died and was reborn (*à la* Albert Hofmann after his first purposeful dose of LSD). First noticed during the heyday of mid-century psychedelic research, some physicians cited their patients' experiencing a "oneness with God."[12] For many, it can feel like the ego has dissolved into a perfect state of heavenly afterlife supra-consciousness, formerly enshrined in the psychedelic cliché "we are all One," sung in poetic verse by a Wook bogarting your joint at a festival. One mid-century doctor put it rather bluntly: "disintegration of the ego under LSD leads to a beneficial effect deriving from the experience of belonging to and being accepted by a higher mind behind the universe."[13]

While this phenomenon had been noticed earlier in the 1950s, the first researchers to take the idea of ego loss into some very far out places were the folks in Timothy Leary's group during the 1960s. Relating the psychedelic experience to the death experience as outlined in Leary's *The Psychedelic Experience: A Manual Based on The Tibetan Book of the Dead* (1964) came from the spiritual philosophies of the East. The original *Tibetan Book of the Dead* was to be read to the deceased, those with no ego whatsoever. Leary adopted this protocol. He would decorate his medi-

12. Quoted in Erika Dyck, "Flashback: Psychiatric Experimentation with LSD in Historical Perspective," *Canadian Journal of Psychiatry*, 50, no. 7 (July 2005), p. 385.
13. Joyce Martin, "Schizophreniform Reactions under Day Hospital L.S.D. Therapy," *Congress Report Vol II* (Zurich: Orell Fussli, 1959), p. 320. Dr. Charles Savage would echo these sentiments a few years later: "[t]he person is at one with the universe. In his mystic selflessness he awakens with a feeling of rebirth, often physically felt, and he is provided with a new beginning, a new set of values"; see Savage, "LSD, Alcoholism . . ." (1962), pp. 432–43.

cine space with Eastern tapestries, play Eastern music, and read from his *Manual* to guide a person under a high dose of LSD through a death/rebirth-simulacrum to achieve ego loss.

Since Leary was instrumental in shaping modern psychedelic culture, the ego loss (or death/rebirth) experience has gained popular appeal among psychenauts. Though often overlooked or ignored in the psychedelic Renaissance is a truth that used to be taken for granted when the first tests with LSD began in earnest in the 1950s: namely, that—far from dissolving the ego—psychedelics can *inflate* the ego. Or rather, while one may feel like the ego has dissolved under a high dose of LSD or mushrooms—and I have no doubt that it does—such dissipation is only temporary. Once a person has returned to baseline, the ego can very much recalcify into something bigger and stronger. There is nothing ego-lossy about a college student taking ayahuasca in the Peruvian Amazon, coming back to the States, and believing it is her job to save the world.

Dr. Charles Savage, one of the first American doctors to work with LSD, believed that the ego-inflation caused by that chemical could serve as a way to help those with low self-esteem.[14] But the doctors had to be careful. One British patient took on the identity of the emperor Nero and turned into a psychopath, delighting in telling his doctors his plans to commit mass murder.[15] Psychedelic psychotherapists like Robert Masters and Jean Houston also noted post-LSD session ego inflation including "heightened aggressiveness, an impression of greater self-confidence, and probably better self-esteem."[16]

I contend that it is how and why we choose to work with psychedelic medicines that determines if our egos will inflate or deflate. Being aware that such inflations are possible—and indeed *very* likely—is a good place to start.

---

14. Charles Savage, "LSD, Alcoholism . . ." (1962), p. 433.

15. Joyce Martin, "A Case of Psychopathic Personality with Homosexuality Treated by LSD," in Richard Crocket and Ronald Sandison (eds.), *Hallucinogenic Drugs and Their Psychotherapeutic Use: Proceedings of the Quarterly Meeting of the Royal Medico-Psychological Association* (London: H. K. Lewis and Co., 1963), p. 114.

16. Robert Masters and Jean Houston, *The Varieties of Psychedelic Experience: The Classic Guide to the Effects of LSD on the Human Psyche* (VT: Park Street Press, 2000), p. 200.

Some queer psychedelic SJWs reject the "we are all oneness" of psychedelia.[17] In their article for *Psychedelic Justice*, "Why Oneness Is Not Incompatible with Identity Politics," authors Costello and Cassity take issue with the fact that the Mystical Experience Questionnaire (MEQ), which is used by some psychedelic-psychotherapists to determine if a person has had a healing experience with substantia, leaves far too many options off the table. For example, instead of producing stats that show the healing ratios of those who experience "encounters with spirit guides, powerful somatic-based energetic experiences, reparative rational experiences, connections with nature, and strong sensory or even sensual experiences," the MEQ instead focuses solely on "oneness."[18] I agree with Costello and Cassity entirely. Meeting and conversing with entities, feeling an orgasmic kinship with nature, and having strong somatic experiences with psychedelics are quite powerful, and have certainly helped heal many of my own traumas (along with countless others). Oneness need not be favored above the rest.

But for Costello and Cassity there is a much deeper problem with oneness. They believe that to say "we are all one" means to say "we are all the same."[19] I dare say that in the quarter century I have studied psychedelia (at the time of this writing), I have never once heard "we are all one" referred to as "we are all the same" (Costello's and Cassity's article aside). "We are all one" typically refers to a metaphor meaning that we are all made from the same cosmic mechanisms (frequently referred to as "Source" by your local quantum energy healer). For the spiritual psychenaut, Source (or oneness) represents the embodiment of all love, kindness, blessings, and safety, a place of perfect bliss where there is no suffering or pain of any kind—what your grandmother might call Heaven. "We are all one" is meant to remind us of that sacred and unifying viewpoint. The subtext being that we should all be kinder to each other; for when we harm the other, we harm ourselves. The lovely philosophy of oneness derives from the East, specifically the *brahman* of Hinduism. *New World Encyclopedia* offers us a definition for *brahman* that's as good as any: "the supreme cosmic power, ontological ground of being, and the

17. Costello and Cassity, "Why Oneness . . .," in Labate and Cavnar (2021), p. 128.
18. Costello and Cassity, "Why Oneness . . .," in Labate and Cavnar (2021), pp. 127–8.
19. Costello and Cassity, "Why Oneness . . .," in Labate and Cavnar (2021), p. 127.

source, goal and purpose of all spiritual knowledge." The *atman* (or soul) of every person is but a mere piece of the larger *brahman*; in other words, "we are all one." By mistaking "we are all one" for "we are all the same," Costello and Cassity have unintentionally erected a straw-nonbinary person argument.

Costello and Cassity also wonder if "White, cisgender, heterosexual men who developed and propagated the discourse of oneness . . . are more likely to have that experience than queer or trans people."[20] They recommend developing a study on that topic that might help us sort it out. The idea is that if more queer people were involved in mid-century psychedelic research, the movement would look radically different today due to the influence of the queer identity perspective. Only queer people *did* use psychedelics, and in a very real way influenced the culture (including "oneness"). Dr. Richard Alpert (1931–2019) co-authored the *Manual* with Timothy Leary and Ralph Metzner (1936–2019). He took to these Eastern concepts in such a profound way that he changed his name to *Ram Dass* (meaning "Servant of God") while traveling through India in 1967. Allen Ginsberg (1926–1997) wrote of his first LSD experience in this way: "I long for a Yes of Harmony to penetrate, to every corner of the universe, under every condition whatsoever, a Yes there Is . . . a Yes I am . . . a Yes You Are . . . *a We*. . . . [A]n image of the Universe in miniature conscious sentient part of the *interrelated machine*."[21] Gerald Heard (1889–1971) complemented these cosmic ideas of oneness with his own thoughts on mysticism.[22] Alpert, Ginsberg, and Heard were all homosexuals and participated in the development and propagation of "oneness" with psychedelics, an experience they all held in high esteem. And who knows how many other queer people who took LSD in the 1960s and 1970s also had such experiences.

The concept of ego loss achieved through psychedelics isn't even a Western thing. It's an Eastern thing mixed with a Western thing. For now, we can say with a fair degree of certainty that sexual identity did not matter to a person's ability to experience oneness with psychedelics or influence the culture in noticeable ways. If oneness is a factor of priv-

20. Costello and Cassity, "Why Oneness . . .," in Labate and Cavnar (2021), p. 129.
21. Allen Ginsberg "Lysergic Acid"; *italics* mine.
22. Stephen J. Novack, "LSD before Leary: Sidney Cohen's Critique of 1950s Psychedelic Drug Research," *Isis*, 88, no. 1 (1997), p. 93.

ilege, as Costello and Cassity maintain, then such privilege exist broadly between even the two most unlikely demographics: ancient, emaciated mystics meditating in the mountains of India, and mid-century gay, white American, intellectuals. Between those two extremes, it seems we have plenty of room for inclusion of contemporary queer people to experience oneness should they so desire.

Psychedelic Gay Conversion Therapy

The psychedelic Gender Narrative invokes past oppression to claim victimhood in the present. For example, the queering psychedelia crowd will rightfully point out that during the 1950s and 1960s medicines like LSD were seen as potential "cures" for homosexuality and claim that such bygone incidents somehow cause distress for queer people today. What they don't say, however, is that these homosexual patients *sought out* doctors to give them LSD to rid them of what both parties considered a mental disorder. A typical request might read something like a letter Richard Alpert received: "I am primarily an overt acting-out homosexual and I don't want to be anymore. I've heard about LSD and I think it could help me. Would you work with me?"[23] Alpert accepted, although he offered no "guarantee" of any lasting changes. In this case, which unfolded over the course of four LSD sessions, the man was reporting steady intercourse with women a year later. Whether or not he ever slept with men again (besides two in the first year to see "whether or not the changes were real") is lost to time.[24]

In fairness, we do know of the inhumane, forced psychedelic gay conversion (coupled with electroshock) therapy of two teenage boys living in France.[25] But there is no evidence of anything like that happening anywhere else in the West. Moreover, LSD coupled with electroshock

23. Quoted in Richard Alpert, "LSD and Sexuality: Review of a Case of Homosexuality Treated Therapeutically with LSD and Description of a Male-Female Psychedelic Session Program," *Psychedelic Review*, No 10 (1969), p. 22.
24. Alpert, "LSD and Sexuality . . ." (1969), p. 23.
25. See Zoë Dubus, "High Dose Psychedelic Shock Therapy with LSD and Mescaline: The Conversion Treatment of a French Doctor on Two Homosexual Adolescents in the 1960s," in Alex Belser, Clancy Cavnar, and Beatriz C. Labate (eds.), *Queering Psychedelics: From Oppression to Liberation in Psychedelic Medicine* (2022).

therapy wasn't reserved only for homosexuals, but was a technique employed on heterosexuals as well. Not that that excuses any of it.

Gay conversion therapy rode on the heels of a new theory of psychology called "behaviorism," the idea that compulsions (sexual or otherwise) were learned over the course of a person's life. Should that be true, the doctors reasoned, perhaps homosexuality was just another adopted behavior that could be unlearned. Today, we know that isn't true. But in the 1950s or 60s (or any time before) no one was any the wiser.

We know of a certain gay man, Ben, who "despised" his homosexuality. This distress made it difficult for Ben to maintain employment and real relationships to the point that he became suicidal. Desperate, he made an appointment with Dr. Joyce Martin (1905–1969), one of very few doctors to attempt gay conversion therapy with psychedelics during the 1950s. LSD, Ben told Dr. Martin, was his "last hope."[26] But in some cases, the LSD treatment only caused further distress. Ben was, in fact, the patient mentioned earlier who took on the identity of the Emperor Nero and regaled the hospital staff with his homicidal plans. (Note that the psychedelic Gender Narrative does not factor Ben's disconcerting antics into the queer perspective.)

Wanting to pinpoint where in his consciousness this disgust towards his sexuality originated, Ben recalled memories from his childhood—his mother often left him in the care of sex-workers at a bar while she was away. The sex-workers often commented upon young Ben's private areas and teased him about sex and his body. With no parental guidance in life, Ben began exposing himself to little girls his own age, which we can imagine didn't end well.

Dr. Martin's attempts at LSD gay conversion therapy with Ben was a compassionate response to complex childhood sexual trauma that was little understood at the time. Perhaps we can find some grace for Dr. Martin within the larger cultural context in which she lived. The only thing she was really guilt of was an inability to see 20 years into the future. Homosexuality was seen as a mental disorder in those days, and

26. Joyce Martin, "A Case of Psychopathic Personality . . .," in Crocket and Sandison (1963), p. 112.

Dr. Martin did her best to alleviate it (even if we now know such a perspective was erroneous). Like Drs. Carter, Belser, and Lucas, Dr. Martin acted in good-faith.

In her article "Can Psychedelics 'Cure' Gay People?," Chacruna Institute co-founder Clancy Cavnar not only takes aim at Dr. Martin, but also calibrates her scope squarely on psychedelic therapists Drs. Jean Houston and Robert Masters, who, in the mid-1960s, gave peyote to three homosexuals. Cavnar overlooks that Houston and Masters were not trying to convert their volunteers into a heterosexual lifestyle.

The real basis behind Drs. Houston and Master's test was to challenge criticism against what was termed "instant psychotherapy" by their detractors.[27] At that time, many therapists marveled at the way psychedelic medicines shortened the psychotherapeutic process. They met resistance from other therapists who were wary of such claims of instant psychotherapy. Drs. Houston and Masters had a handful of gay volunteers who gravitated towards the theory of changing their sexual preferences with a single dose. They merely obliged these men's desires within the larger context of confirming or denying instant psychotherapy.

Cavnar also recalls a study conducted by Drs. Houston and Masters that included 14 homosexual men; similar to Dr. Martin's gay volunteers, the men in Houston and Masters's study tapped the doctors (not the other way around). And theirs was no psychedelic gay conversion therapy program either. Their real reason for the study was to "examine various aspects of homosexual psychology and problems of social adjustment."[28] In other words, they were trying to alleviate the distress their patients suffered daily by living secret lives in homosexually-repressive times. If attempting to convert to a heterosexual lifestyle was part of any individual volunteer's plans, how much are Drs. Houston and Masters to blame? To turn away a person suffering from a sexual orientation that was considered a disorder within a larger anti-homosexual society would have made Houston and Masters the villains. They were less trying to

27. Masters and Houston (2000), p. 187.
28. Masters and Houston (2000), p. 193.

convert their volunteers than they were trying to stop them from committing suicide; acting no more homophobic for abiding by their clients' wishes to turn heterosexual than they were depression-phobic because they were trying to cure a patient's depression.

Cavnar focuses on one particular case (who Houston and Masters call "S"), a black American economics professor. S was a typical case in those days—a closeted gay man who was nonetheless married. S despised "effeminate" gay men (identity perspective?). Houston and Masters focused on S because "he expected no changes at all [from peyote] and had no motivation whatever to relinquish his homosexuality." Two notes on that: first, this does not mean that Houston and Masters were trying to relinquish it for him; second (and far more important for our purposes), such an admission challenges Cavnar's allegation that S was some kind of gay conversion therapy patient. Like many gay men trapped in those times, S was confused, desperate, emotionally isolated, and seeking a solution for his suffering. And while Houston and Masters contemplated that perhaps S's homosexuality was related to his body dysmorphia, they found no solid connection. Their speculation came from 12 out of the 14 homosexual men who entered their clinic and also reported body dysmorphia.[29]

Here we find a possible nugget for the claim of identity perspectives around which the psychedelic Gender Narrative rallies. Perhaps homosexual men do have poorer views of their body than heterosexual people? S certainly did. So did eleven others. The question then becomes: should we develop psychedelic tests that measure the ratio of body dysmorphia between hetero- and homosexuals? Seems like a worthy pursuit. Although we need not step too lively. After all, S's reaction to peyote was *radically different* from the experiences of the other two gay men in his peyote circle.[30] There does not seem to have been any kind of gay identity perspective among the participants of any of those early tests.

The unspoken truth among psychedelic gender activists is that psy-

29. Masters and Houston (2000), p. 199. Psychedelic gay conversion therapy was so rare that they had little with which to compare their data.
30. Masters and Houston (2000), p. 193.

chedelic gay conversion therapy occupies only the tiniest sliver of the overall history of mid-century psychedelic research. Which is why it's surprising that therapist Jeanna Eichenbaum references "intense 1950s experiments" that tried to convert gay people to straighthood using psychedelics. Calling the few handfuls of cases of attempted gay conversion therapy with psychedelics "intense" is quite the exaggeration. Ignoring that the psychedelic therapists did not solicit any of their patients (save two in France) only adds unneeded tension. Cavnar's article, "Can Psychedelics 'Cure' Gay People?," rests at a short four and a quarter pages. The meat of the article, a subsection titled "Sexual Minorities and Treatment with Psychedelics," wherein Cavnar discusses this history, is only two pages long.[31] May that serve as a reminder (and a relief) as to how "intense" psychedelic gay conversion therapy was during the 1950s and 60s. Perhaps most welcome, there isn't anyone seriously considering opening a psychedelic gay conversion therapy clinic today.

And yet, it almost doesn't matter. In the erratic world of critical social justice, loose definitions of oppression count as social currency, with those like Eichenbaum looking to cash in. She implies that the experiences of queer people are akin to those of "Black, Brown, Native, [and] Asian people."[32] This is to desire victimhood on a whole new level. Growing up outside heteronormativity, I was well aware that my proclivities could be covered up at will. I could hide. A black American man running from a lynch mob had no such option. A Japanese family could not avoid the internment camp. And what Chinese person could dodge the Chinese Exclusion Act of 1882? The harsh experiences and bullying that I (and no doubt, Eichenbaum) endured simply do not hold a candle to the experiences of black and Latin Americans, First Nations peoples, or Asians who suffered under past systemic white supremacy.

But oppression is sorely needed by psychedelic gender activists if they desire a seat at the table of grievance (which, somewhat ironically, represents the ultimate social privilege). And so, besides grossly exaggerating the extent of psychedelic gay conversion therapy in the 1950s and 60s, the queering psychedelia advocates will point to Timothy Leary,

31. Clancy Cavnar, "Can Psychedelics 'Cure' Gay People?" in Labate and Cavnar (2021), p. 116–18.
32. Jeanna Eichenbaum, "Queer Voices Speak to the New Psychedelia," in Labate and Cavnar (2021), p. 106.

who certainly believed that LSD could straighten a person out. During an interview with *Playboy Magazine* in 1966,[33] Leary told the reporter that "LSD is a specific *cure* for homosexuality." In fact, to Leary, homosexuality, along with "impotence and frigidity," were nothing more than "symbolic screw-ups."[34]

Timothy Leary Was Gay

I once found myself in a conversation with a psychedelic SJW colleague about Leary's anti-homosexual comments. My colleague was lamenting that while Leary is revered in psychedelic circles, his views on homosexuality were nothing more than "white male patriarchy." I explained that Leary was a man of his time, no different from most anyone else. To hold him accountable to modern sensibilities is anachronistic. But that wasn't good enough . . . "Leary should have known better," he replied. Seeing that I was getting nowhere, I politely told him about Dr. Joyce Martin, a British doctor of Middle Eastern descent who was at the forefront of psychedelic gay conversion therapy.

My colleague quickly changed his tune. *Middle Eastern female*? The gender math didn't compute. Dr. Martin had two whole oppression points (female, Middle Eastern) while any white American homosexual man would only have one oppression point. Such intersectional blasphemy caused a severe bout of cognitive dissonance in his mind. Dr. Martin should not have been in the "oppressor" role. How could a Middle Eastern woman not join up with her homosexual patients in an intersectional identity cabal to take down the white male patriarchy? My colleague hemmed and hawed and eventually concluded that obviously Dr. Martin was just a woman of her time, so we shouldn't really hold her accountable for her views.

Indeed, why would we hold her accountable for anything? Her clients *came to her* seeking a treatment for a lifestyle that society had wrongfully deemed inappropriate, a cultural taboo which Dr. Martin

---

33. Costello and Cassity place the publication date in September 1996, three months after Leary died; Costello and Cassity "Why Oneness . . .," in Labate and Cavnar (2021), p. 130.
34. "Playboy Interview: Timothy Leary" *Playboy* (September 1966), unpaged; *italics* in original; Psanctum Timothy Leary Collection, Box 1, The Psanctum Psychedelic Library.

had nothing to do with creating. In the eyes of my colleague, Leary's real crime was simply not having enough intersectional points.

And Leary's true sexuality is far more nuanced than casting him as a bigot. Leary was himself bisexual and engaged in homosexual activities in his youth. In his adult life, he had at least one known relationship with Hubert Coffey, faculty advisor for his doctoral dissertation at the University of Alabama. Fearing exposure, the two men broke off their affair. Sadly, Coffey went looking for love in all the wrong places after the breakup and got himself arrested for engaging in sexual acts in a public bathroom. This chilled Leary's spine. In those days, conservatives, not leftists, led the "cancellation" mob. Coffey's career was over. Would Tim's be next? "[Tim] wasn't devastated. He was *terrified* . . . He thought he would be exposed," recalls Mary della Cioppa (a woman with whom Leary also had an affair).[35] This traumatic experience could easily account for Leary's later rejection of his own bisexuality, which he made sure to hide once he became a public figure.

Perhaps Leary wasn't a bigot. Maybe he was just afraid and acted in the face of that fear. He responded through his wounds. He certainly didn't have any problems with his friend, beat poet Allen Ginsburg's homosexual lifestyle, nor that of his even closer friend and research and writing partner, Richard Alpert. Leary was also acquainted with Aldous Huxley's best friend Gerald Heard.[36] All four of these men were queer in one respect or another, and all four had a tremendous impact on psychedelic history and culture. And part of that impact included shaping the very idea of oneness that is allegedly the sole province of the heteronormative. We should be celebrating, not ignoring, that contribution.

We've thankfully moved well beyond the age of miscategorizing sexual orientations outside of heteronormativity as mental disorders. Ho-

---

35. Quoted in Robert Greenfield, *Timothy Leary: A Biography* (FL: Harcourt, Inc., 2006), pp. 94–5.
36. In a confusing sentence, Jeanna Eichenbaum refers to Aldous Huxley's "probably queer" friend "Gerald Humphrey [*sic*]." It took a few moments to realize that Eichenbaum had smelted Gerald Heard and Humphry Osmond—two different people—into a singular person that never existed. Also, Heard was not "probably queer," he was openly gay. See Eichenbaum, "Queer Voices . . .," in Labate and Cavnar (2021), p. 105.

mosexuality was removed from the American Psychological Association's diagnostic manual in 1973. And so, the queering psychedelia contingent fixes its crosshairs on small matters like whether or not psychedelic clinical trials factor in a person's gender identity or sexual orientation, or ask for preferred pronouns upon arrival.[37] (Which is odd. Have you ever met a gender ideologue who did not make pronouns an immediate topic of conversation?) For Dr. Belser, despite lacking any explanation as to why, this amounts to "homophobia and transphobia."[38] Smart as he is, one wonders if Dr. Belser knows what the word "phobia" means.

And the grievances do not end there. Eichenbaum insists that "queer people are not used to being [understood] by straight, establishment people and institutions."[39] Here, Eichenbaum rests her faith in the myth of the identity perspective. For my tenure in the field, I can say I have never once felt the sting of heterosexual bigotry from anyone with whom I have ever worked or even simply met in the psychedelic Renaissance. I have never felt misunderstood due to my orientation. This, of course, does not mean that the memories of high school bullies slamming my head into a locker while calling me a "fag" don't come to my mind every now and then. And I'm sure such treatment was and is far worse for my queer sisters and brothers living in more conservative areas throughout the West. My experience, of course, is just that—nothing more. It is quite possible that some gay researchers have felt ostracized in psychedelic spaces. Should that be the case, the solution requires individual, not social, justice. And I support any initiatives—psychedelic or otherwise—that try to heal the trauma experienced by my fabulous countryfolk. I just do not wish to be included in Eichenbaum's, or anyone else's, abstraction.

But there is another side to this conversation. This much-needed mental health protocol for the queer population, at times, can feel like something different. It sometimes feels like a ruse that compels us to agree that identity perspectives serve as some kind of innate knowledge mark-

37. I agree that knowing a person's sexual orientation can be helpful in therapy. I also agree that in some cases—specifically when it comes to measuring narcissism—gender identity can serve a useful purpose in therapy too.

38. Belser, "10 Calls to Action . . .," in Labate and Cavnar (2021), p. 123.

39. Eichenbaum, "Queer Voices . . .," in Labate and Cavnar (2021), p. 106.

er about a topic. Such a rule applies within psychedelia. I don't want anyone to consider my ideas based on my sexual orientation. I want my ideas to be considered on their merits (or lack thereof). If someone told me that he liked my work because #supportqueerauthors, I'd tell him to go fuck himself. Nor would I ever "demand," as Eichenbaum does, that someone listen to me simply because I was on the receiving end of bullying in high school.[40] I'm not sure what qualifications I received through that experience that entitles me to such a privilege. Since Eichenbaum offers no explanation, we may assume that her demand comes from a belief that her identity perspective gives her an insight into the psychedelic experience to which we should all listen. And yet, there exists a fatal flaw in her demand. According to the identity perspective, all the heteronormative people who listen to Eichenbaum would not be able to comprehend her experiences anyway. Neither will gay men, straight and lesbian women, and a host of others whose identities do not perfectly align with that of Eichenbaum. Again, the identity perspective eats itself.

We all develop over a lifetime of triumphs and traumas, and we will all respond to them differently. Those who deal with gender dysphoria need compassion, not ridicule. They need friends and communities that love them. And love includes, above all else, honesty. Perhaps instead of using mushrooms to affirm the impossible, they can be used to find love in a person's heart for those who do not agree with her. And may those who are missing it, also find love in themselves, beyond any divisive ideology.

We don't know the sexual orientations for most of the people who took LSD in a clinical setting or recreationally over the better part of the last half-century. There simply isn't enough information to make even an educated guess. Of those known gay LSD researchers who greatly impacted psychedelic culture, identity perspective does not seem to have played any role in their development of "oneness"; and if it did in some to be determined way, then psychedelia was already "queered" half a century ago (whatever that means to you). Nonetheless, I hope we can all get on board with the idea of using psychedelics to help heal the trauma that

40. Eichenbaum, "Queer Voices . . .," in Labate and Cavnar (2021), p. 105.

comes with living an "alternative" lifestyle in more conservative areas of the West—a program that might have benefitted a closeted bisexual like Timothy Leary should it have existed in his day. As we move through new areas of understanding, let's make sure to hold grace for those who came before us, doing the best they could, in the face of their own cultural wounds.

Conclusion

Psychedelic Exceptionalism: A Roadmap for Change

I would ask any person to sit down and graph the overdose rate for heroin and the overdose rate for cannabis . . . and struggle for more than a nanosecond with why they are different.[1]

—Keith Humphreys

All Cops?

On our drive back to Portland from British Columbia for the 2022 Spirit Plant Medicine Conference, my business partner Eden and I were stopped and searched at the border. No big deal, we thought.

About a month before we made our way up to Canada for SPMC, we were busily running our weekly Psanctum Open Mic. Since entry is donation based, we have received some interesting payments in the past. One night we received a carton of eggs. Other times we received cannabis or mushrooms as admission. Such a thing happened one Monday

1. Quoted in Michael Shellenberger, *San Fransicko: Why Progressives Ruin Cities* (NY: HarperCollins, 2021), p. 70.

night about a month or so before SPMC. Eden accepted a donation of two thin psilocybin mushrooms stems nestled in a small, blue earplug case. When we left the venue, Eden put the case in the center consol of her car and ultimately forgot about them. I forgot about them too.

The feds at the border reminded us.

We sat in the border patrol station for hours. Since no women were on staff that night, Eden wasn't searched (because gender isn't real); I, however, was searched . . . *everywhere* (because patriarchy?). Eventually, the local sheriff of Sumas County police arrived (border patrol works in unison with the local PD). The feds took the sheriff into a back office for a chat. They all came out about twenty minutes later; Eden and I sat there in fear, waiting to hear our fate. The sheriff looked at us and began to speak. I soon realized that, even though he was facing our direction, he wasn't really talking to Eden and me—he was *really* talking to the feds when he said, "I have buddies on the force who are former military. These guys come home with all kinds of PTSDs, anxiety, depression—really messed up. They tell me that the only thing that actually works for them are these little mushrooms here. Point is, I know these things for the medicines they are. I have no jurisdiction over what these guys [meaning the feds] do, but I'm not going to bust you. I hope you get home safely tonight."

I'm paraphrasing here. He actually spoke much longer and flowerier and really drove home the point that psychedelic mushrooms are beneficial to the individual and society. That they help dig people out of some of the darkest places they can go. Most importantly, they heal our veterans who come home to a government that couldn't care less about them. It is time we let those who guard us while we sleep have access to these life-saving medicines.

An argument can be made that the sheriff was racist, and had Eden and I been black American, he would have busted us. It's a fair hypothetical, one that I certainly do not deny. However, this is also the 21st century, and an equally fair hypothetical might imagine the sheriff as a black American[2] with a nightstick up his ass about white Americans due

2. In fact, had there been a border-stop in Whatcom County, WA, and Eden and I had crossed there, we would have dealt with a black American sheriff, Donnell "Tank" Tanksley.

to DEI training. What if he truly believed that Eden and I were "born into not being human," as DEI instructor Ashleigh Shackelford garbles?[3] Perhaps he would have smiled as we were carted away.

While counting our blessings on the drive back to Portland around 4 a.m., I had a thought that manifested a small grin across my face. A little over twenty years earlier I was sitting in lockup because I was with someone who had a negligible amount of cannabis on him. This time, I had mushrooms in my possession and the police let me go.

Not all cops are bastards. That Sumas County sheriff was fucking awesome! Unapologetically spreading the Good News to his comrades and helping us beat the rap in the process.

The fed that had his finger up my asshole?

That guy's a bastard.

While psychedelic medicines are not magic bullets, I believe society will be made better through their mainstream acceptance. And I fear that, should the introduction of these medicines come with a critical social justice message, we will push both the psychedelic Renaissance and the country into becoming even more divisive. We need a psychedelic Renaissance based in truth, forgiveness, and love—not the opposite of our better angels found in identity politics. As critical social justice is more and more exposed as the disruptive and harmful scam that it is and slowly fades from Western Civilization, may it not see a resurgence piggybacked on these sacred medicines. Through bogus ideas like unconscious bias and microaggressions, misunderstandings of police shooting and crime statistics, and an unapologetic dismissal of all the Western advancements that make all our lives better (including innovations in psychedelic therapy), Chacruna Institute, Psymposia, and the recently mushrooming psilocybin-facilitator industry in Oregon recycle division and distrust of the other throughout the Renaissance.

Whether any of them intend to or not.

3. Quoted on John Stossel, "Diversity, Equity & Inclusion: DEI Training's Unintended Consequences" (March 21, 2023).

Naked Apes

In the US Bill of Rights (1791), we find the first attempt by any people in history to enshrine what political scientists call negative rights. Negative rights are those rights that limit governmental authority over the individual (they are the opposite of positive rights—those rights the government grants). We may think of negative rights as those *natural* rights you would enjoy as a naked ape walking through a rainforest. Should you find yourself in such a position, you could declare, scream, or swear anything you like. You could create any religious beliefs you desired, and you could hang out with any other naked apes discussing whatever was on your naked ape minds. As linguistically inclined, socially and spiritually attuned naked apes, these are the natural rights of life, religious belief, and assembling with other apes, all preserved as a negative right in the First Amendment to the US Constitution. Likewise, should you find yourself walking as a naked ape through a rainforest and someone or something tries to attack you, you have the natural right to defend yourself (as outlined in its negative right form in the Second Amendment).

Those are the rights that conservatives seem to gravitate toward, but they have a blind spot in one area: if you were a naked ape walking through a rainforest, you have the natural right to pick any plant or mushroom and eat it for food, medicine, or to explore your own consciousness. Conservatives might consider that the right to alter one's conscious stands proudly beside other natural rights like the right to speech and the right to defend oneself against attack. LSD celebrity Timothy Leary borrowed this concept of a "fifth freedom—the right to manage your own nervous system," from Allen Ginsberg.[4] Only this freedom isn't really a fifth freedom. It falls under the larger umbrella of the negative right outlined in the Fourth Amendment, the natural right to be left alone by the government if you aren't causing any problems. Exactly *what* social problems arise when a group of spiritually-minded people convene to eat mushrooms in religious ceremony?

---

4. Timothy Leary, *Flashbacks: A Personal and Cultural History of an Era* (NY: J.P. Putnam's Sons, 1990), p. 50.

Spiritual Apes

Notwithstanding Francine Douglas's gaffe, there is still something spiritually profound about the psychedelic experience that leads this writer to believe that outside forces, or energies, or deities (or whatever you want to call them) are an objective reality that can be reached through plant medicines. I have many friends and colleagues who have had these kinds of experiences and I've had a few of them myself. I'll tell you one of my favorites: a few years ago, two friends (Casey and Morgan) drove with Eden and me south from Portland to Williams, Oregon, to drink the sacred vine, ayahuasca. As we sat in a large circle of about 20 or so people with a small altar in the center, we imbibed the medicine and nestled into the space. Some of us lay back on our mats, while others remained seated upright. I was one of those lying down; Morgan was lying to my right. At one point, what I can only describe as a *spirit*[5] entered the room and possessed Morgan, a young woman lying down a few folks over to my left, and me. We three rose from our mats and headed to the altar. Mind you, this wasn't a Morgan got up, then I got up, then the other woman got up situation. The three of us rose like Manchurian candidates from our mats *simultaneously* and walked to the altar. We proceeded to dance around the altar like planets orbiting the sun. We could see the spirit moving us. We collapsed into it, surrendering our bodies and souls to that majestic dance. Soon after, we all returned to our respective mats at the same time.

None of that was planned. Neither Morgan nor I even knew the other woman.

As I have argued elsewhere, I believe phenomena like that merit our attention. Some are already working on the question, like Greenwich University psychologist Dr. David Luke.[6] If indigenous elders have something to add to it, I am happy to listen. Today's indigenous methods are beautiful, egalitarian, and healing. But they aren't all that ancient. They show clear signs of specifically Western influence in some areas; for example, a liberal/egalitarian approach to facilitation and the idea of

5. For lack of a better term.
6. See David Luke and Rory Spowers, *DMT: Entity Encounters* (VT: Park Street Press, 2021).

treating various mental health issues with these medicines.[7]

Snow and Ice

Europeans were no saints either though. They burned witches, murdered Jews, and tried animals in criminal courts—all in the name of a loving God. Much like their First Nations counterparts, Europeans didn't exactly improve morally through their use of a variety of plant medicines.

White Americans equally fell short of sainthood. The deplorable racism and demonization of the other, the cruelty of Jim Crow, the insane injustice of lynch mobs, Japanese internment camps—none of that should ever be overlooked or excused either. During the United States' racist past, white Americans also engaged in a variety of plant medicine usage like cannabis, opium, mescaline, peyote, and others to little positive racial effect. Although, I am aware of one trip report (from the 1950s) that discusses the tripper's thoughts on race, and certainly to a positive effect. Betty Eisner (1915–2004) was a late 1950s LSD researcher. In those days it was not only common, but encouraged, for the doctor to take the medicine. During one of Eisner's first experiences, she came face to face with her own racism:

> I was made to feel the coldness . . . of the myth that Nordic people are superior to others. I realized that this had been built into me from earliest childhood. I felt its austerity and its coldness—anyone who must be superior pays the price of snow and ice. And through these symbols I released the racial intolerance back and down to my childhood where I was brought up in the South—and I loosened part of my own need for feeling superior.[8]

---

7. I would also argue that both the Winnebago and the Delaware probably discovered the therapeutic properties of peyote independent of Western contact. However, without Western forms of mass communication and transportation, such medicines would have likely stayed with both the Winnebago and the Delaware. Further still, the use of plant medicines like cannabis to understand mental health issues predates the Winnebago and the Delaware.

8. Betty Eisner, *Remembrances of LSD Therapy Past* (2002), unpublished manuscript, pp. 17–18.

Well, there's good news! We now know we have a choice. The Betty Eisner route or the JEDI route. What I like about the Betty Eisner route is that it leads to open dialogue, sharing perspectives, learning, and bettering ourselves. It also leads to working together, which will be necessary if we really want to heal the most amount of our sisters and brothers through our Renaissance. Eisner's experience highlights an interesting point. Within psychedelic circles, we often speak of dose, set, and setting. To recap, dose meaning how much medicine we take; set meaning our mindset, and setting referring to the environment in which a person has her journey. While in the past, using psychedelics didn't cure anyone's bigotry, it would seem that positive change can occur when dose, set, and setting weave the microcosm with the macrocosm. Hear me out. The West's slow evolution towards a more egalitarian society ("setting"), provided the backdrop for the LSD ("dose"), to change the mind of Betty Eisner ("set"). Eisner's shift in her racist perspective represented a historical merging of dose, set, and setting on a grand scale!

That's why it's so important that we pause before promoting any other divisive and authoritarian programs in psychedelia. Right now, we have the power within us all to change the tide of history towards a more compassionate, redemptive future. Right now, we can have good-faith conversations about these ideas and decide which is the proper course: love and understanding or JEDI and divisiveness.

It's quite possible that there will always and forever be a stigma attached to all drugs in the West. It's easy for me (living in the Pacific Northwest) to overlook that psychedelics are hardly safe to experience in some uber-conservative parts of the States (and other areas). It is oppressive in the face of our natural right, but this oppression reaches across color lines. People in those places have every right to use these substances under protection of the 4th Amendment. Instead of regurgitating outdated narratives, we should work together to share a more useful message, one of which I hope many of us can agree: that psychedelic use is both a natural right and a spiritual right. And that they are a *good* thing for a lot of people when used responsibly.

But responsibility seems lost on many psilocybin facilitator schools in the Portland area that bypass real education for critical social justice ideology. Their programs are contentious and ill-equipped to produce mindful medicine facilitators. This does not mean that all facilitators are subpar—most of them are excellent. But their excellence comes from other places than their psilocybin-facilitator training schools (e.g., earlier therapy training, psychology degrees, having an innate tenderness about them, and, in some cases, years of service in the entheogenic underground).[9] Students are taught that the Aztecs employed psilocybin mushrooms in their religion and the Spanish willingly tried to erase its use. They are not taught that Aztec psychedelic rites were misogynistic, elitist, and involved human sacrifice and cannibalism—and that *that* was what irked the Spaniards. The students are hectored to mimic (but somehow not appropriate) indigenous healing traditions—but, as we saw, psychedelic therapeutic models are Western in origin.

Perhaps a misunderstanding of psychedelic history does not matter when it comes to facilitating medicine. I can understand that. But I also hope that this book helps us all find a common unity in the barbarisms of our ancestors, so that we can all be kinder to each other today. And I think that certainly has a role to play in medicine facilitation. Moreover, teaching facilitators little more than white guilt through the bogus IAT offers little chance of them actually relating to clients who might look different from them. These medicines are revolutionary because they connect us with something deeper about our common humanity—and *no*, that connection isn't "we are all the same."

Black Americans of the past were barred from engaging in psychedelic research, a clear historical tragedy. How many brilliant minds were sacrificed on the altar of systemic racism, we will never know. However, that does not mean that by dint of skin color a black American living *today* has something worthwhile to say about psychedelics any more than anyone else of any other skin color. A person can't both be oppressed and expect special privileges for her oppression. Oppressed people typically do not receive bonuses for being oppressed.

The same rule applies to me. I am not a psychedelic-therapist sim-

9. This last group more or less paying a $10,000 formality fee so they could facilitate above ground.

ply because some of my Italian predecessors worked with LSD. Skin tone and heritage have nothing to do with whether or not a researcher is bringing *ideas* to the table. A demand for recognition today because someone else was denied recognition in the past doesn't add up. Worse more, to exploit real past oppression for present personal gain, as some of our colleagues do, feels more like egotism than any real effort to bring positive change into the world.

Conscientious Capitalism

We often hear that money is the root of all evil. But that is only part of what the letter of 1 Timothy, found in the New Testament, says. The full line reads "*For the love of* money is the root of all evil" (1 Tim. 6:10).[10] Money can be used for positive outcomes. Greed is the problem. The question here is not: is capitalism good (indeed, people have done good things in the spirit of capitalism); nor is the question is capitalism bad (indeed, people have done bad things in the spirit of capitalism). The question is: how do we harness capitalism so that it benefits the most people? Proper psychedelic use can increase empathy in a person, which is much needed in tomorrow's business leaders.[11] How will teaching our future business leaders to discriminate based on racist and discordant JEDI mind tricks benefit anyone?

What if, instead of tearing down or breaking the system (as Dr. NiCole Buchanan recommends),[12] the psychedelic Renaissance commits itself to conscientious capitalism and benevolently rewrites those parts of the system that need correction? Why demolish an entire house simply because one of the bedrooms needs a new coat of paint? And does Buchanan's plan include the university system, of which she has made a comfortable and lucrative career for herself? Perhaps it should. It's no secret that much of the elite university system is corrupt from top to bottom. And is it not the very ideas Dr. Buchanan espouses (i.e.,

---

10. *Italics* mine.
11. Psilocybin seems to influence emotional empathy more so than it does cognitive empathy. See, Kush V. Bhatt and Cory R. Weissman, "The Effect of Psilocybin on Empathy and Prosocial Behavior: A Proposed Mechanism for Enduring Antidepressant Effects," *Nature*, *Mental Health Research*, 3, no. 7 (February 20, 2024).
12. See epigram on page 41 of this book.

unconscious bias, microaggressions, and other JEDI rubbish) that corrupted the university system in the first place? On the legal end, is it not "equitable" law, which Dr. Buchanan also supports, that has resulted in unsafe neighborhoods throughout minority communities? Moreover, Dr. Buchanan does not offer a single solution (or even hopeful recommendation) as to what we would replace our current system with after we use plant medicines to break it. We are all to look upon the rubble of our fallen civilization and ask ourselves, "Now what?" Why eradicate free markets when greed is the problem? Why eradicate the justice system when equitable law and bastard cops are the problem? What if, instead of encouraging division, we taught compassion and understanding to future leaders of all kinds? We could raise our progeny to see capitalism as a way that enriches others, not just themselves.

Psychedelic Exceptionalism

Some within the psychedelic intelligentsia oppose so-called psychedelic exceptionalism, a belief shared by many that plant medicines serve as positive-behavior reinforcing tools.[13] For the psychedelic exceptionalist, plant medicines are preferable over heavy alcohol use, cocaine, heroin, speed, opiates/opioids, and the like. And while cocaine and heroin *do* derive from plants—and in their natural forms are not quite as harmful as they are in their processed forms—by the time they reach the user on the street there is the possibility of any number of adulterants contaminating their purity.

One of the more vocal intellectuals against psychedelic exceptionalism is Dr. Carl Hart. And while I agree with him in many areas, I find we part company when he claims: "Let people know that 'shit, your psilocybin or LSD use is just like my crack use.'"[14] For Dr. Hart, it's all just different preferences for getting high in one form or another.

I respectfully disagree.

True, there is nothing wrong with using psychedelics just to get high recreationally, but that's not the only way to do it (and is not the thrust

13. Hart (2021), p. 178.

14. Quoted in Madison Margolin, "Inside the 'Psychedelic Exceptionalism' Debate: Should all Drugs be Legal, or Just Pot and Psychedelics?" *Double Blind Mag* (July 25, 2022).

of the psychedelic Renaissance). Many psychenauts prefer using these medicines not in recreational "just getting high" ways, but rather to probe our minds, hearts, and souls in ceremonial settings. We examine the unexplored areas of ourselves and others through the lens of the cosmos, and work to integrate the experience into our lives once the journey has ended.

That's not "just getting high." That is a regiment—a roadmap to a better quality of life, which makes society better overall.

Dr. Hart is echoed by Madison Margolin, who states, "So the question becomes: Should psychedelics be treated so differently from other drugs, given that any substance may have the power to soothe or scorch the human psyche, and body, too? That's the crux of the psychedelic exceptionalism debate."[15]

First, that is *not* the crux of the psychedelic exceptionalism debate. The crux of the debate has to do with the levels of addiction among various substances and the violence that follows to meet that dependance, i.e., the degrees of harm that a drug can cause a person and society. During the wave of drive-by shootings, gang rapes, and deadly beatings that swept the inner cities in the 80s and 90s (and today), Dr. Hart and Margolin might consider that psilocybin mushrooms surprisingly count for very little of it. Addictive drugs like crack account for almost all of it. And yet, Dr. Hart asks that we pretend crack and mushrooms are more or less the same thing, while Margolin alludes to such a comparison.

We cannot cure that which we misdiagnose.

Second, psychedelics like mushrooms, LSD, ayahuasca, peyote, and others do *not* scorch the body. This incessant need to make highly questionable associations between addictive drugs and entheogens is why I find it difficult to take anti-psychedelic exceptionalism arguments seriously. And to compare a person who might be having a bad trip as having her mind "scorched," as if to say that LSD has the same kind of deteriorating effects on consciousness and the brain as fentanyl and meth have over time, is without foundation. LSD, ayahuasca, and mushrooms have little to no deleterious effects on the body.

I've never even heard of such a thing.

Like affiliates at Chacruna Institute, Dr. Hart and Margolin are

15. Margolin, "Inside the Psychedelic . . ." (2022).

leaving out a major part of this story—namely, the violent crime that comes with certain drug cultures. The crack epidemic of the mid- to late 1980s and early 1990s reached a level of intensity that, as Thomas Sowell put it, "You were more likely to die in the streets than you were to die fighting in World War II."[16] In one instance, a crew gang-raped a seventeen-year-old girl in front of her boyfriend. They then shot off her boyfriend's dick.[17] He slowly bled out overnight, eventually succumbing to what could have only been a truly agonizing death.

You don't typically see that kind of violence in a 5 MeO-DMT circle.

In my home state of Oregon, voters passed two ballot initiatives in 2020, Measure 109 and Measure 110 (mentioned in the previous chapter) in an attempt to compassionately change drug laws. Measure 109 made psilocybin-assisted therapy more or less legal (it's kind of a gray area) for therapeutic purposes in the state. Measure 110 decriminalized all drugs, which has led to "open-air drug markets," i.e., places to score addictive and dangerous drugs with few legal ramifications.[18]

Decriminalization in Oregon was an absolute failure. So much so that we are experiencing the city's largest exodus of taxpaying residents and a staggering influx of people who need empathy and help, not incentives to keep living destructive lives on the streets.[19]

The reason decriminalization failed is obvious: during the campaign for Measure 110, we weren't allowed to say what we all knew to be true for fear of sounding politically incorrect: that fentanyl, crack, and meth have a far higher potential for abuse, gang violence, and death than do mushrooms, ayahuasca, and LSD. Oregon decrim advocates (well, not Eden and me) took the postmodern relativist approach: *nothing* (in this case, drugs) *is better or worse than anything else, it's all just different.* We are now seeing the results of that misstep.

Anti-psychedelic exceptionalists will often point to Portugal, where

16. Thoams Sowell, *The Quest for Cosmic Justice* (NY: Simon and Schuster, 1999), p. 8.
17. Godwin (1978), p. 203.
18. Shellenberger (2021), p. 77.
19. Anthony Effinger, "More Oregonians Left in 2022 than Arrived, Reversing a Long-Standing Trend," *Willamette Week* (September 14, 2023).

all drugs have been decriminalized since 2001.[20] They will say that Portugal doesn't have the social problems we see in America's decriminalized cities. And that's true, it doesn't. But it's not an apt comparison. Portugal does not allow open-air drug markets. In Portugal a person will be arrested for using drugs publicly in a way that she will not be in Portland, Oakland, Seattle, and Denver. According to Stanford University addiction expert Keith Humphreys, "Portugal is a conservative culture where drug use is looked down upon. . . . All of these cities [San Francisco, Portland, Seattle] are libertarian in their views about drugs and alcohol. In Portugal they put pressure on people to go to treatment. It's social pressure and pressure toward making people change their behavior."[21]

That's why decriminalization works in Portugal. Those struggling with addiction are urged to seek help and regain control of their lives. We do the opposite in the States, which is why decriminalization doesn't work here.[22]

So to those good folks living in areas working to decriminalize *everything*, here's a head's up from someone who lives in the first state to do so: if you do not draw a fine line between psychedelics and other, more dangerous substances, and decrim passes, you aren't going to get stoned hippies in the park throwing a Frisbee, you're going to get randos on your porch smoking fentanyl trying to start fights with passersby. Followed by the mass exodus of the very people who keep a city alive—taxpayers.

We are told to have compassion. And I agree. Compassion is paramount here. But allowing people to destroy their lives is not compassionate. Allowing them to ruin the lives of their family and friends is not compassionate. Allowing women to live in open-air drug markets, where they are at greater risk of sexual assault, is not compassionate. Leaving piles of used needles in parks where kids play is not compassionate. And allowing people to slowly die on the streets is not compassionate.

---

20. Margolin, "Inside the Psychedelic . . ." (2022).

21. Quoted in Shellenberger (2021), p. 49.

22. But it wasn't all just the dangerously lax penalties for destructive drug use. Addiction centers, promised through our municipalities via Measure 110, never opened. Our city released the floodgates by acting as a beacon for safe drug use without ensuring lifeboats were in place. No one who supported Measure 110 was responsible for that.

Dr. Hart makes no secret that he sometimes enjoys an evening of heroin and methamphetamine use to no ill-effect.[23] Is that because heroin and methamphetamine aren't addictive, *or* is it because Dr. Hart is an exceptionally smart, responsible, and capable person? He is a bestselling author and an Ivy League professor. I have no doubt that such an exceptional man can take pleasure in an evening at home enjoying some smack or *scante* and not come to ruin. When he runs out of his supply, he doesn't need to acquire heroin through dangerous avenues. I would also imagine that the heroin in which he partakes is much cleaner than what a desperate person, jonesing for the needle, finds on the streets. And I personally know recreational heroin users who certainly are not strung-out junkies robbing old ladies to satisfy a crippling addiction. They are good people who have steady jobs and careers, work hard, hold deep and meaningful relationships, and do not cause any problems in society.

To show no favoritism, I will relate a heresy among psychenauts about my favorite plant to ever evolve on Earth, cannabis, of which I enjoy regularly. Cannabis simply hasn't affected me in any discernable negative way. And it's not just me. Go to any psychedelic conference and you will meet some of the brightest people science, psychology, and law have to offer; the majority of those people also smoke cannabis regularly to no ill-effect. But (and here's the heresy) cannabis can also be addicting and destructive for some people, even if it isn't for my colleagues and me. I would be disingenuous if I didn't mention that I have known cannabis smokers who overused in their youth and became lazy, uninspired, and burnt out in adulthood—far worse off than the recreational heroin users I know today. So I fully agree with Dr. Hart that there are more factors wrapped in this equation beyond just comparing one substance to another. Still, show me a cannabis smoker sitting at home binge-watching *Seinfeld* shoving snacks down her throat, and I'll show you a person who isn't likely to aim a gun at a man's penis and squeeze the trigger.

To deny that heroin and meth (or fentanyl, which is currently rotting out Rose City) are no more addicting and/or potentially dangerous than mushrooms and ayahuasca—that it's all just relative—is simply unrealistic. Heroin, crack, methamphetamine, speed, and a host of opioids (if over-prescribed), and some of the violent crime that comes along with

23. Hart, (2021), p. 14 (for heroin); pp. 181–82 (for methamphetamine).

them, are not only different from mushrooms, cannabis, LSD, ayahuasca, and other entheogens but are so obviously more potentially harmful to the human body, mind, and essence that for Dr. Hart (or anyone else) to claim otherwise seems, in the very least, unhelpful.

Dr. Hart's analysis of the Trayvon Martin shooting (outlined in chapter 10 of this book) should have led him to reconsider psychedelic exceptionalism. Does he really believe that psilocybe mushrooms are just as dangerous as lean? Would LSD have damaged Trayvon Martin's liver in such a noticeable way? Would ayahuasca have caused his violent behavior? Does Dr. Hart believe that honoring the Divine Feminine through entheogenic sacraments is no different than referring to women as "bitches" and "hoes" while trashed on purple drank? I can find agreement that drugs—in and of themselves—are not always the problem (as Dr. Hart's safe and responsible heroin and meth use testifies), but it seems evident that certain *cultures* tied to certain drugs are a big part of the issue. But without social pressure, what chances do we have of actually changing the culture positively? And how do we guarantee that someone in the throes of an intense heroin withdrawal isn't going to harm someone on the streets to obtain her fix?

Yes, drug laws need to be reformed. *Yes*, users of addictive drugs deserve respect and should enter rehab and treatment programs, not prisons. *Yes*, cities like Oakland and Portland demonstrate that decriminalizing everything without any social pressure for personal improvement is not a viable solution. And *yes*, honoring the Sacred Feminine is way better than objectifying women.

I'll take Gaia and mushrooms over misogyny and lean any day.

The Divine Masculine

Peppered throughout this book I have made mention to the concept of the Divine Masculine, dropping a few spores along the way for the curious to follow. As we come to a conclusion, I'd like to fully outline what I have been referring to this whole time. The Divine Masculine is what all men (and women, if they choose) should strive to embody. The Divine Masculine is assertive but not forceful; detailed, but not long-winded; intellectual, but not snooty; stoic, but not unfeeling; visionary, but grounded; discerning, but not prejudiced; firm, but not unyielding; confident, but humble; industrious, but not exploitive. Above all, the Divine Masculine *serves.* Serves his family, serves his community, and serves himself in a way that is not self-serving. The Divine Masculine lives well by doing good. The Divine Masculine brought men out of barbarism, taught them fidelity, compassion, enlightenment, and to care about those outside themselves. The Divine Masculine is a gentleman, manhood perfected. I think a rekindling of the Divine Masculine (along with the Sacred Feminine) might serve us well. Whether a person is uber conservative and despises occult ideas or is a critical social justice activist that isn't sure women exist, we should all agree that mentally healthy people are good for society.

We have all fallen short of these values from time to time in our lives. And we will again in the future. But if we keep the Divine Masculine at the forefront of our minds and hearts, we, over time, ignite the alchemy within us that leads to positive change. Ordinary roads seldom lead to extraordinary places, and only the Divine Masculine can walk an extraordinary road. Rekindle the Sacred Feminine and the Divine Masculine in the West and watch so many of our problems vanish.

The Most Racist Phrase

There is a phrase that, while common in the West, you might have noticed is almost entirely absent from this book. I have never written this phrase or said this phrase out loud up until now because it is the most racist phrase I have ever heard.[24] I break my silence in this moment because I believe it is important. The phrase I'm referring to is "people of color." The phrase has several shortcomings, one of which I touched upon earlier when discussing Dr. Monnica Williams's misunderstanding of historical lynching. People of color were not the majority of those lynched. Black American men were.[25] That most racist phrase muddles the issues.

The phrase also sets up a false identity perspective of experience

24. Notwithstanding one instance earlier when I was quoting someone else (see p. 198).
25. Although, the largest mass lynching took place in New Orleans in 1891, and all eleven were Italian Americans. Though, this does not compare at all to the 3,446 black American men who were lynched between the years 1882 through 1968. See Tuskegee University, "Lynchings: By State and Race, 1882–1968."

for far too many people by completely erasing cultures and individuals. "People of color" is the *opposite* of diversity. A wealthy Southeast Asian kid and an impoverished black American kid can barely be said to have shared similar "people of color" experiences. And Thomas Sowell doesn't seem to have much in common with Michael Eric Dyson—at least in terms of their ideas. Furthermore, I'd wager that an impoverished white American kid has more in common with his black American neighbor than he has with any upper-class white American kid.

The more damaging aspect of the term serves the same purpose as the dreaded N-word by reducing a person to skin tone instead of allowing who she is as a person to breathe.

Imagine the following conversation:

> Harris: "How shall we refer to this woman?"
>
> Johnson: "How about we call her a 'person of honesty'?"
>
> Harris: "No, Johnson! 'Honesty' tells us something about her character. Try again."
>
> Johnson: "What about 'person of integrity'?"
>
> Harris: "Same problem! You are telling me about her character. We need a construct—not a human being! This must stop at once."
>
> Johnson: "What about 'person of . . . *color*'? "
>
> Harris: "That's it! 'Person of color' tells me nothing about this woman at all!"

That most racist phrase instantly otherizes and makes an abstraction of the individual. It insists that a person's immutable traits say more about her than her morals, values, beliefs, and accomplishments. I recall going to a party once where some of the other attendees and I were in a conversation about climate change. One of the more Woke people in the conversation called a Southeast Asian man over to our group, saying, "You're a person of color! What's your perspective on climate change as a person of color?" As if the man's melanin level was any reflection of his personal beliefs. The cringe was felt by a few of us. The phrase people of color serves the opposite purpose of Dr. Martin Luther King Jr.'s revolutionary admonishment: that we treat each other based on the content of character, not the color of skin. So long as we make a person's immutable traits the most important thing about her, we will forever be running around in circles playing grab-ass, stubbing our toes, wondering why racism is seemingly everywhere.

So I'd like to end this subchapter with a prediction: in 50 to 70 years (or so), people of the future will look back on those of us today who use the term "people of color" the same way we look back and wince at white Americans who used the N-word 50 to 70 years ago.

If I Were a Psychopath

Where does this leave us? Psychedelics are nonspecific amplifiers. They require a certain mindset and environment to be most effective. Distrust, grievance, and resentment of millions of people the psychedelic SJW has never met are probably not the best things to amplify. We have to have conversations about these highly nuanced and serious issues before psychedelics go mainstream. Psychedelic researchers took to the universities to try to legitimize these medicines. But the universities are now captured by this regressive CSJ ideology. And authoritarianism was never part of the plan for the psychedelic Renaissance. Yes, psychedelics can heal us; but no, not if our institutions are being run by psychopaths. And that is not hyperbole on my part.

It's provable.

For example, if I were a psychopath, my first order of business would be to turn friends into enemies based on immutable characteristics. I would use every opportunity, every crisis, every virus, to sow hatred and division, whereby creating an easy transition from liberty to authoritarianism. I would reward blind obedience and punish good-intentioned dissent.

I would sanctify corporate hold of the government.

If I were a psychopath, I would entrance the masses to be glued to their devices; I'd entice them to pay any price. Even the freedom to a private life. I would brainwash the masses to worship abstractions, consume endless distractions, and make dystopian narratives the main attraction. I'd only promote the horrors of one, while pretending the others had never been done.

If I were a psychopath, I'd insist we put the opposition in submission. I'd poison minds with JEDI division. I'd keep them glued to screens while I'd feed the daily hate into the machine. I'd break up families and incentivize mothers to marry the state as their new lovers. I'd excuse the fathers who abandon their kids—in fact, I wouldn't even mention it.

If I were a psychopath, I would pretend I was not othering the other, by creating false analogies to scramble cognitive function. I would install new language as linguistic mandates, deny biological reality, and shut down debate. I would criminalize thinking by calling it "hate." Make people afraid to converse and relate.

If I were a psychopath, I would kill basic freedoms, objective reality, and speech. I would demonize anyone with the courage to speak. To keep the narratives tight, I'd train doctors and teachers to professionally gaslight. I would hypnotize the population with the ontological lie that questioning these narratives causes intellectual genocide. With their misguided minds now weaponized, I would terrorize all who rose to defy, and beleaguer them until they complied.

If I were a psychopath, that's what I'd do.

If you were a psychopath, wouldn't you?

This moment is paramount. Western culture is leading the way against racial bigotry in the modern world just as psychedelics are gaining more mainstream acceptance. The convergence of these separate culture wars is creating fertile ground for either a new future where bigotry of all kinds is shunned, or a dystopian regression wherein we replay the pitfalls of the past. Outside our beautiful psychedelic Renaissance there is a whole world of people interested in these medicines, eager to know what those of us who have dedicated our lives to these questions have to say. I urge my colleagues to export growth, understanding, compassion, *some hard truths*, and good will. We are doomed to fail if: first, our main exports are false accusations of uncaring racism and transphobia. And second, if we are not allowed to question those, or any other, claims. I'm not dismissing the very pressing issues outlined in this book like the abuse of First Nations peoples, the history of systemic racism in the United States, or mistreatment of homosexuals. I'm asking that we come together to try to solve contemporary issues without all the blind hatred confusing the better angels of our nature.

I do not consider the psychedelic SJW the enemy. Nor do I consider conservatives the enemy. I consider our dishonest media, our government that abuses such dishonesty, corporatism, racism, and sexism the enemy. At base, I agree with those of Chacruna Institute. There *is* a revolution to be had.

May ours be a revolution where we cast aside the shackles of surface differences and all the social pitfalls that come with them. May ours be a revolution where we wake up from the misinformation and lies pumped out by the legacy media and shared relentlessly on social media. May ours be a revolution where we put aside our egos and listen to each other in good faith. May ours be a revolution in which intellectuals again value teaching students how to think, not what to think. A revolution where business leaders hold the same care for their employees that they hold for their kin. A revolution where we snuff out racism instead of perpetuating it through JEDI mind tricks. A revolution that unites First Nations with Western psychedelic models.

May ours be a revolution of radical unity.

A revolution of radical love.

Bibliography

"80-Year-Old California Store Owner Who Shot Robbers Dies," *Associated Press* (December 27, 2022); accessed via: https://www.yahoo.com/news/80-old-california-store-owner-011844759.html.

"Across the Border," *The Oasis*, July 15 (1899), unpaged; accessed via: https://chroniclingamerica.loc.gov/lccn/sn85032933/1899-07-15/ed-1/seq-6/#words=marihuana+marijuana+mariguana+ Indian+hemp+cannabis+dope.

Adler, William M., *Land of Opportunity: One Family's Quest for the American Dream in the Age of Crack* (Ann Arbor: University of Michigan Press, 2021).

"A History of Black Americans in California"; accessed via: https://www.nps.gov/parkhistory/online_books/5views/5views2.htm#:~:text=Within%20the%20decade%20of%20the,both%20northern%20and%20southern%20counties.

Ahmed-Jones, Keeno and Ava Daeipour, "An Open Letter and Call to Action for MAPS Canada"; accessed via: https://www.psymposia.com/magazine/psychedelics-diversity-maps-canada-open-letter/.

Albertus Magnus, *De Vegetabilibus Libri VII. Historiæ Naturalis Pars XVIII* (Berolini: Typis Et Impensis Georgii Reimeri, 1867).

Amanita Dreamer, *Dosing Amanita Muscaria and What to Expect* (GA: Amanita Dreamer Publishing, 2023).

Anslinger, Harry J., *The Protectors: Our Battle Against the Crime Gangs* (NY: Farrar, Strauss, and Company, 1964).

Anslinger, Harry J. and Courtney Ryley Cooper, "Marijuana: Assassin of Youth," *The Reader's Digest* (February 1938); accessed via: https://www.druglibrary.org/schaffer/history/e1930/mjassassinrd.htm.

Arfu Staff, "Psychedelic Privilege: Are DMT Entities Racist?" *arfru.com* (undated), accessed via: https://afru.com/ dmt-entities-beings-racist/.

"Articles of Incorporation of Multidisciplinary Association for Psychedelic Studies, Inc."; accessed via: https://maps.org/wp-content/uploads/2010/04/articlesofincorporationandamendment.pdf.

AZ BlueMeanie, "Update on Protestor with Assault Rifle at Obama Event in Phoenix," *Blog for Arizona* (August 22, 2009); accessed via: https://blogforarizona.net/update-on-guns-at-obama-event-in-phoenix/.

Akerlof, George A. and Janet L. Yellen, "An Analysis of Out-of-Wedlock Births in the United States," Brookings Institute (August 1, 1996); accessed via: https://www.brookings.edu/articles/an-analysis-of-out-of-wedlock-births-in-the-united-states/.

"Alexandra Chasin Discusses Assassin of Youth: A Kaleidoscopic History of Harry J. Anslinger's War on Drugs," Cambridge Community Television (January 6, 2017); accessed via: https://www.youtube.co m/channel/UCZT3Pf-bqdGqkHnSt-OISv8Q.

Alfonseca, Kiara, "Police Have Killed More than 100 Children Since 2015 in US, Data Shows," *ABC News* (April 28, 2021); accessed via: https://abcnews.go.com/US/police-us-killed-100-children-2015-data-shows/story?id=77190654.

Alpert, Richard, "LSD and Sexuality: Review of a Case of Homosexuality Treated Therapeutically with LSD and Description of a Male-Female Psychedelic Session Program," *Psychedelic Review*, No 10 (1969): 21–24.

Alvarez, Lizette, "At Zimmerman Trial, Victim's Friend Is Pressed on Her Story," *The New York Times* (June 27, 2013); accessed via: https://www.nytimes.com/2013/06/28/us/at-zimmerman-trial-victims-friend-is-pressed-on-her-story.html.

——"Defense in Trayvon Martin Case Raises Questions About the Victim's Character," *The New York Times* (May 23, 2013); accessed via: https://www.nytimes.com/2013/05/24/us/zimmermans-lawyers-release-text-messages-of-trayvon-martin.html.

"American College of Pediatricians Statement on Gender," *Toronto Sun* (June 10, 2024); accessed via: https://www.youtube.com/watch?v=e0LrP3Tc4K8.

"Ancient Sources on Nubia and Ethiopia," accessed via: https://factsanddetails.com/world/cat56/sub371/entry-6156.html.

Anderson, Elijah, *Streetwise: Race, Class, and Change in an Urban Community* (IL: University of Chicago Press, 1995).

Anderson, Elisha, "Police Sergeant Fights Tears in Describing Girl's Death," *USA Today* (June 5, 2013); accessed via:https://www.usatoday.com/story/news/nation/2013/06/05/officer-fights-tears-in-testimony-about-girls-death/2394725/.

Angle, Alex, "The Maternal Mortality Crisis in Arkansas," *KNWA Fox 24* (July 10, 2022); accessed via: https://www.nwahomepage.com/news/the-maternal-mortality-crisis-in-arkansas/.

Ashby, Ken, "Michael Brown; Thug or Gentle Giant?" (Letter to the Editor), in *The Dallas Morning News*; accessed via: https://www.dallasnews.com/opinion/2014/08/29/michael-brown-thug-or-gentle-giant/.

Austen, Ian, " 'Horrible History': Mass Grave of Indigenous Children Reported in Canada," *The New York Times*, May 28, 2021; accessed via: https://www.nytimes.com/2021/05/28/world/canada/kamloops-mass-grave-residential-schools.html.

Ayers, Edward L. *Vengeance and Justice: Crime and Punishment in the 19th Century American South* (UK: Oxford University Press).

Balko, Radley, *Rise of the Warrior Cop: The Militarization of America's Police Forces* (NY: PublicAffairs, 2014).

Ball, Dr. Martin, "My Scarlet Letter" (transcript of podcast sent to author).

Barnett, Gordon J., (trans.) Jacques-Joseph Moreau, *Hashish and Mental Illness* (NY: Raven Press, 1973).

Belser, Alexander, "10 Calls to Action: Toward an LBGTQ-Affirmative Psychedelic Therapy," in Bia Labate and Clancy Cavnar (eds.), *Psychedelic Justice: Toward a Diverse and Equitable Psychedelic Culture* (NM: Synergetic Press, 2021).

Bennett, Chris, *Cannabis and the Soma Solution* (OR: Trine Day, 2010).

——*Liber 420: Cannabis, Magickal Herbs, and the Occult* (OR: Trine Day, 2018).

——*Cannabis: Lost Sacrament of the Ancient World* (OR: Trine Day, 2023).

Bhatt, Kush V., and Cory R. Weissman, "The Effect of Psilocybin on Empathy and Prosocial Behavior: A Proposed Mechanism for Enduring Antidepressant Effects" *Nature, Mental Health Research*, 3, no. 7 (February 20, 2024); accessed via: https://www.nature.com/articles/s44184-023-00053-8.

Bing, Leon, *Do or Die: For the First Time, Members of L.A.'s Most Notorious Teenage Gangs—Crips and Bloods—Speak for Themselves* (NY: HarperCollins Publishers, 1991).

Black Lives Matter, "About" (undated). https://blacklivesmatter.com/about/

Blimes, Alex, "Jay-Z on his Music, Politics, and his Violent Past," *GQ Magazine* (June 28, 2017; original, 2005); accessed via:https://www.gq-magazine.co.uk/article/jay-z-interview-music-politi cs-violence.

Boethius, *Consolatio philosophiæ*; accessed via: faculty.georgetown.edu.

Bogadi, Marija and Snježana Kaštelan, "A Potential Effect of Psilocybin on Anxiety in Neurotic Personality Structures in Adolescents," *Croatian Medical Journal*, 62, 5 (October 2020): 528–530.

Boghossian, Peter, and James Lindsay, *How to Have Impossible Conversations: A Very Practical Guide* (NY: Go Hatchette Books, 2019).

Boller, Paul F., *Not So! Popular Myths about America from Columbus to Clinton* (UK: Oxford University Press, 1996).

Bonnie, Richard J. and Charles H. Whitebread, "The Forbidden Fruit and the Tree of Knowledge: An Inquiry into the Legal History of Marijuana Prohibition," *Schaffer Drug Library*; accessed via: https://www.druglibrary.org/schaffer/library/studies/vlr/vlr4.htm.

Bouquet, Martin, et al., "Acts of the Council in Orleans,"*Recueil des Historiens* (Poitiers: Imprimerie de H. Oudin Frères, 1878).

"Boy, 16, Says Man Sold Narcotic Cigarettes," *The New York Times* (October 7, 1928); accessed via: https://www.nytimes.com/1928/10/07/archives/boy-16-says-man-sold-narcotic-cigarettes-youth-seized-with-alleged.html.

Bronner, David, "End the Racist War on Drugs" (April 20, 2023): accessed via: https://www.instagram.com/p/CrQ43c9MlIy/.

Bruce, Heather, et al., "Between Principles and Practice: Tensions in Anti-Racist Education–2014 Race & Pedagogy National Conference" (2014). Race and Pedagogy Conference; accessed via: https://soundideas.pugetsound.edu/race_pedagogy/23/.

Buchanan, NiCole T., "Curriculum Vitae," p. 3–5; accessed via: https://psychology.msu.edu/_ass ets /pdfs/faculty-cvs/buchanan-cv-2021.pdf.

——"Excising a Virus of the Mind: Individual and Institutional Responsibility for Reducing Implicit Bias," for TEDxMSU at Michigan State University, East Lansing, MI; accessed via: https://youtu.be/b5UUBPA1-FU; Buchanan, N. T. (2016, January).

——"Bias and its Role in Social Inequity. Invited presentation for the forum, Sharper Focus, Wider Lens Symposium on The Nature of Inequality," Michigan State University Honor's College; accessed via: www.youtube.com/watch?v=s6zxPCGI64A.

——"Psychedelic Justice: Creating a Socially Just Psychedelic Renaissance" (August 16, 2021); accessed via: https://chacruna.net/psychedelic_renaissance_social_justice/.

——"Why Psychedelic Science Should Pay Speakers and Trainers of Color," in Beatriz C. Labate and Clancy Cavnar, *Psychedelic Justice: Towards a Diverse and Equitable Psychedelic Culture* (2021).

Campos, Isaac, *Home Grown: Marijuana and the Origins of Mexico's War on Drugs* (NC: University of North Carolina Press, 2012).

——"Mexicans and the Origins of Cannabis Prohibition in the United States: A Reassessment," *Social History of Alcohol and Drugs*, Vol. 32 (2018).

Cardano, Girolamo, *De subtilitate* (Venice: Gulielmum Rouillium, 1551). Facsimile edition available at http://books.google.com.

"Causes of Gestational Hypertension," *Stanford Medicine*; accessed via: https://stanfordhealthcare.org/medical-conditions/womens-health/gestational-hypertension/causes.html#:~:text=The%20cause%20of%20gestational%20hypertension,Kidney%20disease.

Cassidy, Megan "No Charges for Phoenix Officer who Shot Unarmed Man," *The Republic* (April 1, 2015); accessed via: https://www.azcentral.com/story/news/local/phoenix/2015/04/01/phoenix-police-rumain-brisbon-autopsy-release-abrk/70777818/.

——"Unarmed Arizona Man Killed by Cop," *The Arizona Republic* (Dec. 4, 2024); accessed via: https://www.usatoday.com/story/newsnation/2014/12/04/phoenix-police-unarmed-man-killed-by-officer/19878931/.

Chacruna Institute, "Diversity, Culture, and Social Justice in Psychedelics Course" (February 16, 2022); accessed via: https://chacruna.net/chacruna-institutes-course-diversity-culture-and-social-justice-in-psychedelics/.

Chan, Stella, "Black Lives Matter Co-Founder Stepping Down from Organization," CNN (May 28, 2021); accessed via: https://www.cnn.com/2021/05/28/us/black-lives-matter-patrisse-cullors-resigns/index.html.

Chen, Angus, "Why is it So Hard to Test Whether Drivers are Stoned?" *NPR: Health News from NPR* (February, 2016), accessed via:https://www.npr.org/sections/health-shots/2016/02/09/466147956/why-its-so-hard-to-make-a-solid-test-for-driving-while-stoned.

Chakraborty, Titas and Matthias van Rossum, "Slave Trade and Slavery in Asia: New Perspectives," *Journal of Social History*, Vol. 54, Is. 1 (Fall, 2020): 1–14.

Chapkis, Wendy, "What Psychedelic Researchers and Activists can Learn from Medical Marijuana Legalization" (April 21, 2017); accessed via: https://chacruna.net/psychedelic-researchers-can-learn-from-marijuana-legalization/.

"Character of the Mexican: Proper and Improper," *The Sun,* May 17 (1914).

Clegg, Robert, "Percentage of Births to Unmarried Women," *Center for Equal Opportunity* (February 26, 2020); accessed via: https://www.ceousa.org/2020/02/26/percentage-of-births-to-unmarried-women/.

Clement of Alexandria, *Exhortation of the Greeks*; accessed via: newadvent.org.

Cleveland Clinic, "Hemorrhage," accessed via: https://my.clevelandclinic.org/health/symptoms/21654-hemorrhage.

Cohen, Shawn, "Headmaster of Elite NYC School Tells Colleagues he was 'Trapped by a Disgruntled Teacher . . . ,'" *Dailymail* (April 23, 2021); accessed via: https://www.dailymail. co.uk/news/ article-9497375/Headmaster-elite-NYC-school-says-trapped-disgruntled-teacher.html.

Cole, Monica, "Mattel Pushes Transgender Barbie," *American Family Association* (June 24, 2022); accessed via: https://afa.net/the-stand/culture/2022/06/mattel-pushes-transgender-barbie/.

Common Sense Drug Policy, "The Devil Weed and Harry Anslinger" (2003): accessed via: http://www. csdp.org/publicservice/anslinger.htm.

"Conference on Cannabis Sativa Linne," *Schaffer Library of Drug Policy* (January 14, 1937); accessed via: https://druglibrary.net/schaffer/hemp/taxact/canncon.htm.

Coolidge, Calvin, "Address to the National Conference on Outdoor Recreation in Washington, DC: 'The Democracy of Sports,'" The American Presidency Project; accessed via: https://www.presidency.ucsb.edu/documents/address-the-national-conference-outdoor-recreation-washington-dc-the-democracy-sports.

"Correction of a Key Study: No Evidence of 'Gender-Affirming' Surgeries Improving Mental Health," *Society for Evidence Based Gender Medicine* (August 30, 2020); accessed via: https://segm.org/ajp_correction_2020.

"Correction to Bränström and Pachankis," *The American Journal of Psychiatry* (August 1, 2001): 734; accessed via: https://ajp.psychiatryonline.org/doi/10.1176/appi.ajp.2020.1778 correction.

Crocket, Richard and Ronald Sandison (eds.). *Hallucinogenic Drugs and their Psychotherapeutic Use: Proceedings of the Quarterly Meeting of the Royal Medi-*

co-Psychological Association (London: H.K. Lewis and Co., 1963).

Crudele, Mark and Crystal Cranmore, "McDonald's Worker Short in Neck during Dispute in Brooklyn," *Eyewitness News, ABC7* (August 2, 2022); accessed via: https://abc7ny.com/nyc-mcdonalds-shooting-worker-shot/12092742/.

Contreras, Guillermo, "Family of 6-Year-Old Boy Shot and Killed by Bexar Deputies in 2017 Files Lawsuit," San Antonio Express-News December, 2019); accessed via: https://www.express news.com/news/local/article/Family-of-6-year-old-boy-shot-and-killed-by-Bexar-14877045.php.

Crenshaw, Kimberlé, Neil Gotanda, Gary Peller, Kendall Thomas (eds.), *Critical Race Theory: The Key Writings that Formed the Movement* (NY: The New Press, 1995).

Danger. Dallas, "PSA: The Instagram for the Workers is marie_equi_workers_collective"; accessed via: https://www.tiktok.com/@danger.dallas/video/7117080672195464494?lang=en.

"Dangerous Mexican Weed to Smoke," reprinted in *Phillipsburg Herald*, August 18 (1904), unpaged; accessed via: https://chroniclingamerica.loc.gov/lccn/sn85029677/1904-08-18/ed-1/seq-8/#words=marihuana+marijuana+mariguana+Indian+hemp+cannabis+dope.

Davis, Alan K., et al., "Effects of Psilocybin-Assisted Therapy on Major Depressive Disorder: A Randomized Clinical Trial," *JAMA Psychiatry*, 78, 5 (November 4, 2020): 481 – 489.

Davy, Sir Humphrey, *Researches, Chemical and Philosophical* (London: J. Johnson, 1800), p. 496; accessed via: https://archive.org/details/researcheschemic00davy/page/496/mode/2up?q=Tobin&view=theater.

Day, Juliana, "The Role and Reaction of the Psychiatrist in LSD Therapy," *Journal of Nervous and Mental Diseases* 125, no. 1 (Jan–March 1957), pp. 437–38.

Declercq, Eugene and Laurie Zephyrin, "Maternal Mortality in the United States: A Primer" (Commonwealth Fund, December 16, 2020); accessed via: https://www.commonwealthfund.org/publications/issue-brief-report/2020/dec/maternal-mortality-united-states-primer.

DeGue, Sara, et al., "Deaths Due to Use of Lethal Force by Law Enforcement: Findings From the National Violent Death Reporting System, 17 U.S. States, 2009–2012" *American Journal of Preventative Medicine* (2016); accessed via: https://www.ncbi.nlm.nih.gov/pmc/articles/PMC60 80222/.

Delaval, Craig, "Cocaine, Conspiracy Theories, and the C.I.A. in Central America," *Drug Wars* (2014); accessed via: https://www.pbs.org/wgbh/pages/frontline/shows/drugs/special/cia.html.

Deveny, John Patrick, *Paschal Beverly Randolph: A Nineteenth Century Black-American Spiritualist, Rosicrucian, and Sex Magician* (NY: State University of New York Press, 1996).

Diamond, Jared, *Guns, Germs, and Steel: The Fates of Human Societies* (NY: W.W. Norton and Company, 1999).

DiAngelo, Robin, *White Fragility: Why it's so Hard for White People to Talk about Racism* (MA: Beacon Press, 2018).

Dioscorides, *Pharmacorum simplicium req[ue] medicæ, Libri VIII.* Strasbourg: In inclyta Argentorato, 1529. Facsimile edition available at www.biodiversitylibrary.org.

Dolitsky, Alexander B., "Opinion: Neo-Marxism is a Threat to the Country," *Juneau Empire* (January 25, 2023); accessed via: https://www.juneauempire.com/opinion/opinion-neo-marxism-is-a-threat-to-the-country/.

Dorman, Sam, "Adding Wokeness: Oregon Promotes Teacher Program to Subtract 'Racism in Mathematics,'" *New York Post* (February 12, 2021); accessed via: https://nypost.com/2021/02 /12/adding-wokeness-oregon-promotes-teacher-program-to-subtract-racism-in-mathematics/.

Douglas, Francine, "Swoxwiyam and Sqwelqwel: The Power of Indigenous Knowledge and Cultural Ceremonies for All with Francine Douglas," Spirit Plant Medicine Conference, 2022.

Drake, Bruce, "Incarceration Gap Widens between Whites and Blacks," Pew Research Center (September 6, 2013); accessed via: https://www.pewresearch.org/short-reads/2013/09/06/incarceration-gap-between-whites-and-blacks-widens/.

Drange, Matt, "They Called 911 for Assistance. Then the Police used Lethal Force," *Business Insider* (November 22, 2022); accessed via: https://www.businessinsider.com/police-deaths-transgender-people-officer-killings-mental-health-crisis-2022-11.

Drew, Katherine F. (trans. and ed.), *The Laws of the Salic Franks* (Philadelphia: University of Pennsylvania Press, 1991).

"Driver Killed at NSA Identified as Transgender Sex Worker, Friend Says," *Chicago Tribune* (June 22, 2019); accessed via: https://www.chicagotribune.com/2015/04/01/driver-killed-at-nsa-identified-as-transgender-sex-worker-friend-says/.

Dulchinos, Donald P., *Pioneer of Innerspace: The Life of Fitz Hugh Ludlow, Hasheesh Easter* (Autonomedia, 1998).

"Dr. David F. Musto Interview," *Frontline* (Winter, 1997–98); accessed via: https://www.pbs.org/wgbh/pages/frontline/shows/dope/interviews/musto.html.

D'Souza, Dinesh, *The End of Racism: Principles for a Multiracial Society* (NY: The Free Press, 1995).

Dubus, Zoë, "High Dose Psychedelic Shock Therapy with LSD and Mescaline: The Conversion Treatment of a French Doctor on Two Homosexual Adolescents in the 1960s," in Alex Belser, Clancy Cavnar, and Beatriz C. Labate, *Queering Psychedelics: From Oppression to Liberation in Psychedelic Medicine* (2022).

Dunn, Catherine M. (ed.), Henry Cornelius Agrippa of Nettesheim, *Of the Vanitie and Uncertaintie of Artes and Sciences* (Northridge: California State University Foundation, 1974).

Duvall, Chris S., "Decriminalization Doesn't Address Marijuana's Standing as a Drug of the Poor," *The Conversation* (June 30, 2015); accessed via: https://theconversation.com/decriminalization-doesnt-address-marijuanas-standing-as-a-drug-of-the-poor-42345.

Dyck, Erika, "Flashback: Psychiatric Experimentation with LSD in Historical Perspective," *Canadian Journal of Psychiatry*, 50, no. 7 (June, 2005): 381–87.

Dyck, Erika and Chris Elcock, *Expanding Mindscapes: A Global History of Psychedelics* (MA: MIT Press, 2024).

Dyck, Ericka, Patrick Farrell, Beatriz Caiuby Labate, Clancy Cavnar, Ibrahim Gabriell and Glauber Loures de Assis (eds.), *Women and Psychedelics: Uncovering Invisible Voices* (NM: Synergetic Press, 2024).

Effinger, Anthony, "More Oregonians Left in 2022 than Arrived, Reversing a Long-Standing Trend," *Willamette Week* (September 14, 2023); accessed via: https://www.wweek.com

Eichenbaum, Jeanna, "Queer Voices Speak to the New Psychedelia," in Bia Labate and Clancy Cavnar (eds.), *Psychedelic Justice: Toward a Diverse and Equitable Psychedelic Culture* (NM: Synergetic Press, 2021).

Eisner, Betty, *Remembrances of LSD Therapy Past* (2002), unpublished manuscript; accessed via: maps.org.

"Electrocution Death of Murderer," Reefer Madness Museum; accessed via: http://reefermadness museum.org/chap10/GorePart-1.htm.

Epiphanius, "Contra Haereses," 2.2, in George Robert Stowe Mead, *Simon Magus: Essays on the Founder of Simonism Based on Ancient Sources* (Leipzig, Germany: edidit G. Dindorfius, 1859).

Eriacho, Belinda, "Considerations for Working with Indigenous People in Psychedelic Spaces and Guidelines for Inclusion of Indigenous Peoples in Psychedelic Science Conferences," in Beatriz C. Labate and Clancy Cavnar, *Psychedelic Justice: Toward a Diverse and Equitable Psychedelic Culture* (NM: Synergetic Press, 2021).

Evans Shultes, Richard, and Albert Hofmann, *Plant of the Gods: Their Sacred, Healing, and Hallucinogenic Powers* (VT: Healing Arts Press, 1992).

Everitt, Patrick, "The Cactus and the Beast: Investigating the Role of Peyote (Mescaline) in the Magick of Aleister Crowley," M.A. Western Esotericism (Thesis), University of Amsterdam (2014–2016).

Fatsis, Stefan, "No Viet Cong ever Called me Ni[**]er: The Story Behind the Famous Quote that Muhammad Ali Probably Never Said," *Slate* (June 08, 2016); accessed via: https://slate.com/cult ure/2016/06/did-muhammad-ali-ever-say-no-viet-cong-ever-called-me-nigger.html.

Favata, Martin A. and José B. Fernández (trans.), *The Account: Álvar Núñez Cabeza de Vaca's Relatión* (TX: Arte Público Press, 1993).

Feuerherd, Ben, and Bruce Golding, "This 'Black Israelite' from Brooklyn Sparked the Covington Controversy," *New York Post* (January 22, 2019); accessed via: https://nypost.com/2019/01/22/this-hebrew-israelite-from-brooklyn-sparked-the-covington-controversy/.

"Fired San Antonio Police Officer Indicted for Shooting Teen as he Ate Hamburger in McDonald's Parking Lot," *CBS News* (December 2, 2022); accessed via: https://www.cbsnews.com/news/james-brennand-indicted-san-antonio-police-officer-hot-erik-cantu-mcdonalds-parking-lot/.

Fisher, George, "Racial Myths of the Cannabis War," *Boston University Law Review* Vol. 1, Issue 3 (May 2021).

Flanders-Stepans, Mary Beth, "Alarming Racial Differences in Maternal Mortality," *Journal of Perinatal Education*, 9, 2 (Spring 2000); accessed via: https://www.ncbi.nlm.nih.gov/pmc/articles/PMC1595019/#:~:text=The%20leading%20causes%20of%20maternal,%2C%20%26%20Berg%2C%201999).

Flood, Alison, "Richard Dawkins Loses 'Humanist of the Year' Title Over Trans Comments," *The Guardian*, April 20 (2021); accessed via: https://www.theguardian.com/books/2021/apr/20/ /richard-dawkins-loses-humanist-of-the-year-trans-comments.

Formanek, Jared and Ray Sanchez, "Charges Dropped Against 5 Oklahoma City Officers who Fatally Shot 15-Year-Old," CNN (July, 2023); accessed via: https://www.cnn.com/2023/07/29/us/oklahoma-police-shootings-charges-dropped/index.html.

Fox, Alex, "Archaeologists Identify Traces of Burnt Cannabis in Ancient Jewish Shrine," *Smithsonian Magazine*, June 4, 2020; accessed via: https://www.smithsonianmag.com/smart-news/cannabis-found-altar-ancient-israeli-shrine-180975016/.

Frazao, Kristine, "The Black Lives Matter Movement Brought in Millions. So Where is that Money Now?" KATV ABC News 7 (February 21, 2033); accessed via: https://katv.com/news/nation-world/the-black-lives-matter-movement-brought-in-millions-so-where-is-that-money-now.

Freake, James (trans.), Donald Tyson (ed.), Cornelius Agrippa von Nettesheim, *Three Books of Occult Philosophy* (St. Paul, Minn.: Llewellyn Publications, 1992).

From the Community, "Opinion: Letter to the President and Provost: Action Items for Achieving Racial Equity," *The Stanford Daily* (June 19, 2020); accessed via: https://stanforddaily.com/2020 /06/19/letter-to-the-president-provost-of-stanford-university-concerning-a-george-floyd-action-plan/.

Fryer, Roland, "Policing the Police: The Impact of 'Pattern-or-Practice'; Investigations on Crime," *National Bureau of Economic Research* (June 2020).

Fynn-Paul, Jeff, *Not Stolen: The Truth about European Colonialism in the New World* (Bombardier Books, 2023).

George, Jamilah R. and NiCole Buchanan, "Black Lives Matter and Psychedelic Integration" (November 4, 2022); accessed via: https://chacruna.net/black-lives-integration/.

George, Jamilah R., Timothy I. Michaels, Jae Sevelius, and Monnica T. Williams, "The Psychedelic Renaissance and the Limitations of a White-Dominant

Medical Framework: A Call for Indigenous and Ethnic Minority Inclusion," *Journal of Psychedelic Studies*," Vol. 4, 1 (2020): 4–15.

Gieringer, Dale H., "The Origins of Cannabis Prohibition in California," *Schaffer Library of Drug Policy*, Vol. 26, No. 2 (June, 2006), p. 6, n. 17; accessed via: https://www.druglibrary.org/schaffer/history/California_Marijuana_Law_History/California_Marijuana_Law_History_Page2.html.

Ginsburg, Allen, "Howl"; accessed via: https://www.poetryfoundation.org/poems/49303/howl

——"Lysergic Acid"; accessed via: https://oakiedog.substack.com/p/ginsberg-on-acid

Glasgow, James W., Will County Attorney, "Glasgow Announces Jordan Henry Sentenced to 22 Years in Aggravated Vehicular Hijacking on Diversey Parkway in Chicago" (March 2023); accessed via: https://willcountysao.com/2023/03/glasgow-announces-jordan-henry-sentenced-to-22-years-in-aggravated-vehicular-hijacking-on-diversey-parkway-in-chicago/#:~:text=Henry%20currently%20is%20facing%20charges,Public%20Place%20that%20allegedly%20occurred.

Glendinning, Nigel (*trans.*), Julio Caro Baroja, *The World of the Witches* (UK: Pheonix Press, 2001).

Glick, Daniel, "Marijuana Prohibition Began with these Arrests in 1937," *Leafy* (July, 2020); accessed via: https://www.leafly.com/news/politics/drug-war-prisoners-1-2-true-story-moses-sam-two-denver-drifters-became-cannabis-pioneers.

Godwin, John, *Murder U.S.A: The Ways We Kill Each Other* (NY: Ballantine Books, 1978).

Gold, Scott and Andrew Blankstein, "It was a Terrifying Time," *Los Angeles Times* (August 4, 2010); accessed via: https://www.latimes.com/archives/la-xpm-2010-aug-04-la-me-serial-killers-20100804-story.html.

Gold, Veronika, "Reflections on Personal Experiences in Psychedelic Training and Research," *MAPS Bulletin* Vol 29, No 1 (Spring 2019); accessed via: https://maps.org/news/bulletin/reflections-on-personal-experiences-in-psychedelic-training-and-research-spring-2019/.

Goldhill, Olivia, "The World is Relying on a Flawed Psychological Test to Fight Racism," *Quartz* (December 3, 2017); accessed via: https://qz.com/1144504/the-world-is-relying-on-a-flawed-psychological-test-to-fight-racism.

Gould, Stephen Jay, "Nonoverlapping Magisteria," *Natural History*, Vol. 106, No. 2 (January 1997).

Gramlich, John, "Gun Deaths Among U.S. Children and Teens Rose 50% in Two Years," Pew Research Center (April 6, 2023); accessed via: https://www.pewresearch.org/short-reads/2023/04/06/gun-deaths-among-us-kids-rose-50-percent-in-two-years/.

Green, Tiffany L., "The Problem with Implicit Bias Training," *Scientific American* (August 28, 2020); accessed via: https://www.scientificamerican.com/article/

the-problem-with-implicit-bias-training/.

Grassi, Batista, "Il Nostro Agarico Moscario Sperimentato come Aliment Nervoso," *Gazzetta degli Ospitali Milano*, Vol. 1 (188): 961–972.

Gray, Mike, *Drug Crazy: How we got into this Mess and How we Can Get Out* (NY: Random House, 1998).

Grof, Stan, "Stan Grof Interviews Dr. Albert Hofmann, Esalen Institute, Big Sur California, 1984," *MAPS Bulletin*, 11, no. 2 (2001).

G-Twinz, "Skittles and Iced Tea"; accessed via: https://www.youtube.com/watch?v=xaP6HrXY0i0.

Gukasyan, Natalie, et al., "Efficacy and Safety of Psilocybin-Assisted Treatment for Major Depressive Disorder: Prospective 12–Month Follow Up," *Journal of Psychopharmacology* (February 15, 2022): 151–158.

Gussaw, Adam, "The Test: Rethinking Trayvon" in *Southwest Review* (Vol. 106, Issue 2), Southern Methodist University (Summer 2021); accessed via: https://go.gale.com/ps/i.do?id=GALE%7CA671029142&sid=googleScholar&v=2.1&it=r&linkaccess=abs&issn=00384712&p=AONE&sw=w&userGroupName=oregon_oweb&isGeoAuthType=true.

Guth, Steven (trans.), Georg Dehn (ed.), Abraham of Worms, *The Book of Abramelin: A New Translation* (Lake Worth, FL, Ibis Press, 2006.).

Halifax, Joan, *Shamanic Voices: A Survey of Visionary Narratives* (NY: Penguin Press, 1991).

Hansen, Joseph, *Quellen und untersuchungen* (Bonn, Germany: Carl Georgi, 1901).

Harari, Yuval Noah, *Sapiens: A Brief History of Humankind* (Harper Perennial, 2018).

Harding, Lee, "Diversity Training Increases Prejudice an[d] 'Activates Bigotry' Among Participants, New Study Says," *ZeroHedge* (February 13, 2024); accessed via: https://www.zerohedge.com/political/diversity-training-increases-prejudice-activates-bigotry-among-participants-new-study.

Harner, Michael (ed.), *Hallucinogens and Shamanism* (UK: Oxford University Press, 1973).

Hart, Carl, *Drug Use for Grown-Ups: Chasing Liberty in the Land of the Free* (2021).

Haskell, David Millard, "What DEI Research Concludes about Diversity Training: It is Divisive, Counter-Productive, and Unnecessary," *Aristotle Foundation for Public Policy* (February 12, 2024); accessed via: https://aristotlefoundation.org/reality-check/what-dei-research-concludes-about-diversity-training-it-is-divisive-counter-productive-and-unnecessary/.

Hemarajata, Peera, "Revisiting the Great Imitator: The Origin and History of Syphilis," *American Society for Microbiology* (June 17, 2019); accessed via: https://asm.org/articles/2019/june/revisiting-the-great-imitator,-part-i-the-origin-a#:~:text=There%20is%20still%20debate%20over,following%20exploration%20of%20the%20Americas.

Henning, SA Doug and SA Christopher Olson, "Interview of Officer Jeronimo Yanez," *Minnesota Department of Public Safety Bureau of Criminal Apprehen-*

sion Transcript; accessed via: https://www.ramseycounty. us/sites/default/files/County%20Attorney/Yanez%20BCA%20 Interview%20Transcript%20 7.7.16.pdf.

Herer, Jack, *The Emperor Wears No Clothes* (HEMP/Queen of Clubs Publishing, 1995).

Herzstein, Robert E., *Henry R. Luce, Time, and the American Crusade in Asia* (Cambridge, United Kingdom: Cambridge University Press, 2005).

Hillman, David, *The Chemical Muse: Drugs Use and the Roots of Western Civilization* (Thomas Dunne Books, 2014).

Hoff Sommers, Christina, "6 Feminist Myths that Will Not Die," Time Magazine (June 17, 2016); accessed via: https://time.com/3222543/wage-pay-gap-myth-feminism/.

——"The Gender Wage Gap Myth," *American Enterprise Institute* (February 3, 2014); accessed via: https://www.aei.org/articles/the-gender-wage-gap-myth/.

Hofmann, Albert, *LSD: My Problem Child: Reflections on Sacred Drugs, Mysticism, and Science* (CA: MAPS, 2009).

Hollinshed, Denise, "Outing at St. Louis Park Turns to Tragedy as Bullets Fly, Killing 6-Year-Old Boy" (March 12, 2015); accessed via: https://www.stltoday.com/news/local/crime-courts/outing-at-st-louis-park-turns-to-tragedy-as-bullets-fly-killing-6-year-old/article_4c0a7015-e591-5c8b-8ec0-9781e2472c30.html.

Hooker, Sir William Jackson, "Echinocactus Williamsii," in *Curtis's Botanical Magazine* (London: Reeve, Benham and Reeve, King William Street, Strand, 1847), Vol. III, Third Series.

Horizons Northwest: Perspectives on Psychedelics, Portland Art Museum (September 15–18, 2022).

Horowitz, Michael and Cynthia Palmer, *Moksha: Aldous Huxley's Classic Writings on Psychedelics and the Visionary Experience* (VT: Park Street Press, 1999).

Howard, Jacqueline, "Black Men Nearly 3 Times as Likely to Die from Police Use of Force, Study Says," CNN (December 20, 2016); accessed via: https://www.cnn.com/2016/12/20/health/ black-men-killed-by-police.

Howard, James H., "The Mescal Bean Cult of the Central and Southern Plains: An Ancestor of the Peyote Cult?" *American Anthropologist*, Vol. 59, No. 1 (Feb, 1957): 75–87.

"Indonesia: New Criminal Code Disastrous for Rights: Provisions Harmful to Women, Minorities, Free Speech," Human Rights Watch (December 8, 2022); accessed via: https://www.hrw.org/news/2022/12/08/indonesia-new-criminal-code-disastrous-rights.

Ingraham, Christopher, "Officer who Shot Philando Castile said Smell of Marijuana Made Him Fear for His Life," in *The Washington Post* (June 21, 2017); accessed via: https://www.washingt onpost.com/news/wonk /wp/2017/06/21/officer-who-shot-philando-castile-said-smell-of-marijuana-made-him-fear-for-his-life/.

"Insanity Caused by Hindoo Drug," *Los Angeles Herald*, May 14 (1905), p. 3; accessed via: https://chroniclingamerica.loc.gov/lccn/sn85042462/1905-05-14/ed-1/seq-3/.

"Is the Mexican Nation 'Locoed' by a Peculiar Weed?" in *Ogden Standard*, unpaged (September 25, 1915), accessed via: https://mexfiles.net/2018/01/21/reefermadness/.

"'It's Morning Again in America . . .' and the Birth of Political Ads," *American Association of Advertising Agencies* (2023); accessed via: https://www.aaaa.org/timeline-event/morning-america-dawn-first-political-ads/?cn-reloaded=1.

Jakowski, Lara and Patrick Belem, "Eskawata Kayawai: The Spirit of Transformation" (2023).

James, William, *The Varieties of Religious Experience* (New York: Signet Classic, 2003).

Janiger, Oscar. "Personal Statement by Oscar Janiger," *Bulletin of the Multidisciplinary Association for Psychedelic Studies*, 9, no. 1 (Spring 1999).

"Janitor Selling Marijuana to High School Students," *Reefer Madness Museum*; accessed via: http://reefermadnessmuseum.org/chap10/GorePart-1.htm.

Jaschik, Scott, "Florida State Fires Professor Over 'Extreme Negligence' in His Research," Inside Higher Ed. (July 20, 2023); accessed via: https://www.insidehighered.com/news/quick-takes/2023/07/20/florida-state-fires-professor.

Jay, Mike, *Emperors of Dreams: Drugs in the Nineteenth Century* (UK: Dedalus, 2005).

Jesso, James W., Facebook post (April 6, 2021); accessed via: https://www. facebook.com/profile/502104195/search/?q=Psymposia.

"John Good's Testimony" (March 20, 2012); accessed via: https://famous-trials.com/images/ftriatrials.com/images/ftrials/zimmerman/documents/Zimmerman-Document-C.pdf.

Jones, Christopher M., "Patterns and Characteristics of Methamphetamine Use Among Adults — United States, 2015–2018," Centers for Disease Control and Prevention (March 27, 2020); accessed via: https://www.cdc.gov/mmwr/volumes/69/wr/mm6912a1.htm.

Jordan, Don, and Michael Walsh, *White Cargo: The Forgotten History of Britain's White Slaves in America* (NY: New York University Press, 2007).

Juan-Tresserras, Jordi, "La Arqueología de las Drogas en la Península Ibérica: una síntesis de las Recientes Investigaciones Arqueobotánicas," *Complutum*, 11 (2000).

Kachnowski, Vera M., et al., "Weighing the Impact of Simple Possession of Marijuana: Trends and Sentencing in the Federal Justice System," *United States Sentencing Commission* (January 2023).

Kane, H.H., *Drugs that Enslave: The Opium, Morphine, Chloral, and Hashisch Habit* (PA: Presley Blakiston, 1881).

Kavanaugh, Shane Dixon, "How a Portland 'Lesbian Bar for Everyone' Closed After One Day," (August 10, 2022); accessed via: https://www.oregonlive.com/portland/2022/08/how-a-portland-lesbian-bar-for-everyone-closed-after-one-day.html.

Kendi, Ibram X., *How to be an Antiracist* (NY: One World, August 13, 2019).

Kent, James, "Wonderland Miami Exposes Growing Rift in Psychedelic Community," *Psychedelic Spotlight*, November 8, 2022; accessed via: https://psychedelicspotlight.com/wonderland-miami-exposes-growing-rift-in-psychedelic-community/.

Khan, Amanda J., et al., "Psilocybin for Trauma-Related Disorders," *Current Topics in Behavioral Neurosciences*, 56 (2022): 319–332.

King, Dante, "Diagnosing Whiteness and Anti-Blackness: White Psychopathology, Collective Psychosis and Trauma in America," lecture presented at UC San Francisco (February 8, 2024); accessed via: https://www.facebook.com/watch/?v=770047187929114.

Kluckhohn, Clyde and Dorothea Leighton, *The Navaho* (MA: Harvard University Press, 1974).

Klug, H. (trans.), Van Arsdall et al., "The Mandrake Plant and its Legend: A New Perspective" Old Names—New Growth: Proceedings of the 2nd ASPNS Conference, University of Graz, Austria, 6–10 June 2007.

Komp, Ellen, "Mark Twain's 'Hashish' Experience in San Francisco," *San Francisco Gate* (Oct. 2, 2011); accessed via: https://www.sfgate.com/opinion/article/Mark-Twain-s-hasheesh-experience-in-S-F-2328992.php.

Koger, Larry, *Black Slaveowners: Free Black Slave Masters in South Carolina, 1790–1860* (NC: McFarland & Company, 2012).

Krauthamer, Barbara, *Black Slaves, Indian Masters: Slavery, Emancipation, and Citizenship in the Native American South* (NC: University of North Carolina Press, 2013).

Kriegman, Zac, "BLM Spreads Falsehoods That Have Led to the Murders of Thousands of Black People in the Most Disadvantaged Communities"; accessed via: https://kriegman.substack.com/ p/post-leading-to-termination-blm-falsehoods.

Kritikos, P.G., and S.P. Papadaki, "The History of the Poppy and of Opium and their Expansion in Antiquity in the Eastern Mediterranean Area," United Nations Office on Drugs and Crime (January 1, 1967); accessed via: https://www.unodc.org/unodc/en/data-and-analysis/bulletin/bulletin_1967-01-01_3_page004.html.

Labate, Beatriz C., Clancy Cavnar, Thiago Rodrigus (eds.), *Drug Policies and the Politics of Drugs in the Americas* (Switzerland: Springer, 2016).

——"Prohibition and the War on Drugs in the Americas: An Analytical Approach," *Drug Policies and the Politics of Drugs in the Americas* (Switzerland: Springer International Publishing, 2016).

Labate, Beatriz C. and Clancy Cavnar (eds.), *Psychedelic Justice: Toward a Diverse and Equitable Psychedelic Culture* (NM: Synergetic Press, 2021).

Labate, Beatriz C. and NiCole Buchanan, "Hate and Social Media in Psychedelic Spaces," in *Psychedelic Justice: Toward a Diverse and Equitable Psychedelic Future* (NM: Synergetic Press, 2021).

LA Parent Union, "Food Neutrality"; accessed via: https://twitter.com/UTLAUncensored/status/1569179938334601217?ref_src=twsrc%5Etfw%7Ctwcamp%5Etweetembed%7Ctwterm%5E1569898242292465664%7Ctwgr%5E885ecd84838cdaa00074ec192bd76899a182f1f6%7Ctwcon%5Es3_&ref_url=https%3A%2F%2Fcaliforniaglobe.com%2Farticles%2Fla-unified-school-district-posts-bizarre-video-about-food-neutrality%2F.

Lawrence, Anne, "Shame and Narcissistic Personality Disorder in Autogynephilic Transexuals," *Archives of Sexual Behavior*, 37 (April 23, 2008): 457–61.

Leary, Timothy, *Flashbacks: A Personal and Cultural History of an Era* (NY: J.P. Putnam's Sons, 1990).

Le Barre, Weston, *The Peyote Cult* (OK: University of Oklahoma Press, 1989).

Leduff, Charlie, "What Killed Aiyana Stanley-Jones?" *Mother Jones* (Nov.-Dec. 2010); accessed via: https://www.motherjones.com/politics/2010/09/aiyana-stanley-jones-detroit/.

Lee, Martin A., *Smoke Signals: A Social History of Marijuana* (NY: Scribner, 2012).

Lemon, Lara S., et al., "Prepregnancy Obesity and the Racial Disparity in Infant Mortality," *Obesity* (Sliver Spring), 24, 12 (December 1, 2016); accessed via: https://www.ncbi.nlm.nih.gov /pmc/articles/PMC5130106/.

Lemons, Stephen, "Christopher Broughton's Pastor Steven Anderson Prays for President Obama's Death," *Phoenix New Times* (August 26, 2009); accessed via: https://www.phoenixnewtimes.com/news/christopher-broughtons-pastor-steven-anderson-prays-for-president-barack-obamas-death-6500993.

Leon, Kat, "Queer Community Reacts to Portland's New Lesbian Bar," *PSU Vanguard* (May 4, 2022); accessed via: https://psuvanguard.com/queer-community-reacts-to-portlands-new-lesbian-bar/.

Leovy, Jill, *Ghettoside: Investigating a Homicide Epidemic* (London: Penguin Random House, 2014).

Letcher, Andy, *Shroom: A Cultural History of the Magic Mushroom* (NY: HarperCollins, 2007).

Levitt, Steven D., "Understanding Why Crime Fell in the 1990s: Four Factors that Explain the Decline and Six that Do Not," *Journal of Economic Perspectives*, Vol. 18, No. 1 (Winter, 2004); accessed via: https://pricetheory.uchicago.edu/levitt/Papers/LevittUnderstandingWhyCrime2004.pdf.

Lewis, Nancy and Sari Horowitz, "Hundreds Flee Fatal Shootout Near SE Club," *Washington Post* (October 28, 1988); accessed via: https://www.washingtonpost.com/archive/politics/1988/10/28/hundreds-flee-fatal-shootout-near-se-club/f39e436f-32b1-4eb1-904c-db0f57919049/.

Lilly, Christiana, "Miami Schools Police Chief Charles Hurley Accused of Baker Acting Students to Decrease Crime Stats," *The Huffington Post* (May 17,

2012); accessed via: https://www.huffpost.com/entry/chief-charles-hurley-baker-act_n_1519015.

Limbong, Andrew, "Microaggressions are a Big Deal: How to Talk Them Out and When to Walk Away" (June 9, 2020); accessed via: https://www.npr.org/2020/06/08/872371063/microaggressions-are-a-big-deal-how-to-talk-them-out-and-when-to-walk-away.

Lindsay, James A., *Race Marxism: The Truth about Critical Race Theory and Practice* (FL: New Discourses, 2022).

Lindsay, James A., et al., "Academic Grievance Studies and the Corruption of Scholarship," *Areo Magazine* (February 10, 2018); accessed via: https://areomagazine.com/2018/10/02/academic-grievance-studies-and-the-corruption-of-scholarship/.

Littedale, Richard, *Commentary on the Song of Songs* (London: J. Masters, 1869).

Llwydd, Gwyllm, *The Hasheesh Eater And Other Writings: Illustrations by Gwyllm Llwydd* (CreateSpace, 2018). "Local Hash-Easters: Arabs Near Stockton Growing Indian Hemp and Making the Drug," in *San Fracisco Caller*, June 24 (1895); accessed via: https://chroniclingamerica.loc.gov/lccn/sn85066387/1895-06-24/ed-1/seq-7/.

Los Angeles Department of Public Health, Injury and Violence Prevention Program, "Gang Homicides in Los Angeles County, 1980–2008," Compiled from info from LA Sheriff Dept., LA Police Dept, LA Dept of Coroner, CA Dept of Health Services–Center for Health Statistics, Death Statistical Master File (April 21, 2011); accessed via: http://www.publichealth.lacounty.gov/ivpp/injury_topics/GangAwarenessPrevention/Gang%20Homicide%20Chart%20Apr%2021%202011%20chart.pdf.

Lowe, Peggy, "Missouri has the Highest Black Homicide Rate in America—and Some of the Loosest Gun Laws," KCUR (April 26, 2023); accessed via: https://www.kcur.org/news/2023-04-26/missouri-has-a-gun-problem-study-says-that-drives-the-countrys-highest-black-homicide-rate.

Lucas, Phillippe, "Psychedelic Use in Canada: Results of the Canadian Psychedelic Survey," Spirit Plant Medicine Conference (2022); accessed via: https://spiritplantmedicine.com/video/psychedelic-use-in-canada-results-of-the-canadian-psychedelic-survey-with-phillippe-lucas/.

Luke, Daivd and Rory Spowers, *DMT: Entity Encounters* (VT: Park Street Press, 2021).

Lumholtz, Carl, *Unknown Mexico: A Record of Five Years' Exploration Among the Tribes of the Western Sierra Madre* (NY: Charles Scribner's Sons, 1902).

Luscombe, Belinda, "Workplace Salaries: At Last, Women on Top," *Time* (September 1, 2010); accessed via: https://content.time.com/time/business/article/0,8599,2015274,00.html.

Mac Donald, Heather, *The War on Cops* (NY: Encounter Books, 2017).

——"CNN Fans More Hatred of Cops, in Touting Flawed Study," Manhattan Institute (December 22, 2016); accessed via: https://manhattan.institute/article/cnn-fans-more-hatred-of-cops-in-touting-flawed-study.

——"Courts v. Cops: The Legal War on the War on Crime," in *City Journal* (Winter, 2013; accessed via: https://www.city-journal.org/article/courts-v-cops.

"Man Charged in Shooting of McDonald's Worker over French Fries also Charged in 2020 Murder," *Eyewitness News, ABC7* (August 3, 2022); accessed via: https://abc7ny.com/michael-morgan-nyc-mcdonalds-shooting/12096330/.

Malanga, Steven, "The Rainbow Coalition Evaporates," *City Journal* (Winter 2008); accessed via: https://www.city-journal.org/html/rainbow-coalition-evaporates-13062.html?wallitnosession=1.

Manheim, Ralph (trans.), Carl Kerényi, *Dionysos: Archetypal Image of Indestructible Life* (NY: Princeton University Press, 1976).

"Man who Shot, Killed 19-Year-Old Burger King Worker in Harlem Indicted for Murder," *Eyewitness News, ABC7* (Marh 3, 2022); accessed via:https://abc7ny.com/winston-glynn-burger-king-shooting-east-harlem-kristal-bayron-nieves/11618297/.

MAPS "Article Three: Revisions adopted October 17, 2019"; accessed via: https://maps.org/wp-content/uploads/2021/12/2019_10_17-Amendment-MAPSArticlesofIncorporation-2020.pdf.

MAPS Canada, "Policies"; accessed via: https://www.mapscanada.org/policies/.

M., Donna, "Yes, Your Kid's Trans Thing is a Phase," *New Discourses* (September 18, 2021); accessed via: https://newdiscourses.com/2021/09/yes-your-kids-trans-thing-phase/.

"Marc Lamont Hill Interviews Key Opponent of Critical Race Theory," theGrio Politics; accessed via: https://www.youtube.com/watch?v=ihnuYXKBGZg.

Marcuse, Herbert, *An Essay on Liberation* (1969); accessed via: https://www.marxists.org/reference/archive/marcuse/works/1969/essay-liberation.pdf.

Margolin, Madison, "Inside the 'Psychedelic Exceptionalism' Debate: Should all Drugs be Legal, or Just Pot and Psychedelics?" *Double Blind Mag* (July 25, 2022); accessed via: https://doubleblindmag.com/psychedelic-exceptionalism/.

Markel, Howard, "An Alcoholic's Savior: God, Belladonna or Both?" *New York Times* (April 9, 2010).

Marriott, Alice, and Carol K. Rachlin, *Peyote: An Account of the Origins and Growth of the Peyote Religion* (NY: Thomas Y. Crowell Company, 1971).

Martin, Joyce, "A Case of Psychopathic Personality with Homosexuality Treated by LSD," Richard Crocket and Ronald Sandison (eds.), *Hallucinogenic Drugs and Their Psychotherapeutic Use: Proceedings of the Quarterly Meeting of the Royal Medico-Psychological Association* (London: H. K. Lewis and Co., 1963).

——"Schizophreniform Reactions Under Day Hospital L.S.D. Therapy," *Congress Report Vol II* (Zurich: Orell Fussli, 1959).

Masters, Robert and Jean Houston, *The Varieties of Psychedelic Experience: The Classic Guide to the Effects of LSD on the Human Psyche* (VT: Park Street Press, 2000).

McCabe, Sean Esteban, et al., "Race/Ethnicity and Gender Differences in Drug Use and Abuse Among College Students," *The Journal of Ethnicity and Substance Abuse* (May 13, 2008); accessed via: https://www.ncbi.nlm.nih.gov/pmc/articles/PMC2377408/.

McCarthy, Ciara, "Alabama Man with Spoon Killed by Officer had a 'Mental Episode,' Police Say," in *The Guardian*; accessed via: https://www.theguardian.com/us-news/2015/aug/24/alaba ma-man-spoon-killed-police.

McCoy, Terrence, "The Story of How a White Phoenix Cop Killed an Unarmed Black Man," *The Washington Post* (December 5, 2014); accessed via: https://www.washingtonpost.com/news/morning-mix/wp/2014/12/05/how-a-white-phoenix-cop-killed-an-unarmed-black-man/.

"McDonald's Worker Stabbed while Defending Coworkers in East Harlem," *Eyewitness News, ABC7* (March 9, 2022); accessed via: https://abc7ny.com/mcdonalds-worker-stabbed-stabbing-east-harlem-nypd/11634939/.

McLaughlin, Gerald T., "Cocaine: The History and Regulation of a Dangerous Drug," *Cornell Law Review*, Vol. 58, Issue 3 (March 1973).

McWilliams, John C., *The Protectors: Harry J. Anslinger and the Federal Bureau of Narcotics 1930–1962* (Newark: University of Delaware Press, 1990).

McWhorter, John, *Woke Racism: How a New Religion has Betrayed Black America* (NY: Portfolio/Penguin, 2021).

"Medicine: St'elmexw"; trailer accessed via: https://medicine.movie/.

Melechi, Antonio, "Drugs of Liberation: From Psychiatry to Psychedelia," *Psychedelia Britannica: Hallucinogenic Drugs in Britain* (London: Turnaround, 1997).

Metcalfe, Anna-Jayne, "Trans Murder Monitoring Update" (September 30, 2023); accessed via: https://transrespect.org/wp-content/uploads/2023/11/TvT_TMM_TDoR2023_Table.pdf.

"Mexican Arrested here for Selling Marihuana Plants," *Tulsa Tribune* (September 9, 1929); accessed via: http://reefermadnessmuseum.org/chap04/Oklahoma/OK_RFNewspaper.htm.

"Michael Shellenberger's Guide to Escaping the Woke Matrix," University of Austin (June 26, 2023); accessed via: https://www.youtube.com/watch?v=Ey-7iWsDYnJ8&t=2130s.

Miller, Joshua Rhett, "BLM Site Removes Page on 'Nuclear Family Structure' amid NFL Vet's Criticism," *New York Post* (September 24, 2020); accessed via: https://nypost.com/2020/09/24/blm-removes-website-language-blasting-nuclear-family-structure/.

——"Store Owner Craig Cope, 80, who Shot Robber Armed with AR-15 Rifle Says it was 'Him or Me,'" *New York Post* (August 2, 2022); accessed via: https://nypost.com/2022/08/02/california-store-owner-recalls-shooting-would-be-robber/.

Milonakis, Andy, "Red Lean, Purple Lean" (June 20, 2011); accessed via: https://genius.com/ Andy-milonakis-red-lean-purple-lean-lyrics.

Mocerino, María, "This is Not Native American History, This is US History with

Belinda Eriacho," October 2, 2020); accessed via: https://chacruna.net/belinda_eriacho_ native_american s/.

Mohan, Pavithra, "What it's Like to Date and Marry out of Your Social Class," *Fast Company* (October 22, 2018); accessed via: https://www.fastcompany.com/90250775/what-its-like-to-date-and-marry-out-of-your-social-class.

Mondelez International, "The Fifth Annual State of Snacking: Global Consumer Trends Study"; accessed via: https://www.mondelezinternational.com/.

Money, John and Anke A. Ehrhardt, *Man and Woman, Boy and Girl: The Differentiation and Dimorphism of Gender Identity from Conception to Maturity* (MA: Johns Hopkins University Press, 1972).

Mooney, James, *Cherokee Shamanism* (Simplicissimus Book Farm, 2015).

Mora, George, et al. (eds., trans.), Johannes Weyer, *Witches, Devils, and Doctors in the Renaissance* (Binghamton, NY: Medieval and Renaissance Texts and Studies, 1991).

Morice, Jane, "Akron Police Officer's Fatal Shooting of Accused Armed Robber Ruled Justified," *Cleveland.com*; accessed via: https://www.cleveland.com/akron2016/07/fatal_ akron_police_officer-inv.html.

Morin, Rich, et al., "Behind the Badge," Pew Research Center (January 11, 2017); accessed via: https://www.pewresearch.org/social-trends/2017/01/11/behind-the-badge/.

Morrison, Aaron, "BLM's Patrisse Cullors to Step Down from Movement Foundation," *AP News* (May 27, 2021); accessed via: https://apnews.com/article/ca-state-wire-george-floyd-philanthropy-race-and-ethnicity-0a89ec240a702537a3d89d281789adcf.

Mulukom, Valerie van, Ruairi E. Patterson, Michiel van Elk "Broadening Your Mind to Include Others: The Relationship between Serotonergic Psychedelic Experiences and Maladaptive Narcissism," in *Psychopharmacology (Berl)*, May 2020: 2725–2737; accessed via: https://pure.coventry.ac.uk/ws/portalfiles/portal/31285090/Binder3.pdf.

Munn, Henry (*trans.*), Álvaro Estrada, *María Sabina: Her Life and Chants* (CA: Ross-Erikson, 1981).

Muraresku, Brian C., *The Immortality Key: The Secret History of the Religion with No Name* (NY: St. Martin's Press, 2020).

Murray, Douglas, *The War on the West* (NY: Broadside Books, 2022).

Myburgh, James, "The Hunting of George Zimmerman," *Politicsweb* (August 14, 2013); accessed via: https://www.politicsweb.co.za/news-and-analysis/the-hunting-of-george-zimmerman.

Myers, Anthony, "Skittles Devotes its Platforms to Provide Visibility for LGBTQ+ Artists, Influencers, and Creators," *Confectionary News* (June, 2021); accessed via: https://www.confectionerynews.com/Article/2021/06/07/Skittles-devotes-its-platforms-to-provide-visibilty-for-LGBTQ-artists-influencers-and-creators.

NAACP, "The Origins of Modern Day Policing," accessed via: https://naacp.org/

find-resources/history-explained/origins-modern-day-policing.

"Narcotic Cigarettes Seized as 3 are Held," *The New York Times* (October 8, 1934).

"Narcotic Garden Found in Brooklyn," *The New York Times* (October 18, 1934).

National Black Women's Justice Institute, "Black Women, Sexual Assault, and Criminalization" (April 11, no year stated in original); accessed via: https://www.nbwji.org/post/black-women-sexual-assault-criminalization.

National Center for Health Statistics, "Infant Mortality Rates by State," *Centers for Disease Control and Prevention* (2017); accessed via: https://www.cdc.gov/nchs/pressroom/sosmap/infan t_mortality_rates/infant_mortality.htm.

"Native American Elder Nathan Phillips on Confrontation: 'I Forgive Him,'" *Today* (January 29, 2019); accessed via: https://www.youtube.com/watch?v=h-9-qmN0Hmw.

Nalewicki, Jennifer, "Before Being Ritually Sacrificed, This Nazca Child was Drugged with Psychedelics," *Science Alert* (Nov 1, 2022); accessed via: https://www.sciencealert.com/before-being-ritually-sacrificed-this-nazca-child-was-drugged-with-psychedelics?utm_content=sked638745c56429ed155b9e6ae2&utm_medium=social&utm_name=sked&utm_source=facebook&fbclid=IwAR1wJYN0qFXPs-umo0aQs6bRcGuRnlY-q3ltclQurE96-oLwUFcxxaUkIdR4#1b4t5vwmwgp5mikoje.

National Geographic, "Witch Trials in the 21st Century" (2024) accessed via: https://education.nationalgeographic.org/resource/witch-trials-21st-century/.

Newcomb, W.W., *The Indians of Texas: From Prehistoric to Modern Times* (TX: University of Texas, 1980).

Nickels, David, "We Need to Talk about MAPS Supporting the Police, the Military, and Violent White Supremacism," *Psymposia* (July 17, 2020); accessed via: https://www.psymposia.com/ma gazine/acab/.

NORML (June 13, 2020); accessed via: https://twitter.com/norml/status/1271916399326367747.

Novack, Stephen J., "LSD before Leary: Sidney Cohen's Critique of 1950s Psychedelic Drug Research," *Isis*, 88, no. 1 (1997): 87–100.

"Number of People Shot to Death by the Police in the United States from 2017 to 2023, by Race," *Statista*; accessed via: https://www.statista.com/statistics/585152/people-shot-to-death-by-us-police-by-race/.

Nynauld, Jean de, *De la lycanthropie, transformation et extase des sorciers* (Paris: Chez Jean Millot, 1615); reprint of the original edition Éditions Frénésie, Paris, France (1990).

Observer Newsroom, "California Adopts New Mathematics Framework Focused on Equity and Social Justice" (July 14, 2023); accessed via: https://sacobserver.com/2023/07/california-adopts-new-mathematics-framework-focused-on-equity-and-social-justice/.

Office of the Law Revision Counsel United States Code, 18 U.S. Code § 922 – "Unlawful Acts."

Office of the Medical Examiner Florida, Districts 7 & 24, "Medical Examiner Report" (February 27, 2012); accessed via: http://i2.cdn.turner.com/cnn/2012/images/05/17/martin.autopsy.pdf.

"Officer Convicted of Manslaughter in Shooting Death of Boy, 6," CBS News (March 24, 2017); accessed via: https://www.cbsnews.com/news/derrick-stafford-convicted-of-manslaughter-in-shooting-death-of-jeremy-mardis/.

Ogden, Daniel, *Magic, Witchcraft, and Ghosts in the Greek and Roman Worlds* (UK: Oxford University Press, 2009).

O'Kane, Caitlin, "Mattel's First Transgender Barbie Designed after Laverne Cox," CBS News (May 27, 2022); accessed via: https://www.cbsnews.com/news/laverne-cox-barbie-mattel-transgender-doll/.

Olvera-Hernández, Nidia, "We Must Continue Calling the Cannabis Plant 'Marijuana'" (February, 2018); accessed via: https://chacruna.net/why-continue-calling-cannabis/.

"Open Letter Concerning Abuses by Octavio Rettig and Gerry Sandoval," DMT-Nexus (2019); accessed via: https://www.dmt-nexus.me/forum/default.aspx?g=posts&t=86872.

O' Reilly, David, et al. "Cough, Codeine, and Confusion," in *British Medical Association* (December 7, 2015); accessed via: https://www.ncbi.nlm.nih.gov/pmc/articles/PMC4691881/.

Orwell, George, *1984* (NY: A Signet Book: New American Library, 1952).

Osbourne, Thomas, *Collection of Voyages and Travels, Consisting of Authentic Writers in Our Own Tongue, Vol. 1.* (London, 1745).

O'Shaughnessy, W.B., *The Bengal Dispensary and Companion to the Pharmacopeia* (London: W. H. Allen and Co., Leadenhall Street, 1842).

Palmer, Cynthia and Michael Horowitz (eds.), *Sisters of the Extreme: Women Writing on the Drug Experience* (VT: Park Street Press, 2000).

Paoletti, Jo B., *Pink and Blue: Telling the Boys from the Girls in America* (IN: Indiana University Press, 2012).

Pathfinder; accessed via: https://www.pathfinder.org/

Pearson, Michael and David Mattingly, "Gun, Drug Texts Feature in New Trayvon Martin Shooting Evidence"; accessed via: https://www.cnn.com/2013/05/23/justice/florida-zimmerman-defense/index.html.

Petrullo, Vincenzo, *The Diabolic Root: A Study of Peyotism, The New Indian Religion Among the Delawares* (PA: University of Pennsylvania Press: The University Museum, 1934).

"Playboy Interview: Timothy Leary" *Playboy* (September, 1966); Psanctum Timothy Leary Collection, Box 1.

Pluckrose, Helen, *The Counterweight Handbook: Principled Strategies for Surviving and Defeating Critical Social Justice—at Work, in Schools, and Beyond* (NC: Pitchstone Publishing, 2024).

Pluckrose, Helen and James Lindsay, *Social Injustice: Why Many Popular Answers to Important Questions of Race, Gender, and Identity are Wrong—and How to*

Know What's Right (NC: Pitchstone Publishing, 2022).
Plutarch, *Conjugalia Praecepta*; accessed via: perseus.tufts.edu.
——*De defectu oraculorum*; accessed via: http://www.perseus.tufts.edu.
Powell, Michael, "New York's Private Schools Tackle White Privilege. It has not Been Easy," *The New York Times* (August 27, 2021); accessed via: https://www.nytimes.com/2021/08/27/us/new-york-private-schools-racism.html.
Press Release, "Presidential Task Force on Missing and Murdered American Indians and Alaska Natives Release Status Report," Office of Public Affairs, US Department of Justice (December 10, 2020); accessed via: https://www.justice.gov/opa/pr/presidential-task-force-missing-and-murdered-american-indians-and-alaska-natives-releases.
"Protesters Interrupt Rick Doblin at MAPS Psychedelic Science 2023 Closing Ceremony"; accessed via: https://www.youtube.com/watch?v=7LJmfWNvscE.
Psymposia, "David Nickels"; accessed via: https://www.psymposia.com/author/david-nickles/.
"Racism, Weed, and Jazz: The True Origins of the War on Drugs," *News Beat* (August, 2017); accessed via: https://usnewsbeat.medium.com/racism-weed-jazz-the-true-origins-of-the-war-on-drugs-8e6fd4ef813.
Ramaswamy, Vivek, *Woke Inc.: Inside Corporate America's Social Justice Scam* (NY: Center Street, 2021).
Ramirez, Jose F., *Historia de las Indias de Nueva-Espana, y Islas de Tierre Firme por El Padre Fray Diego Duran* (Mexico: Imprenta de J. M. Andrande y F. Escalante,1807); accessed via: https://ia800200.us.archive.org/8/items/historiadelasind01dur/historiadelasind01dur.pdf.
Randazzo, Sara, "To Increase Equity, School Districts Eliminate Honors Classes," *Wall Street Journal* (Feb 17, 2023); accessed via: https://www.wsj.com/articles/to-increase-equity-school-districts-eliminate-honors-classes-d5985dee.
Randolph, Paschal Beverly, "The Ansairetic Mystery: A New Revelation Concerning SEX," in Deveney (1996).
Rathge, Adam R., "Mapping the Muggleheads: New Orleans and the Marijuana Menace, 1920–1930," *Southern Spaces* (Oct. 23, 2018); accessed via: https://southernspaces.org/2018/mapping-muggleheads-new-orleans-and-marijuana-menace-1920-1930/.
"Rayquan Borum Found Guilty of 2nd-degree Murder in Fatal Shooting during Charlotte Riots," WBTV; accessed via: https://www.wbtv.com/2019/03/08/rayquan-borum-found-guilty-nd-degree-murder-fatal-shooting-during-charlotte-riots/.
Rebel Wisdom, "Psychedelic Capitalism and the Sacred"; accessed via: https://youtube.com/watch?v=rf7S0PcfsA4&t=1655s.
Reed, Betsy, "Sweden Passes Law Lowering Age to Legally Change Gender from 18 to 16," *The Gurdian* (April 17, 2024); accessed via: https://www.theguardian.com.

Reefer Madness Museum, "Is it the 'War on Drugs' or the 'War on Blacks'?; accessed via: http://reefermadnessmuseum.org/chap04/Oklahoma/OK_RF-Newspaper.htm.

Reilly, Katie, "The Viral Lincoln Memorial Confrontation Shows We're Ill-Equipped to Deal with Online Disinformation," *Time* (January 23, 2019); accessed via: https://time.com/5509832/covington-catholic-nathan-philips-social-media-division/.

Reilly, Wilfred, *Hate Crime Hoax: How the Left is Selling a Fake Race War* (DC: Regnery Publishing, 2019).

Reiman, Amanda, Mark Welty, and Perry Solomon, "Cannabis as a Substitute for Opioid-Based Pain Medication: Patient Self-Report," *Cannabis and Cannabinoid Research*, 2, 1 (2017): pp. 160–166.

Rinkel, Max "Experimentally Induced Psychosis in Man." In *Neuropharmacology: Transactions of the 2nd Conference* (May 25–27, 1955), edited by Harold Abramson, p. 240.

Riverside County, "[Archived] Attempted Armed Commercial Robbery–Update," Riverside County Sheriff (August 4, 2022); accessed via: https://www.riversidesheriff.org/CivicAlerts.aspx?AID=3610&ARC=5847.

Rodriguez, Leah, "Why Maternal Mortality is so High in Sub-Saharan Africa," *Global Citizen* (August 6, 2021); accessed via: https://www.globalcitizen.org/en/content/maternal-mortality-sub-saharan-africacauses/#:~:text=Women%20in%20sub%2DSaharan%20Africa,200%2C000%20maternal%20deaths%20a%20year.

Rosenthal, Ellena, "Who Crushed the Lesbian Bars? A New Minefield of Identity Politics" *Willamette Week* (November 30, 2016); accessed via: https://www.wweek.com/culture/2016/11/30/who-crushed-the-lesbian-bars-a-new-minefield-of-sexual-politics/.

Rouillard, Jacques, "In Kamloops, Not One Body Has Been Found," *The Dorchester Review*, January 11, 2022; accessed via: https://www.dorchesterreview.ca/blogs/news/in-kamloops-not-one-body-has-been-found.

Ruck, Carl A.P., *Sacred Mushrooms of the Goddess: Secrets of Eleusis* (CA: Ronin Publishing, 2006).

——"The Wild and the Cultivated: Wine in Euripides' Bacchae," *Journal of Ethnopharmacology*, 5 (1982).

Ruck, Carl A.P., et al., *The Road to Eleusis: Unveiling the Secret of the Mysteries* (CA: North Atlantic Books, 2008).

Rythmia (September 1, 2020); accessed via: https://www.facebook.com/rythmia.

Savage, Charles, "LSD, Alcoholism, and Transcendence," *The Journal of Nervous and Mental Diseases* (Vol 135 Nov 1962): 429–435.

Savage, Charles, James Terrill, and Donald D. Jackson "LSD, Transcendence, and the New Beginning," *The Journal of Nervous and Mental Diseases*, Vol. 13, no. 5 (1962): 425–439.

"The Resolution and Subsequent Remobilization of Resistance by LSD in Psychotherapy," from the Round Table "Psychodynamic and Therapeutic Aspects of Mescaline and Lysergic Acid Diethylamide," held at the annual meeting of the American Psychiatric Association, May 3, 1956. Transcripts reprinted in *Journal of Nervous and Mental Diseases* 125, no. 1 (January– March 1957).

"Screen Writer Bandit Killed," *Los Angeles Times* (June 17, 1925).

"Seattle Public Schools K-12 Math Ethnic Studies Framework" (August 20, 2019); accessed via: https://www.k12.wa.us/sites/default/files/public/socialstudies/pubdocs/Math%20SDS%20ES%20Framework.pdf.

Sedacca, Matthew and Georgia Worell, "Accused Burger King Killer Winston Glynn Compares himself to Jesus and Mandela," *New York Post* (November 26, 2022); accessed via: http://nypost.com/2022/11/26/accused-burger-king-killer-winston-glynn-compares-self-to-jesus/.

Selk, Avi, "Gun Owners are Outraged by the Philando Castile Case. The NRA is Silent," *The Washington Post* (June 27, 2017); accessed via: https://www.washingtonpost.com/news/post-nation/wp/2017/06/18/some-gun-owners-are-disturbed-by-the-philando-castile-verdict-the-nra-is-silent/

"Senseless Brutality: A Mexican Priest Flogs the Corpse of a Dead Wizard," *The Memphis Appeal*, Vol. XLVII, No. 1, April 25 (1887); accessed via: https://chroniclingamerica.loc.gov/lccn/sn84024448/1887-04-25/ed-1/seq-1/#words=marihuana+marijuana+mariguana+Indian+hemp+cannabis+dope.

Sergis, Manolis, "Dog Sacrifice in Ancient and Modern Greece: From the Sacrifice Ritual to Dog Torture," *Folklore*, 45 (2010).

Schlein, Lisa, "UN: Most Child, Maternal Deaths Occur in Sub-Saharan Africa," *VOA News* (September 19, 2019); accessed via:https://www.voanews.com/a/africa_un-most-child-maternal-deaths-occur-sub-saharan-africa/6176106.html.

Schmidlin, Kyle, "Column: 'War on Drugs' Merely Fights the Symptoms of a Faulty System," CBS News (September 13, 2008); accessed via: https://www.cbsnews.com/news/column-war-on-drugs-merely-fights-the-symptoms-of-a-faulty-system/.

Schlosser, Eric, *Reefer Madness: Sex, Drugs, and Cheap Labor in the Black Market* (NY: Houghton Mifflin Company, 2003).

Schwartz, Joel, "Roots of Unconscious Prejudice Affect 90 to 95 Percent of People, Psychologists Demonstrate at Press Conference," *University of Washington News* (September 29, 1998); accessed via: https://www.washington.edu/news/1998/09/29/roots-of-unconscious-prejudice-affect-90-to-95-percent-of-people-psychologists-demonstrate-at-press-conference/.

Sharpe, Alex, "Review of Helen Joyce's *Trans: When Ideology Meets Reality* . . . ; and Katherine Stock's *Material Girls: Why Reality Matters for Feminism* . . .," *Critical Legal Thinking* (October 8, 2021); accessed via: https://criticallegalthinking.com/2021/10/08/review-of-helen-joyces-trans-when-ideology-meets-reality-london-oneworld-2021-pp-311-rp-16-99-and-kathleen-stocks-material-girls-why-reality-matters-for-feminism-london-fle/.

Shaw, Jazz, "Yes, the NRA (and all of us) Should be Speaking out on the Philando Castile Shooting (June 21, 2017); accessed via: https://hotair.com/jazz-shaw/2017/06/21/yes-nra-us-speaking-philando-castile-shooting-n246393.

Shellenberger, Michael, *San Fransicko: Why Progressives Ruin Cities* (NY: HarperCollins, 2021).

——"The WPATH Files: A New Report Exposing Dangerously Pseudoscientific surgical and hormonal Experiments on Children, Adolescents, and Adults" (March 5, 2024); accessed via: https://www.cga.ct.gov/2024/gaedata/TMY/2024SJ-00004-R000318-Gerber,%20M-Opposes-TMY.PDF.

Shepard, Alicia, "The Iconic Photos of Trayvon Martin & George Zimmerman & Why You May Not See the Others," *Poynter* (March 30, 2012); accessed via: https://www.poynter.org/reporting-editing/2012/the-iconic-photos-of-trayvon-martin-george-zimmerman-why-you-may-not-see-the-others/.

Shingler, Benjamin, "Investigations Launched after Atikamekw Woman Records Quebec Hospital Staff Uttering Slurs Before her Death," CBC News (September 30, 2020); accessed via: https://www.cbc.ca/news/canada/montreal/quebec-atikamekw-joliette-1.5743449.

Singal, Jesse, "The Creators of the Implicit Bias Association Test Should get their Story Straight," *Intelligencer* (December 5, 2017); accessed via: https://nymag.com/intelligencer/2017/ 12/iat-behavior-problem.html.

Singh, Devita, Susan J. Bradley, Kenneth J. Zucker, "A Follow-Up Study of Boys with Gender Identity Disorder," *Frontiers in Psychiatry*, Vol 12 (March 28, 2021); accessed via: https://www. frontiersin.org/journals/psychiatry/articles/10.3389/fpsyt.2021.632784/full#note3a.

Singh, Manvir, "Psychedelics Weren't as Common in Ancient Cultures as we Think," *Vice* (December 10, 2020); accessed via: https://www.vice.com/en/article/4adngq/psychedelic-drug-use-in-ancient-indigenous-cultures.

Sit, Ryan, "Trump Thinks Only Black People are on Welfare, But Really, White Americans Receive Most Benefits," *Newsweek* (January 12, 2018); accessed via: https://www.newsweek. com/donald-trump-welfare-black-white-780252.

Sitkoff, Harvard, *The Struggle for Black Equality: 1954–1992* (NY: Hill and Wang, 1993).

Skeptic Research Center, "How Informed are Americans about Race and Policing?" CUPES007 (2021).

Sloman, Larry, *Reefer Madness: A History of Marijuana* (NY: St. Martin's Griffin, 1998).

Slotkin, James Sydney, *The Peyote Religion: A Story in Indian-White Relations* (Il: University of Chicago, 1956).

Smith, Grover (ed.), *Letters of Aldous Huxley* (New York: Harper and Row, 1969).

Smith, Laura, "How an Axe Murderer Helped Make Weed Illegal," *FEE Stories* (August, 2017); accessed via:https://fee.org/articles/how-an-axe-murderer-

helped-make-weed-illegal/
——"How a Racist Hate-Monger Masterminded America's War on Drugs," *Timeline* (Feb 17 2018); accessed via: https://timeline.com/harry-anslinger-racist-war-on-drugs-prison-industrial-complex-fb5cbc281189.

Smith, R.C., "Report of the Investigation in the State of Texas Particularly Along the Mexican Border," Department of Agriculture, Bureau of Chemistry (April 15, 1917); accessed via: http://reefermadnessmuseum.org/TexasReport1917/TexasReport1917.htm.

Smith-Thompson, Toni and Yusuf Abdul-Qadir, "How Legalizing Cannabis Makes the Case for Reparations" (April 9, 2021); accessed via: https://www.nyclu.org/en/news/how-legalizing-cannabis-makes-case-reparations.

Snowden, Jr., Frank M., *Before Color Prejudice: The Ancient View of Blacks* (MA: Harvard University Press, 1983).

Solomon, Daniel J., "WATCH: That Time Ben Shapiro Called Transgender People Delusional," Forward (December 7, 2016); accessed via: https://forward.com/news/356431/watch-that-time-ben-shapiro-called-transgender-people-delusional/.

Sondern, Frederic, *Brotherhood of Evil: The Mafia* (NY: Farrar, Straus and Cudahy, 1959).

Sowell, Thomas, *Conquests and Cultures: An International History* (Basic Books, 1999).

Spano, John, "L.A. Man Guilty of 11 Deaths" *Los Angeles Times* (May 1, 2007): accessed via: https://www.latimes.com/archives/la-xpm-2007-may-01-me-turner1-story.html.

SpectraDIVERSITY, "CRT and DEI" (February 6, 2023); accessed via: https://www.spectradiversity.com/2023/02/06/crt-and-dei/.

Spectrum News Staff, "NYPD: McDonald's Worker Stabbed while Defending Coworker in East Harlem," Spectrum News NY1 (March 9, 2022); accessed via: https://www.ny1.com/nyc/manhattan/news/2022/03/09/mcdonald-s-worker-stabbed-in-east-harlem.

St. Basil of Caesarea, *Letters*; accessed via newadvent.org.

Staff Writer, "Family Sues Akron Police for Killing Unarmed Man William Lemmon they Suspected of Robbery," *Akron Beacon Journal* (September 26, 2016): accessed via: https://www.beaconjournal.com/story/news/local/2016/09/26/family-sues-akron-police-for/10659295007/.

Statement of Frederick P. Hitz Inspector General Central Intelligence Agency before the Committee on Intelligence, United States House of Representatives, "Regarding Investigation of Allegations of Connections between the CIA and The Contras in Drug Trafficking to the United States, Vol I: The California Story," Congressional Hearings, Intelligence and Security (16 March 1998); accessed via: https://irp.fas.org/congress/1998_hr/980316-ps.htm.

"Statement of H. J. Anslinger," Hearings on H.R.6385, *The Washington Post*, Nov. 23, 1936; accessed via: https://www.druglibrary.org/schaffer/hemp/taxact/

anslng1.htm.
"Statement of H.J. Anslinger," *House Ways and Means Committee*; accessed via: https://www.druglibrary.org/schaffer/hemp/taxact/anslng1.htm
"State of California in 1860; accessed via: https://www2.census.gov/library/publications/decenni al/1860/population/1860a-06.pdf p. 26.
"Statistics Tell the Story: Fathers Matter," National Fatherhood Initiative (2024); accessed via: https://www.fatherhood.org/father-absence-statistic.
Sterk, Claire E., *Fast Lives: Women who Use Crack* (PA: Temple University Press, 1999).
Stern, Ray, "Guns at Obama Protest Scare Folks, but Cops Say no Laws were Broken," *Phoenix New Times* (August 17, 2009); accessed via: https://www.phoenixnewtimes.com/news/guns-at-obama-protest-scare-folks-but-cops-say-no-laws-were-broken-6626833.
Stevens, Jay, *Storming Heaven: LSD and the American Dream* (Grove Press, 1986).
Stewart, Omar, *Peyote Religion: A History* (OK: University of Oklahoma Press, 1994).
Stolaroff, Myron, *Thanatos to Eros: 35 Years of Psychedelic Exploration* (Berlin: VWB, 1994).
Stoll, Werner, "Ein Neues in sehr Kleinin Mengen Wirksames Phantastikum" *Protocolo de la 108th assemblée les 22 et 23 novembre 1947 in Zurich;* reprinted in *Schweizer Archiv fur Neurologie und Psychiatrie.*
Stone, Daniel, "Guns at Obama Rallies: Where's the Outrage?" *Newsweek* (August 18, 2009); accessed via: https://www.newsweek.com/guns-obama-rallies-wheres-outrage-211492.
Stossel, John, "Diversity, Equity & Inclusion: DEI Training's Unintended Consequences" (March 21, 2023); accessed via: https://www.youtube.com/watch?v=D2KX8wXzc78.
Strabo, *Geography of Strabo*, Book II, Chap. V, Vol. I; accessed via: http://penelope.uchicago. edu.
Stuckey, Mike, "Guns near Obama Fuel 'Open-Carry' Debate," *NBC News* (August 24, 2009); accessed via: https://www.nbcnews.com/id/wbna32492783.
"Sworn Statement of Deanna Fox-Williams," Miami-Dade Police Department (2012); accessed via: https://www.scribd.com/document/135692728/Affidavit-From-Commander-Deanna-Fox-Williams.
"Sworn Statement of Sergeant William Tagle," Miami-Dade Police Department (2012); accessed via: https://www.scribd.com/document/135564937/Sergeant-William-Tagle-Internal-Affairs-Investigative-Report.
Tarleton, John, "Interview with Michael Niman"; accessed via: http://www.johntarleton.net/nima n.html.
"Taxation of Marijuana," Hearing Before a Subcommittee of the Committee on Finance, United States Senate, Seventy-Fifth Congress, First Session, *United States Government Printing Office* (July 12, 1937).
"The Iran Contra Affairs"; accessed via: https://www.brown.edu/Research/

Understanding_the_Iran_Contra_Affair/iran-contra-affairs.php.

"The State of Maternal Mortality in Sub-Saharan Africa," *Giving Compass* (August 9, 2021); accessed via: https://givingcompass.org/article/th-state-of-maternal-mortality-in-sub-saharan-africa?gclid=EAIaIQobChMIjd-Pv-bzt-gIVNCCtBh2bPAAkEAAYAyAAEgL99vD_BwE.

"The Well-Baked Man," accessed via: https://www.angelfire.com/ca/ca/Indian/WellBakedMan.html.

Thomas, Ben, "How America's First Drug Czar Made Cannabis a Racial Issue," *Ember: A Journal of Cannabis Culture* (February 2022); accessed via: https://medmen.com/blog/travel-culture/how-americas-first-drug-czar-made-cannabis-a-racial-issue-harry-j-anslinger-war-on-drugs.

Thomas, Hugh, *The Slave Trade: The Story of the Atlantic Slave Trade: !440* – 1870 (NY: Simon and Schuster Paperbacks, 1997).

Theodorate of Cyrus, *On Divine Province* (NJ: Paulis Press, 1988).

Time Staff, "Millennials: The Me Me Me Generation," *Time* (May 20, 2013); accessed via: https://time.com/247/millennials-the-me-me-me-generation/.

Toliver, Aesia, "Court Docs: Suspect asked, 'Are You a Boy or a Girl?' Before Fatal Hampton Shooting," *Wavy* (April 15, 2022); accessed via: https://www.wavy.com/news/local-news/hampton/court-docs-are-you-a-boy-or-a-girl-suspect-asked-before-fatal-hampton-shooting/.

Touleimat, Aref, "Ayahuasca: A Plea for the Decolonization of Psychedelic Studies," *Open Foundation*, June 27, 2022; accessed via: https://open-foundation.org/ayahuasca-decolonization/.

"Trayvon Martin Shooting: New Details Emerge from Twitter Account, Witness Testimony" *The Cutline* (March 26, 2012); accessed via: https://news.yahoo.com/blogs/cutline/trayvon-martin-shooting-details-emerge-facebook-twitter-accounts-180103647.html.

"Trayvon Martin's 'NO–LIMIT – NI[**]A' Tweets," *The Daily Caller*, accessed via: https://www.scribd.com/doc/86809463/Trayvon-Martin-s-NO-LIMIT-NI[**]A-Tweets-The-Daily-Caller.

Troike, Rudolph C., "The Origins of Plains Mescalism," *American Anthropologist*, 64 (1962).

Tuskegee University, "Lynchings: By State and Race, 1882–1968"; accessed via: https://archive.tuskegee.edu/archive/handle/123456789/511.

"Two Seized for Selling Opiate to Troops: Two Accused of Peddling Loco Weed Cigarettes Daily on Governors Island," *New York Times* (January 23, 1935); accessed via: https://druglibrar y.net/schaffer/hemp/history/nytimes/012335.htm.

University of the Fraser Valley, "Faculty: Sarah Beaulieu"; accessed via: https://www.ufv.in/programs/faculty/sarah-beaulieu/.

"Use for Deadly Weed," *The Florida Star*, October 16 (1908); accessed via: https://chroniclingamerica.loc.gov/lccn/sn96027111/1908-10-16/ed-1/seq-3/#words=marihuana+marijuana+mariguana+Indian+hemp+cannabis+dope.

"Use of Marijuana Spreading in West," *The New York Times* (September 16, 1934).

Vela, Enrique, "Tízoc, 'He Who Makes Sacrifice' (1481–1486)," reproduced in *Arqueología Mexicana*; accessed via: https://arqueologiamexicana.mx/mexico-antiguo/tizoc-el-que-hace-sacrificio-1481-1486.

Vitiello, Michael, "The War on Drugs: Moral Panic and Excessive Sentences," *Cleveland State Law Review*, Vol. 26, Issue 2 (2021).

"War on Marijuana Smoking," *The Sun*, Second Section, unpaged (May 26, 1907); accessed via: https://chroniclingamerica.loc.gov/lccn/sn83030272/1907-05-26/ed-1/seq-17/#words=marijuana+marijuana+mariguana+Indian+hemp+-cannabis+dope.

Washington, Booker T., *My Larger Education: Being Chapters from my Experience* (NY: Doubleday, 1911).

——*Up From Slavery* (NY: Airmont Publishing Company, Inc., 1967).

Washington, Jesse, "Blacks Struggle with 72 Percent Unwed Mothers Rate," NBC News; accessed via: https://www.nbcnews.com/id/wbna39993685.

Wasson, Robert Gordon, "Seeking the Magic Mushroom: A New York Banker Goes to Mexico's Mountains to Participate in the Age-old Rituals of Indians Who Chew Strange Growths that Produce Visions," *Life* (May 13, 1957).

Wasson, Robert Gordon and Valentina Wasson, *Russia, Mushrooms, and History* (NY: Pantheon Books Inc., 1957).

Wasson, Valentina P., "The Sacred Mushroom," *This Week* (May 19, 1957).

Waters, Frank, *Book of the Hopi: The First Revelation of the Hopi's Historical and Religious World-view of Life* (NY: Ballantine Books, 1971).

Watts, Alan, "Psychedelics and Religious Experience," *California Law Review,* 56, no. 1 (1968).

Waxman, Olivia B., "The Surprising Link Between U.S. Marijuana Law and the History of Immigration," *Time* (April, 2019); accessed via: https://time.com/5572691/420-marijuana-mexican-immigration/.

Webb, Simon, *The Forgotten Slave Trade: White European Slaves of Islam* (Pen and Sword History, 2021).

——*The Slave Trade in Africa: An Ongoing Holocaust* (Pen and Sword History, 2023).

Weiner, Rachel, "Arlington Prosecutor Promises Data-Driven Reduction in Racial Disparities," *The Washington Post* (April 24, 2021); accessed via: https://www.washingtonpost.com/local/legal-issues/arlington-prosecutor-racial-disparities/2021/04/24/49655384-a1e5-11eb-a774-7b47ceb 36ee8story.html.

Welliver, Mrs. Andy, "Wokova," *Nevada Historical Society Quarterly*, Vol. XI, No, 2 (Summer, 1968).

West, Carolyn M. and Kamilah Johnson, "Sexual Violence in the Lives of African American Women: Risk, Response, and Resilience," *The National Online Resource Center on Violence Against Women, National Resource Center on Domestic Violence* (March 2013); accessed via: https://vawnet.org/material/sexual-violence-lives-african-american-women-risk-response-and-resilience.

"Westchester Hunts Marijuana Sources," *The New York Times* (May 24, 1938).

Wichert, Bill, "Newark Schoolyard Killings: Jose Carranza loses Bid to Overturn Conviction," *NJ.com* (Oct 22, 2014); accessed via: https://www.nj.com/essex/2014/10/newark_schoolyard_killings_jose_carranza_loses_bid_to_overturn_conviction.html.

Wilcox, Walter F., "The Negro Population"; accessed via: https://www2.census.gov/prod2/decennial/documents/03322287no8ch1.pdf.

Williams, Anthony, "#JusticeforPrissy, or How We've Failed our Trans Sisters," *TransMusePlanet* (January 7, 2016); accessed via: https://www.facebook.com/Transmuseplanet/photos/safe-passage-to-our-sister-deonna-mason-aka-prissy-22-of-charlotte-nc-who-was-ki/1050588574991989/?paipv=0&eav=AfZ3acIq2Fz-yzS7xDFQxsnsYFJ1b8IBg3nVqSzMH7mZdPm_Nzneo4l05C0icznU-g&rdr.

Williams, Lauren N., "Trans Activist Speaking up for Victims of Violence and Transgender Women of Color," *Time* (2024); accessed via:https://time.com/collection/american-voices-2017/4573664/american-vocies-cherno-biko/.

Williams, Monnica T., and Beatriz Labate, "Diversity, Equity, and Access in Psychedelic Medicine," *Journal of Psychedelic Studies*, 4, 1 (2020).

Williams, Monnica T., "Curriculum Vitae"; accessed via: https://www.monnicawilliams.com/mtw-CV.pdf.

——"When Feminism Functions as White Supremacy: How White Feminists Oppress Black Women," in Dr. Biatriz C. Labate and Clancy Cavnar (eds.) *Psychedelic Justice: Towards a Diverse and Equitable Psychedelic Culture* (NM: Synergetic Press, 2021).

Williams, Monnica T., Sara Reed, Jamilah George, "Culture and Psychedelic Psychotherapy: Ethnic and Racial Themes from Three Black Women Therapists," *Journal of Psychedelic Studies*, 4, 3 (2020): 125–138.

Winchester, Jake Barlett, *Necromantic Shamanism in 19th Century London* (Wedfty Media Division, 2020).

Winerip, Michael, "Revisiting a Rape Scandal that would have been Monstrous if True," *NY Times* (June 3, 2013); accessed via: https://www.nytimes.com/2013/06/03/booming/revisiting-the-tawana-brawley-rape-scandal.html.

Wing, Nick, "Marijuana Prohibition Was Racist from the Start. Not Much Has Changed," *The Huffington Post* (January 14, 2014); accessed via: https://www.huffpost.com/entry/marijuana-prohibition-racist_n_4590190.

"Woman Billboard was Transphobic and Dangerous," BBC (September 26, 2018); accessed via https://www.youtube.com/watch?v=y8nViKYmEhU.

Wong, Janey, "Lesbian Bar Doc Marie's is Reopening Following its Troubled Start," *PDX Eater* (August 12, 2022); accessed via: https://pdx.eater.com/2022/8/12/23303208/lesbian-bar-doc-maries-reopening.

"WPATH Video Quotes: From WPATH's 'Identity Evolution Workshop held on May 6, 2022,'" *Environmental Progress* (2024); accessed via: https://environmentalprogress.org/big-news/wpath -files.

Yann with Ayahuasca, "An Open Letter to Octavio Rettig and Gerry Sandoval—Here It Is," (April 16, 2019); accessed via: https://yannwithayahuasca.com/2019/04/16/open-letter-to-octavio-rettig-and-dr-gerry-sandoval/.

Yoe, Craig (ed.) et al., *Reefer Madness*, (OR: Dark Horse Books, 2018).

Young, Thomas and Samuel Speed (eds.), Giambattista della Porta, *Natural Magick in XX Books* (London, 1658). Facsimile of original English edition Kessinger (2010).

About the Author

Thomas Hatsis is a public speaker, psychedelic community leader, and author of four books in the field of psychedelic history and practice, including *The Witches' Ointment*. He is also the cofounder of a vibrant psychedelic society, Psanctum, and has the honor of having received the last thirty-four boxes of the Timothy Leary archive to catalogue, digitize, and preserve. He lives in Portland, Oregon.